Teen Health
Course 2

Mary H. Bronson, Ph.D.

Michael J. Cleary, Ed.D.

Betty M. Hubbard, Ed.D., C.H.E.S.

Contributing Author
Dinah Zike, M.Ed.

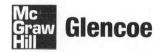 McGraw Hill Glencoe

New York, New York   Columbus, Ohio   Chicago, Illinois   Peoria, Illinois   Woodland Hills, California

Meet the Authors

Mary H. Bronson, Ph.D., has taught health education in grades K–12, as well as health education methods classes at the undergraduate and graduate levels. As health education specialist for the Dallas School District, Dr. Bronson developed and implemented a district-wide health education program. She has been honored as Texas Health Educator of the Year by the Texas Association of Health, Physical Education, Recreation and Dance and selected Teacher of the Year twice, by her colleagues. Dr. Bronson has assisted school districts throughout the country in developing local health education programs. She is also the co-author of the *Glencoe Health* textbook.

Betty M. Hubbard, Ed.D., C.H.E.S., has taught health education in grades K–12 as well as health education methods classes at the undergraduate and graduate levels. She is a professor at the University of Central Arkansas, teaching classes in curriculum development, mental health, and human sexuality. Dr. Hubbard supervises student teachers and conducts in-service training for health education teachers in school districts throughout Arkansas. Her publications, grants, and presentations focus on research-based, comprehensive health instruction.

Michael J. Cleary, Ed.D., is Professor and School Health Education Coordinator at Slippery Rock University. Dr. Cleary taught at Evanston Township High School in Evanston, Illinois, and later became the Lead Teacher Specialist at the McMillen Center for Health Education in Fort Wayne, Indiana. Dr. Cleary has published and presented widely on curriculum development and portfolio assessment in K–12 health education. Dr. Cleary is the co-author of *Managing Your Health: Assessment for Action.* He is a Certified Health Education Specialist.

Dinah Zike, M.Ed., is an international curriculum consultant and inventor who has designed and developed educational products and three-dimensional, interactive graphic organizers for over thirty years. As president and founder of Dinah-Might Adventures, L.P., Dinah is the author of over 100 award-winning educational publications. Dinah has a B.S. and an M.S. in educational curriculum and instruction from Texas A&M University. Dinah Zike's *Foldables* are an exclusive feature of McGraw-Hill textbooks.

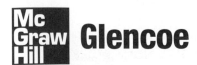

The McGraw·Hill Companies

Send all inquiries to:
Glencoe/McGraw-Hill
21600 Oxnard Street, Suite 500
Woodland Hills, California 91367

ISBN 0-07-861097-4 (Course 2 Student Text)
ISBN 0-07-861098-2 (Course 2 Teacher Wraparound Edition)

Printed in the United States of America.

5 6 7 8 9   071/043   08 07 06 05

Health Consultants

Christine A. Hayashi, M.A. Ed., J.D.
Attorney at Law, Special Education Law
Adjunct Faculty, Educational Leadership and Policy Studies Development
California State University, Northridge
Northridge, California

Patricia Sullivan, M.S., Special Education
Chair, Department of Language Arts
Meade Middle School
Fort Meade, Maryland

UNIT 1
You and Your Health

Kristin Danielson Fink
Executive Director
Community of Caring
Washington, DC

Alice Pappas, Ph.D., R.N.
Associate Professor/ Associate Dean
Baylor University, Louise Herrington School of Nursing
Dallas, Texas

UNIT 2
Keeping Your Body Healthy

Tinker D. Murray, Ph.D.
Professor and Coordinator of the Exercise and Sports Science Program
Southwest Texas State University
San Marcos, Texas

Don Rainey
Instructor, Coordinator of the Physical Fitness and Wellness Program
Southwest Texas State University
San Marcos, Texas

Clayre K. Petray Rowcliffe, Ph.D.
Professor
Department of Kinesiology and Physical Education
California State University, Long Beach
Long Beach, California

Linda Stevenson, Ph.D., R.N.
Assistant Professor
Baylor University, Louise Herrington School of Nursing
Dallas, Texas

Catherine Strain, R.D.
Associate Professor
Marian College
Indianapolis, Indiana

UNIT 3
Understanding Yourself and Others

Stephanie S. Allen
Senior Lecturer
Baylor University, Louise Herrington School of Nursing
Dallas, Texas

Kathleen J. Courtney
HIV/AIDS Education Coordinator
Arkansas Department of Education
Little Rock, Arkansas

Jan King
Teacher
Neshaminy School District
Langhorne, Pennsylvania

UNIT 4
Protecting Your Health

Sally Champlin, C.H.E.S.
Faculty
California State University, Long Beach
Long Beach, California

Sharon Gonzales, R.N.
Nurse
Thomas Grover Middle School
Princeton Junction, New Jersey

Jennifer Weglowski, M.D.
Pediatrician/Senior Pediatric Resident
Children's Hospital of Pittsburgh
Pittsburgh, Pennsylvania

Peggy Woosley
Director of Curriculum
Stuttgart Public Schools
Stuttgart, Arkansas

UNIT 5
Safety and the Environment

Jerry G. Hill
Agency Leadership Team
Arkansas Department of Health
Little Rock, Arkansas

David A. Sleet, Ph.D.
Associate Director for Science
Division of Unintentional Injury Prevention
Centers for Disease Control and Prevention (CDC)
Atlanta, Georgia

Reviewers

Beverly J. Berkin, C.H.E.S.
Health Education Consultant
Bedford Corners, New York

Victoria Bisorca, C.H.E.S.
Lecturer
California State University, Long Beach
Long Beach, California

Beverly J. Bradley, Ph.D., R.N., C.H.E.S.
Assistant Clinical Professor
University of California, San Diego
San Diego, California

Donna Breitenstein, Ed.D.
Professor & Coordinator of Health Education
Director of North Carolina School Health
   Training Center
Appalachian State University
Boone, North Carolina

Julie Campbell-Fouch
Health Teacher, Department Chair
Stanford Middle School
Long Beach, California

Pamela R. Connolly
Subject Area Coordinator for Health and
   Physical Education, Diocese of Pittsburgh
Curriculum Coordinator for Health and Physical
   Education, North Catholic High School
Pittsburgh, Pennsylvania

Roberta Larson Duyff, R.D.
Food and Nutrition Consultant/President
Duyff Associates
St. Louis, Missouri

James Robinson III, Ed.D.
Professor, Assistant Dean for
   Student Affairs
The Texas A&M University System
Health Science Center
School of Rural Public Health
College Station, Texas

Michael Rulon
Health/Physical Education Teacher
Johnson Junior High School
Adjunct Faculty, Laramie County
   Community College
Cheyenne, Wyoming

Jeanne Title
Coordinator, Prevention Education
Napa County Office of Education and Napa
   Valley Unified School District
Napa, California

You and Your Health

1

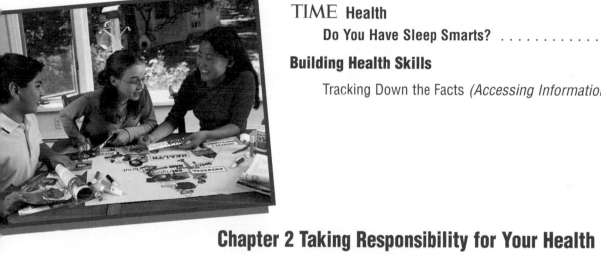

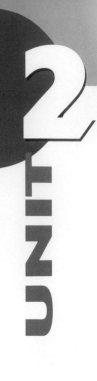

UNIT 2

Keeping Your Body Healthy 50

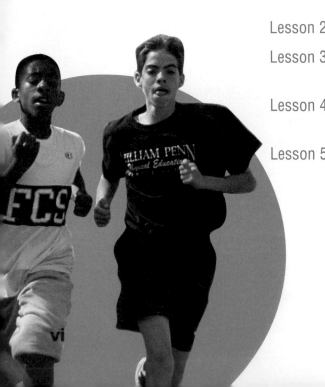

Chapter 5 Personal Health and Consumer Choices   118

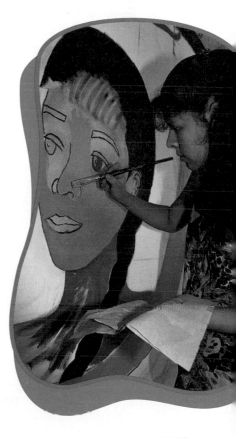

Chapter 6 Growth and Development   152

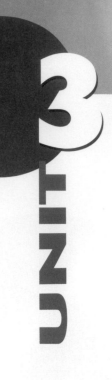

UNIT 3

Understanding Yourself and Others   184

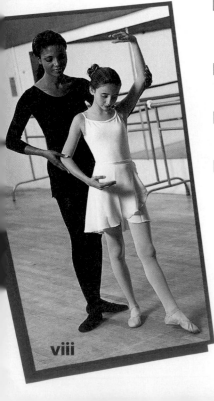

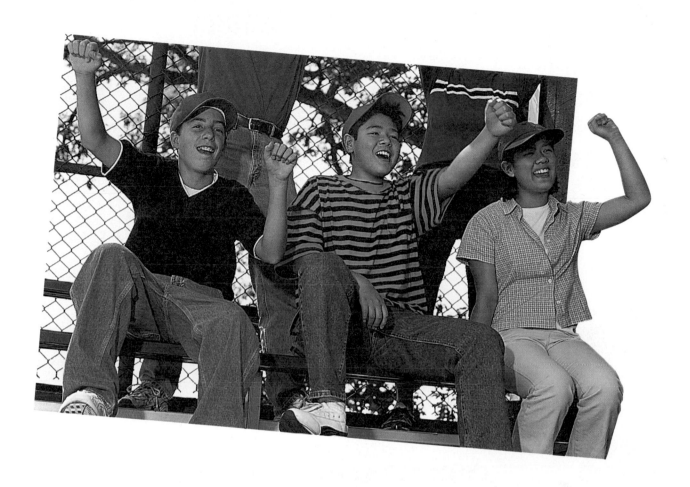

Chapter 9 Resolving Conflicts and Preventing Violence   242

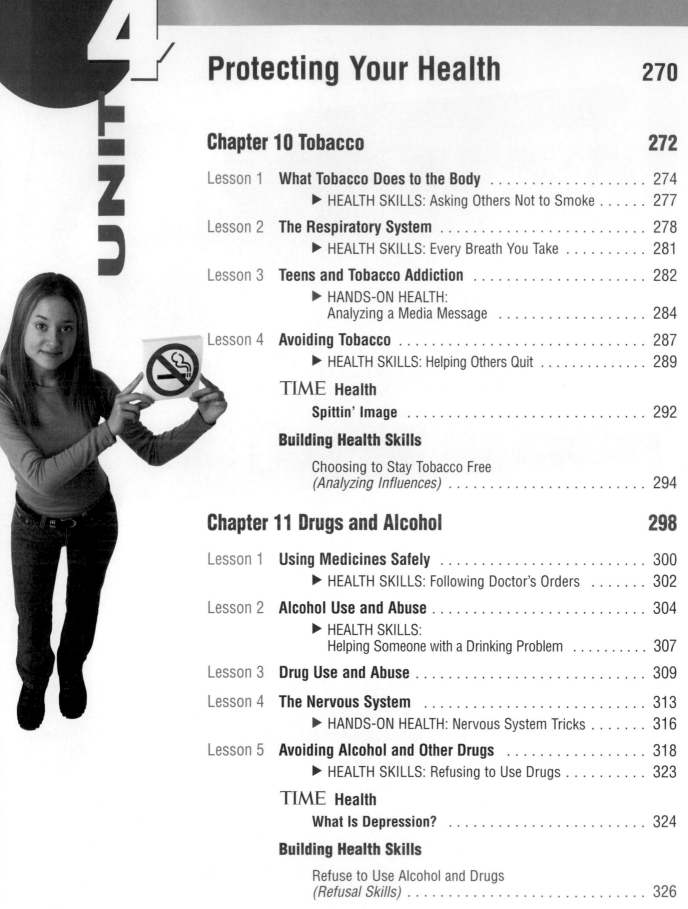

UNIT 4

Protecting Your Health 270

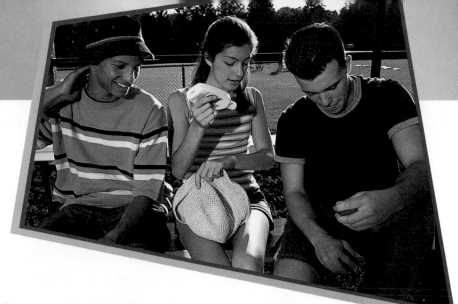

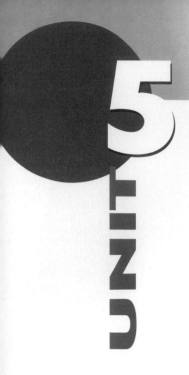

Safety and the Environment   390

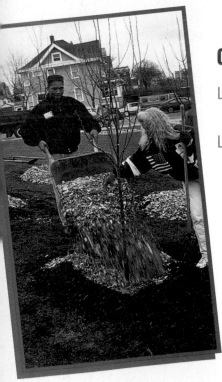

Hands-On Health

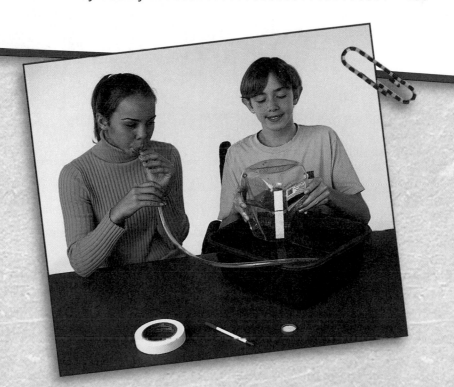

Getting the most out of *Teen* Health

Making healthy and responsible decisions is easy with *Teen Health*. Follow the guidelines below to make the most out of each lesson.

Do the Quick Write

This feature will help you start thinking about the information in a lesson.

Preview the Lesson

Get a preview of what's coming by reading the lesson objectives in the **Learn About....** You can also use this feature to prepare for quizzes and tests.

Review Key Terms

Find each vocabulary term in the text and read its definition. The terms appear in blue so you can locate them easily!

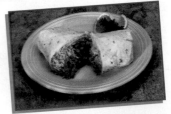

Lesson 1

Nutrients for Health

Quick Write
List the foods you ate yesterday. Do you think that you made healthful choices? If not, what would have been some more healthful choices?

LEARN ABOUT...
- the nutrients your body needs to be healthy.
- how to choose nutrient-rich foods.
- how to read a Nutrition Facts panel.

VOCABULARY
- nutrients
- carbohydrates
- proteins
- fats
- saturated fats
- unsaturated fats
- vitamins
- minerals
- fiber
- cholesterol

The Six Major Nutrients

Eating healthful food helps you feel good and do your best. Nutrients (NOO·tree·ents) are *substances in foods that your body needs in order to grow, have energy, and stay healthy.* The six categories of nutrients are described below.

Carbohydrates, Proteins, and Fats

Carbohydrates (kar·boh·HY·drayts) are *the starches and sugars that provide energy.* Starches are complex carbohydrates. They are found in foods such as rice, pasta, breads, potatoes, beans, and corn. Sugars are simple carbohydrates. They occur naturally in milk, fruit, and honey. Sugar is also added to many foods.

Proteins (PROH·teenz) are *nutrients used to repair body cells and tissues.* Proteins are made up of amino (uh·MEE·noh) acids. Complete proteins contain all the essential amino acids. They are found in foods from animal sources, such as meat, dairy products, and eggs. Plant foods lack one or more essential amino acids, so they're incomplete proteins. However, eating a variety of plant foods, such as beans, nuts, and grains, can provide all the essential amino acids.

Burritos are a good source of several different nutrients, including proteins and carbohydrates.

88 Chapter 4: Food and Nutrition

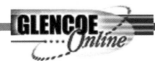

Use Glencoe's Health Web Site to Boost Your Health Smarts!

▶ Rate your health by taking the Health Inventory for each chapter. Jump-start your goals by filling out a Personal Wellness Contract.

▶ Check out Web Link Exercises for fun and interactive games and activities.

▶ Do some detective work on a particular health topic—Health Quests show you how.

▶ Get ready for tests by using the different Online Study Tools to review vocabulary terms and chapter content. E-flashcards, online quizzes, and interactive drag-and-drop games make studying fun!

▶ Building Health Skills features give you another chance to master important skills for wellness.

Reading a Nutrition Facts Panel

Most packaged foods come with a food label that includes a Nutrition Facts panel. The panel lists the product's nutritional value. This information can help you make smart food choices. **Figure 4.1** on page 93 shows how to read the various sections of a Nutrition Facts panel.

The Nutrition Facts panel tells you how large one serving is and the number of calories and amounts of nutrients in a serving. Studying the % Daily Value column will tell you if a food is high or low in certain nutrients. Look for foods that have low daily value percentages (below 5 percent) for fats, cholesterol, and sodium. Choose foods whose labels show high percentages (20 percent or above) of fiber, vitamins, and minerals.

HEALTH SKILLS ACTIVITY

PRACTICING HEALTHFUL BEHAVIORS

Keeping Food Safe

Have you ever felt sick to your stomach and thought to yourself, "It must have been something I ate"? If you handle and prepare foods properly, you will greatly decrease your risk of getting a foodborne illness. To keep food safe, follow these steps:

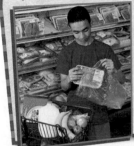

- **CLEAN.** Before you handle food or utensils, wash your hands with warm, soapy water. Wash your hands after handling raw meats, poultry, eggs, and fish as well as everything that comes into contact with these foods. Clean kitchen surfaces as you work.
- **SEPARATE.** Separate raw, cooked, and ready-to-eat foods while buying, preparing, and storing them.
- **COOK.** Make sure that you cook foods to the proper temperature by using a food thermometer. Reheat leftovers thoroughly.
- **CHILL.** Keep perishable foods refrigerated. Thaw frozen foods in the refrigerator.
- **FOLLOW THE LABEL.** Read labels and follow directions such as "Refrigerate after opening."
- **SERVE SAFELY.** Keep hot foods hot and cold foods cold.
- **WHEN IN DOUBT, THROW IT OUT.** Do not eat any food that you think has not been handled or stored properly.

ON YOUR OWN
On a sheet of paper, describe how you would prepare or store each of the following foods to keep it safe:
- Tuna sandwich
- Raw ground beef
- Raw spinach

92 CHAPTER 4: FOOD AND NUTRITION

Try the Health Skills and Hands-On Health Activities

Develop valuable health skills by doing the Health Skills Activities that appear in each chapter. Conduct experiments, create ads, and try the other fun activities in the Hands-On Health features.

Study the Infographics

First, think about the overall message that the infographic is presenting. Then, read each callout carefully and determine what part of the image it is highlighting.

Complete the Lesson Reviews

Completing the lesson reviews can help you see how well you know the material you have just studied. It also gives you a chance to apply what you've learned to different situations, as well as practice a health skill.

FIGURE 4.1

GETTING THE NUTRITION FACTS

Reading Nutrition Facts panels will help you choose healthful food products. *Do you look at the serving size when deciding how much of a food to eat?*

The serving size is the portion most people eat. The amounts listed for calories, nutrients, and food substances are based on one serving of the package's contents.

What is the total amount of fat in the product? How much of that fat is saturated?

The % Daily Value column helps you judge the amounts of the listed nutrients in one serving of the product. The general guideline is that 20 percent or more is a lot and 5 percent or less isn't very much.

This section shows the suggested amounts of nutrients and food substances the average person should aim for each day. Your individual needs may be higher or lower.

How many calories does one serving contain? How many of those calories come from fat?

This shows the percentage of Daily Values for selected vitamins and minerals in one serving of the food.

Lesson 1 Review

Using complete sentences, answer the following questions on a sheet of paper.

Reviewing Terms and Facts

1. **Recall** Identify the six categories of nutrients.
2. **Vocabulary** What are *carbohydrates*?
3. **Discuss** What are *proteins*, and how do they help the body?
4. **Distinguish** Explain the difference between *saturated* and *unsaturated fats*. What food sources contain each of these types of fats?
5. **List** Name three minerals, and explain how each one helps your body.

Thinking Critically

6. **Evaluate** How do the ABCs of good health work together to help you achieve a healthful lifestyle?
7. **Suggest** What would you tell someone who isn't sure how old the leftovers in the refrigerator are? Why?

Applying Health Skills

8. **Accessing Information** Study the Nutrition Facts panel on a package or can of food. Would this food help you fulfill the Dietary Guidelines? Write a short report in which you list your findings and explain the product's nutritional value.

LESSON 1: NUTRIENTS FOR HEALTH **93**

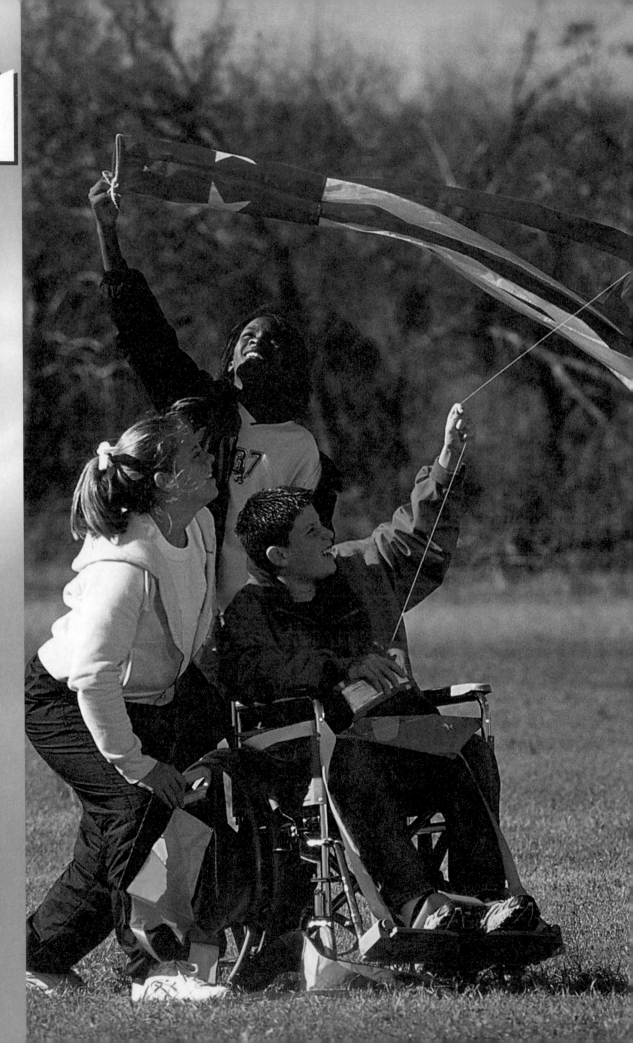

UNIT **1**

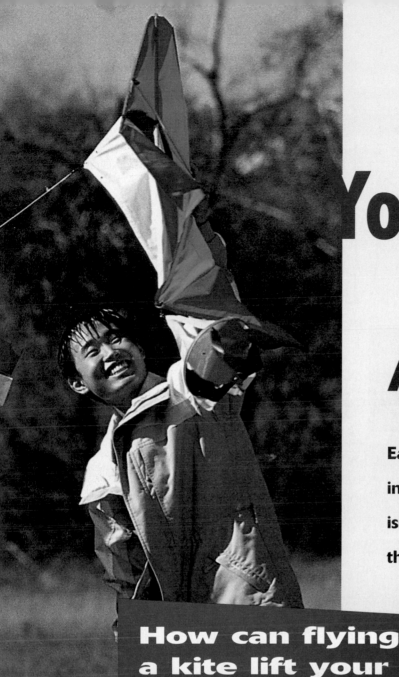

You and Your Health

HEALTH in Action

Eating right and being active are important to good health, but health isn't just physical. Engaging in activities that you enjoy and spending time with your family and friends are also good for your health. When you feel good about yourself, you make better choices and can better meet the goals you set. Your friends and relatives, your talents and activities, and a confident, positive outlook are all parts of the whole that makes you—you!

How can flying a kite lift your spirits?

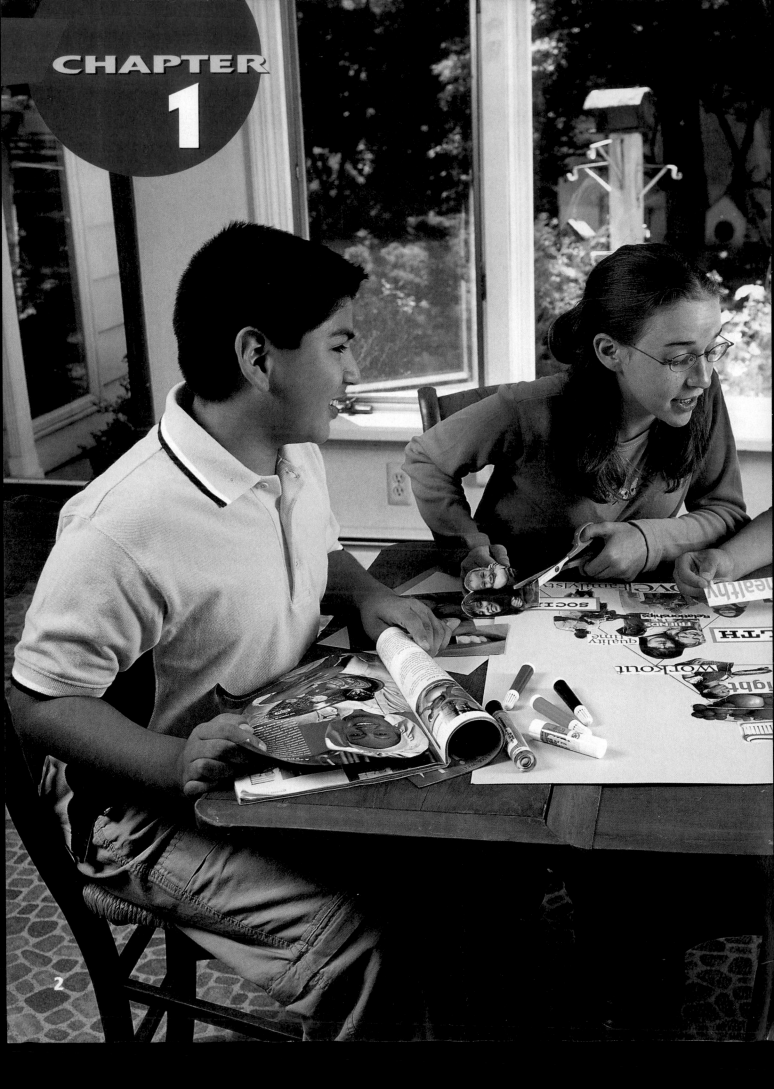

Learning About Your Health

HEALTH *Online*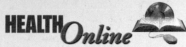

Do you know what it means to be healthy? You'll find out by taking the Health Inventory for Chapter 1 at health.glencoe.com.

FOLDABLES™
Study Organizer

Before You Read

Make this Foldable to record and organize what you learn in Lesson 1 about the three aspects of health. Begin with two plain sheets of 8½″ x 11″ paper.

Step 1

Line up one of the short edges of a sheet of paper with one of the long edges. Cut off the leftover rectangle.

Step 2

Repeat Step 1 with the second sheet. You will now have two squares.

Step 3

Stack the two squares and staple along the fold.

Step 4

Title your journal "Three Parts of Health." Label the inside page spreads *Physical, Mental/Emotional,* and *Social.*

Three Parts of Health

As You Read

On the appropriate page of your journal, take notes on what you learn about each of the three aspects of health, and give examples from your own life.

What Is Health?

Quick Write

Think about some of your habits and everyday activities. Jot down how you think these behaviors contribute to your health.

LEARN ABOUT...

- what it means to be healthy.
- how to balance your physical, mental/emotional, and social health.
- the relationship between health and wellness.

VOCABULARY

- health
- self-assessment
- wellness

Being Healthy

What makes a person healthy? Carl runs every day with the track team. However, he often has trouble controlling his temper. As a result, his friendships don't last very long. Ana often stays up late studying and sometimes skips breakfast. She feels tired a lot of the time. How healthy do you think Carl and Ana are?

Good health involves every part of your life. **Health** is *a combination of physical, mental/emotional, and social well-being.* Think of your health as a triangle with equal sides, as shown in **Figure 1.1** on the next page.

Physical Health

Your physical health involves the condition of your body. There are many things you can do to keep your body strong and healthy.

- Eat a well-balanced diet.
- Participate in regular physical activity.
- Get at least nine hours of sleep every night.
- Have regular health screenings.
- Avoid tobacco, alcohol, and other drugs.
- Understand and follow school rules related to health.
- Avoid unnecessary risks.

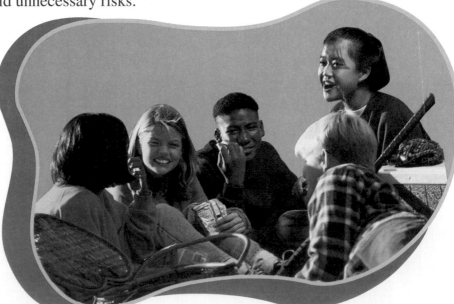

Having good friends is an important part of health.

Mental/Emotional Health

Your mental/emotional health relates to your thoughts and feelings. To keep yourself mentally and emotionally healthy,

- face difficult situations with a positive and realistic outlook.
- identify, express, and manage your feelings appropriately.
- set priorities so that you can handle all of your responsibilities.
- use your talents effectively to achieve your goals.
- be patient with yourself as you learn new skills. If you make a mistake, think about how you can do better the next time.
- accept responsibility for your actions.

Social Health

Social health involves the ways in which you relate to other people. To form strong social connections,

- support and value members of your family.
- have a friendly, open attitude toward other people.
- pay attention to what you say and how you say it.
- be a loyal, truthful, and dependable friend.
- learn to disagree without arguing and show respect for others.
- don't insult others or put them down.

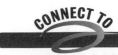

Visual Arts

PICTURE OF HEALTH
Create a poster illustrating the relationships between your physical, mental/emotional, and social health. You can use the image of the health triangle or choose another three-part organization. Your poster may combine original drawings, photos from newspapers and magazines, and computer clip art.

FIGURE 1.1

THE HEALTH TRIANGLE

To achieve and maintain total health, pay attention to all three sides of the health triangle. *If you were in these pictures, what activities would you be doing?*

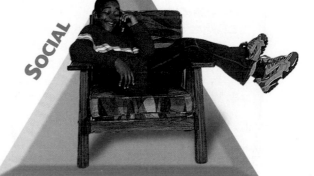

PHYSICAL

MENTAL/EMOTIONAL

SOCIAL

Measuring Your Health

You can't judge how healthy you are just by looking in a mirror. You can get a more complete view through **self-assessment**, or *careful examination and judgment of your own patterns of behavior.* Honest self-assessment can help you judge your current health status. It may reveal areas you can work to improve.

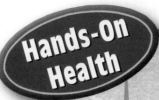

YOUR HEALTH TRIANGLE

Take this survey to recognize how your choices and actions influence your health. Then you can set goals to improve your health.

WHAT YOU WILL NEED
- writing paper and a pen or pencil
- a sheet of graph paper
- scissors

WHAT YOU WILL DO
Part 1: On a sheet of paper, write "yes" or "no," depending on whether each of the statements to the right describes you.

HOW DID YOU DO?
Part 2: You can use graph paper to make a model of your results.
- For each area of health, cut a strip of graph paper. Include one square for each of your "yes" answers.
- Label one of your strips "physical," one "mental/emotional," and one "social."
- Compare the lengths of the strips. Make a triangle with the three strips.

IN CONCLUSION
1. What does your triangle look like? Does it have equal sides, or is it a little lopsided?
2. Is there one area that you are strong in? Is there an area you need to work on?
3. What can you do to improve your health and balance your triangle?

Physical Health
1. I get at least nine hours of sleep each night.
2. I eat a well-balanced diet, including a healthful breakfast each day.
3. I keep my body, teeth, and hair clean.
4. I do at least 60 minutes of moderate physical activity each day.
5. I avoid using tobacco, alcohol, and other drugs.
6. I see a doctor and dentist for regular checkups.

Mental/Emotional Health
1. I generally feel good about myself and accept who I am.
2. I express my feelings clearly and calmly, even when I am angry or sad.
3. I accept helpful criticism.
4. I have at least one activity that I enjoy.
5. I feel that people like and accept me.
6. I like to learn new information and develop new skills.

Social Health
1. I have at least one close friend.
2. I respect and care for my family.
3. I know how to disagree with others without getting angry.
4. I am a good listener.
5. I get support from others when I need it.
6. I say no if people ask me to do something harmful or wrong.

What Is Wellness?

Keeping the three parts of your health triangle in balance is the best way to achieve **wellness**, which is *a state of well-being, or balanced health.* By making wise decisions and practicing healthful behaviors each day, you will be able to achieve a high level of wellness throughout your life.

How are health and wellness related? Your health refers to how you are doing physically, mentally/emotionally, and socially at a particular moment. Your health is constantly changing. For example, you may feel energetic one day and tired the next. Your level of wellness, on the other hand, has to do with how the three aspects of health interact over time. The choices you make every day become part of your long-term level of wellness. You want to make sure that most of the time, you enjoy a high level of wellness— a high level of energy and a feeling of well-being.

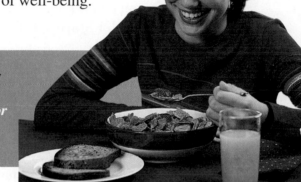

Eating a healthful breakfast every day is a regular behavior that enhances wellness. *Name one behavior you do regularly that contributes to your health and wellness.*

Lesson 1 Review

Using complete sentences, answer the following questions on a sheet of paper.

Reviewing Terms and Facts
1. **Vocabulary** Define the term *health.*
2. **Recall** How can self-assessment help you improve your health?
3. **Explain** What is meant by the term *wellness*? Use it in an original sentence.

Thinking Critically
4. **Apply** Think of two school rules that are related to health. Briefly describe how these rules help protect health and why it's important to follow them.

5. **Analyze** Reread the descriptions of Carl and Ana on page 4, and suggest ways for each of them to improve their personal health.
6. **Analyze** Review the health triangle shown on page 5. Analyze the interrelationships of physical, mental/emotional, and social health.

Applying Health Skills
7. **Goal Setting** Choose an action that would improve your health. Name one barrier that might keep you from taking this action. Describe how you could set a goal to overcome this barrier.

What Influences Your Health?

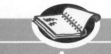
What Affects Your Health?

Both internal (personal) and external (outside) factors affect your health. You have control over many of these factors, but you can't control all of them. For example, you can't change your height, but you *can* improve your posture.

Making healthy choices means understanding and accepting what is beyond your control. It also means making the most of the factors you can control. **Figure 1.2** illustrates all of the factors that affect your health.

FIGURE 1.2

YOUR HEALTH FRAMEWORK

Some factors, such as heredity, are beyond your control. Think of factors like these as the framework of who you are. Inside that framework, you can make personal choices that affect your health. Each of these factors can have a positive or negative influence on health. *Name a health risk associated with each of these factors.*

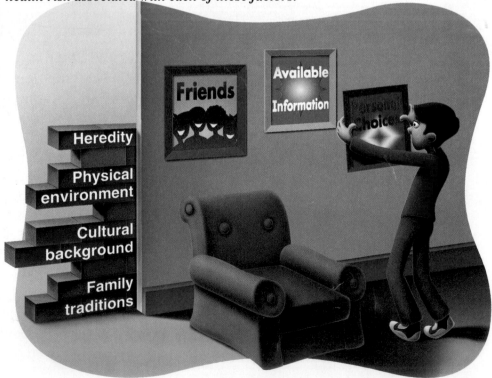

Heredity

Heredity (huh·RED·i·tee) is *the passing on of traits from biological parents to children.* Genetic factors or traits that are passed on through heredity include skin, eye, and hair color; body type and size; growth patterns; and the likelihood of getting certain diseases. Inherited traits are "built in"—you can't choose them or avoid them. However, recognizing the traits that you have inherited from your parents can help you make important decisions about your health. If, for example, members of your family tend to have many cavities, pay special attention to your dental care.

Environment

Your **environment** (en·VY·ruhn·ment) is *all the living and nonliving things that surround you.* It includes physical and social factors that contribute to individual and community health. Social environmental factors include access to education and jobs and presence of gang activity. Physical environmental factors include:

- **your home, neighborhood, and school.** Do you live and go to school in a large city or in a small town? Do you live in an apartment building or in a house?
- **the air you breathe and the water you drink.** Do you live in an area with heavy air pollution? Does your water come from a well, or is it supplied by a public utility?
- **the climate in which you live.** Do you live in a warm or cool climate? Do the seasons change noticeably where you live?

You may not be able to change your environment, but you can still make choices that can help you stay healthy. First, recognize parts of your environment that might harm your health. Then take steps to protect yourself.

Describe your physical surroundings. *What aspects of your environment enhance your health? What aspects pose risks to your health?*

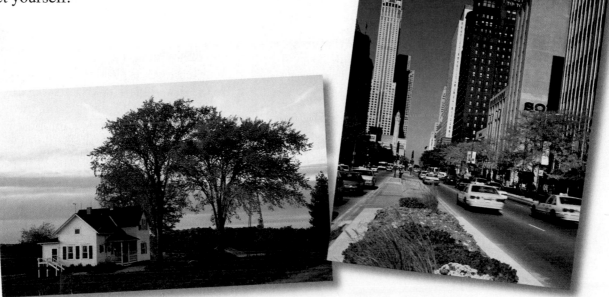

Reading Check
Understand how text is organized. The last sentence of the first paragraph on this page makes a statement. How do the first sentences of the following paragraphs support or expand on that statement?

Your Health Choices

Along with heredity and environment, several other aspects of your life influence your health. When you make a choice, many factors influence your thinking. Your family, friends, and the media can all contribute to your decisions.

Family and Friends

Your family has traditions that influence many aspects of your life, such as the foods you eat, the holidays you celebrate, and the goals you set. Some of these traditions are part of your cultural background. **Culture** is the *beliefs, customs, and traditions of a specific group of people.* Culture is one part of your health framework. You can learn to make wise health choices that help you honor and celebrate your culture. Sometimes, cultural factors can increase your health risks. For example, if your cultural traditions include eating foods that are high in sugar and fat, you may be at increased risk for developing diabetes or heart disease.

HEALTH SKILLS ACTIVITY

ANALYZING INFLUENCES

Class Health Survey

When you recognize the factors that influence your health, you are able to make wise choices about your health and wellness. Such factors may include heredity; the environment; your family, friends, and role models; and the media.

With your class, make a list of at least 15 things that have an impact on your individual and community health. The impact can be positive or negative. Be as specific as possible. For example, *environment* might relate to the air quality or climate where you live. It might mean the social environment, such as feeling safe. Your teacher will write the list on the chalkboard. Then, on a separate sheet of paper, write the five factors from the list that are most important to you. Do not write your name on the paper. Your teacher will collect the papers and tally the class results. What are the top five factors that influence the health of your class?

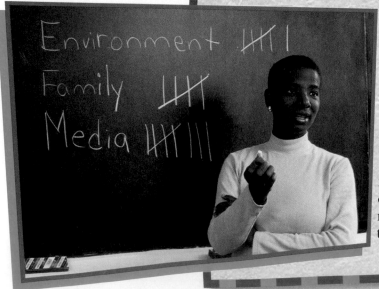

Your friends can also influence your decisions. Their influence can be either positive or negative. A friend who listens to you when you have a problem will probably have a positive influence on your health. A friend who urges you to drink alcohol or smoke cigarettes could have a very negative influence on your health.

The Influence of the Media

Another powerful influence on your individual and community health is the **media**, *the various methods for communicating information.* Media include TV and radio, movies, books, newspapers, magazines, billboards, and the Internet. Media and technology can influence health in various ways. For example, watching too much TV and not getting enough physical activity have created health problems for young people. On the other hand, media and technology can be used to promote important health messages such as antismoking campaigns.

Media sources can be helpful when you gather the information you need to make wise choices. To use these sources effectively, however, you must learn to **evaluate**, or *determine the quality of,* everything you see and hear. A media message often has a specific purpose. Commercials are designed to convince you to buy something, whether it is healthful for you or not. Magazine articles are designed to grab a reader's attention and sell copies.

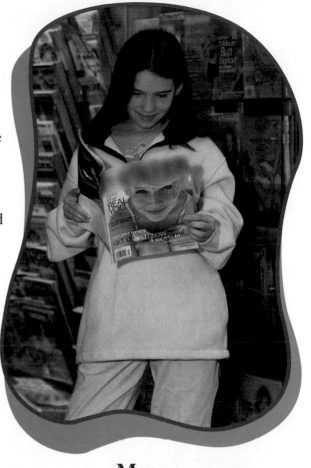

Media messages can be expressed through words, images, or a combination of both. *Which media do you find most helpful and why?*

Lesson 2 Review

Using complete sentences, answer the following questions on a sheet of paper.

Reviewing Terms and Facts

1. **Vocabulary** Define the terms *heredity* and *environment*.
2. **Restate** Describe how you can use information about inherited traits to make health decisions.
3. **List** Identify three factors, other than heredity and physical environment, that can influence a person's health.

Thinking Critically

4. **Evaluate** A friend says, "I don't need to know about my family's health history because there's nothing I can do about it anyway." How might you respond?
5. **Explain** Analyze positive and negative relationships that influence individual and community health, such as families, peers, and role models.

Applying Health Skills

6. **Analyzing Influences** What factor has the most influence on your health? Explain.

Health Risks and Your Behavior

Quick Write

Describe a time when you felt that you were in a risk situation. What did you do? Why? How did it work out? What could you have done to prevent this situation?

LEARN ABOUT...

- what risk behavior is.
- what cumulative risk is.
- how you can avoid health risk behaviors.

VOCABULARY

- risk behaviors
- consequences
- cumulative risks
- subjective
- objective
- prevention
- abstinence

Risk Behaviors

Have you ever seen a small child running toward the street with a concerned parent close behind? The parent was trying to protect the child from the risk of being hit by a vehicle. Risks—the possibility that something harmful may happen to your health and wellness—come in many forms. Since elementary school you have probably been aware of the risks associated with smoking. Did you know, however, that you also take health risks by eating high-fat foods and by not getting enough physical activity or sleep? An important part of taking responsibility for your health is identifying and avoiding **risk behaviors**, *actions or choices that may cause injury or harm to you or to others.*

Some risks are unavoidable. Events are unpredictable; and certain activities, such as playing a sport, can involve some hazards, or potential sources of danger. Risk behaviors, however, are actions that lead you into taking unnecessary risks.

Certain risks carry with them the likelihood that you or someone else will get hurt, now or in the future. For instance, if you pick a fight with another kid at school or in your neighborhood, you face the possibility that you will harm that person. You might cause physical pain, hurt the person emotionally, or affect her or his relationships with others. For these reasons, it is important to realize that your behavior can also affect the health of others.

Wearing a safety helmet will greatly reduce the risk of a serious head injury while cycling. *What other types of protective equipment do you use to avoid the risk of injury?*

The Consequences of Taking Risks

Risk behaviors may lead to a variety of **consequences**, or *the results of actions.* Some consequences affect only you and may not be especially dangerous. Other types of risk behaviors can lead to very serious consequences. **Figure 1.3** shows some of the results of taking unnecessary risks.

FIGURE 1.3

CONSEQUENCES OF HEALTH RISK BEHAVIORS

Every risk can lead to many different kinds of consequences. *Name one risk behavior that could lead to each type of consequence shown here.*

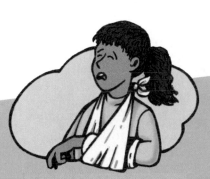

Physical Consequences
You could fall and hurt yourself.

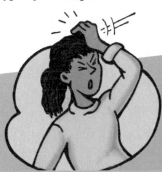

Mental/Emotional Consequences
You could feel upset and angry with yourself.

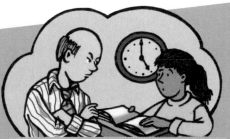

Academic Consequences
You might need to make up for time lost from school because you were injured.

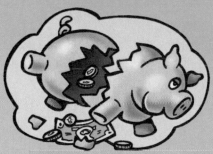

Financial Consequences
You could be forced to pay for damaging something.

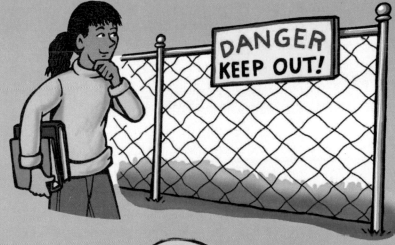

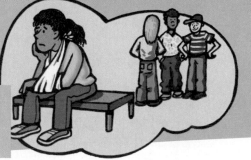

Social Consequences
You could miss out on activities because of injury.

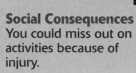

Legal Consequences
You could get in trouble for trespassing.

Types of Risks

Are teens taking risks? The answer seems to be that many people your age are recognizing the danger of engaging in certain risk behaviors. According to a major drug survey conducted by the Department of Health and Human Services, the use of alcohol, tobacco, and other drugs by youths ages 12–17 has either declined or remained the same in recent years. In addition, the Centers for Disease Control and Prevention reported that a large percentage of 12- and 13-year-olds are physically active. Finally, the National Safety Council reported that a large percentage of children ages 5–15 are wearing safety belts when riding in a motor vehicle. See **Figure 1.4**.

Cumulative Risk

Some hazards or risk factors may not seem very dangerous to you. The more risk factors you have, however, the more likely you will be to experience negative consequences. Some groups of risks are referred to as cumulative (KYOO·myuh·luh·tiv) risks. **Cumulative risks** are *related risks that increase in effect with each added risk.* Riding a bicycle without a helmet, for example, is one risk factor. If you are also riding on a busy street and it is raining, your chance of serious injury increases greatly.

FIGURE 1.4

YOUTH RISK BEHAVIOR—ENCOURAGING NEWS

These graphs show that the majority of teens are avoiding risk behaviors. *Do you belong to this majority? If not, how might you begin to change your behavior?*

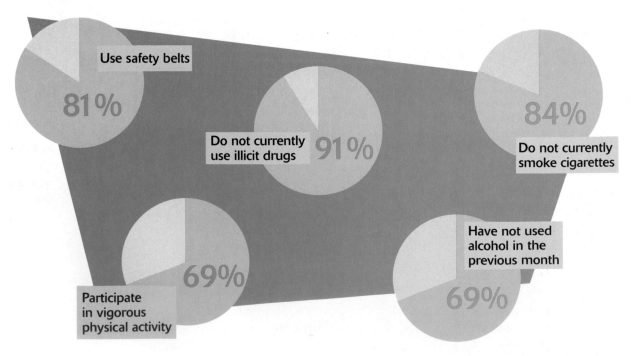

Use safety belts — 81%

Do not currently use illicit drugs — 91%

Do not currently smoke cigarettes — 84%

Participate in vigorous physical activity — 69%

Have not used alcohol in the previous month — 69%

REFUSAL SKILLS

Avoiding Risk Behaviors

Miguel and Jamie have been friends for many years, but lately Jamie has been changing. He has started hanging out with some teens who ride their skateboards in traffic, start fights, and smoke. Miguel has met these guys and feels uncomfortable about hanging out with them. Now Jamie is trying to convince Miguel to skip school with him so that they can spend time at the arcade with these guys. Miguel doesn't want to skip school to hang out with Jamie's friends. How can Miguel refuse Jamie's request?

What Would You Do?

S.T.O.P. is an easy way to remember how to use refusal skills when someone asks you to do something unhealthful or unsafe. With a classmate, role-play a scene in which Miguel uses S.T.O.P. to say no to Jamie.

SAY NO IN A FIRM VOICE.
TELL WHY NOT.
OFFER ANOTHER IDEA.
PROMPTLY LEAVE.

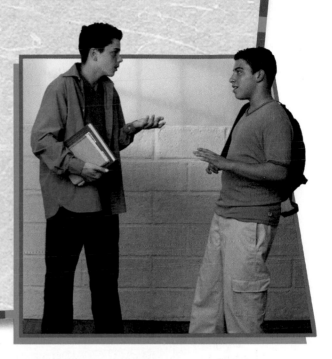

Knowing the Risks

Why do some teens take risks? Some young people take risks because they believe that nothing bad can happen to them. Others may question whether certain actions are really risky. They may believe, for example, that people who have accidents are just unlucky. This idea is **subjective**, which means that it *comes from a person's own views and beliefs, not necessarily from facts.*

When considering risks, it is much better to use **objective** information, which is information *based on facts.* Objective information can help you act responsibly so that you can prevent injuries and illnesses. The following is an example of subjective versus objective thinking:

- *Subjective* (involving a person's own views): "Lots of people smoke cigarettes, so how harmful can it be?"
- *Objective* (based on facts): The average smoker has a risk of dying from cancer of the lung, throat, or mouth that is 14 times greater than that of a nonsmoker.

✔ Reading Check

Distinguish between subjective and objective statements. Write subjective and objective statements about smoking or another risk behavior.

Reducing and Avoiding Risks

One of the most effective strategies to reduce risks or even avoid them entirely is to practice prevention. **Prevention** means *taking steps to make sure that something does not happen.* For example, wearing a helmet can prevent head injuries. Being on the lookout for hazards, or potential sources of danger, is an important part of prevention. If you're aware of hazards, you can protect yourself against them. For example, riding your bike in bad weather is a hazard. You can keep yourself safer by slowing down.

A key element of prevention is **abstinence**, or *not participating in unsafe behaviors or activities.* If you abstain from using tobacco or alcohol or engaging in sexual activity, you can avoid the serious consequences associated with these risk behaviors. **Figure 1.5** shows several ways you can protect yourself from risk.

FIGURE 1.5

Shield Yourself from Risk

Each of these attitudes and actions can help you protect yourself against risks that could threaten your health and even your life. *Which of these do you practice?*

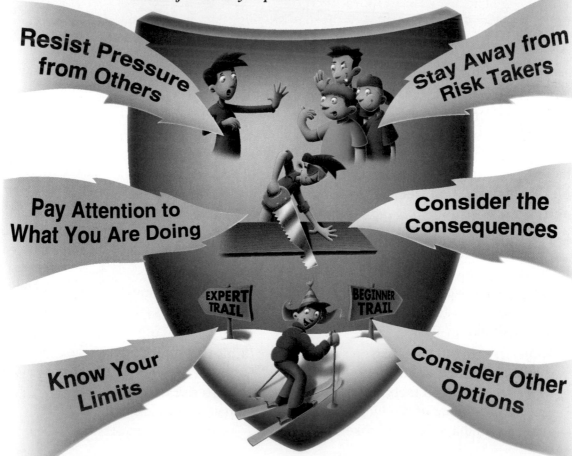

Resist Pressure from Others

Stay Away from Risk Takers

Pay Attention to What You Are Doing

Consider the Consequences

Know Your Limits

Consider Other Options

Keeping Yourself Healthy

You can take an active role in caring for your health. Keeping health and safety in mind will help you enjoy life while protecting your own health and that of others. Most injuries are not caused by bad luck or fate but by poor decision making. If you act responsibly and avoid risks, you can prevent most injuries. By practicing good health habits, you can also prevent many illnesses.

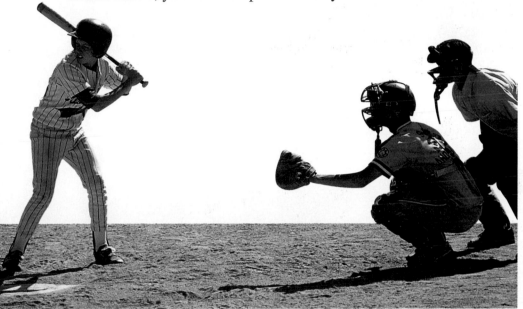

You can avoid most sports injuries by wearing the correct protective equipment and following the rules. *What else can you do to learn how to play a sport more safely?*

Lesson Review

Using complete sentences, answer the following questions on a sheet of paper.

Reviewing Terms and Facts

1. **Vocabulary** Define the term *risk behavior.*
2. **Identify** List six types of consequences that may result from risk behavior.
3. **Vocabulary** Define the term *cumulative risks.* Then give an example of a cumulative risk.

Thinking Critically

4. **Analyze** Explain the role of media and technology in influencing individual and community health.

5. **Describe** Suppose that you were going to spend a day on a boat. What precautions might you take to avoid risks?

Applying Health Skills

6. **Refusal Skills** On hot summer days, you and two of your close friends like to go swimming in a nearby lake. Lately, your friends have been talking about climbing onto some rocks and diving into the water. You think that the plan sounds dangerous. You could get hurt on the rocks or hit your head when you enter the water. Explain how you would use S.T.O.P. to respond to your friends' request.

Do You Have Sleep Smarts?

Take our test to see if you need to wake up your sleeping habits!

Quiz

1. How many hours of sleep does a teen need each night?
a. Five
b. Seven
c. Nine or more

2. You are probably overtired if you
a. sleep until noon on the weekends.
b. can't react as quickly as you used to while playing computer games.
c. don't feel like socializing as much as you have in the past.
d. All of the above

3. Pulling an all-nighter before a big test will usually help you score a better grade than studying and then getting a good night's sleep.
a. True   b. False

4. Sleeplessness in teens is commonly caused by
a. anxiety about school or sports.
b. poor eating habits.
c. a lack of physical activity.
d. All of the above

Answers: 1. c; 2. d; 3. b; 4. d.

Check out the explanations on the next page!

SNOOZE NEWS

THESE sleep facts are interesting enough to keep anyone awake:

HUMANS spend about a third of their lives sleeping.

THE record for the longest period of time without sleep is 18 days, 21 hours, and 40 minutes, which took place during a rocking chair marathon. The record holder experienced hallucinations, slurred speech, blurred vision, and lapses in memory and concentration.

PEOPLE can sleep for a brief period of time with their eyes open—without even knowing they are asleep.

DURING rapid eye movement (REM) sleep, a person's eyes move back and

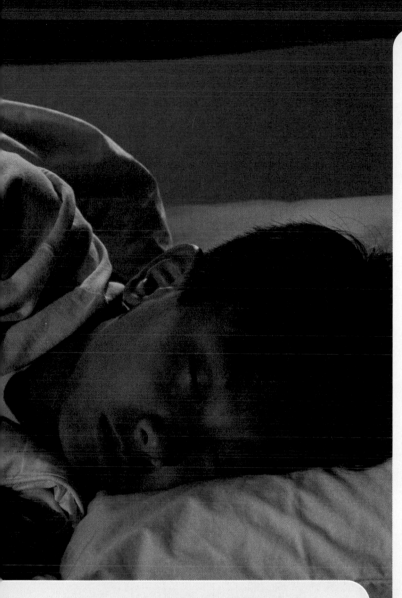

Explanations

1. A teen needs nine or more hours of sleep each night to function at his or her best. **"Research shows that growth hormones are secreted [released] during sleep,"** says sleep expert Amy Wolfson of the College of the Holy Cross in Massachusetts. "The teen years are an important period of growth, so it makes sense that [teens] would need more rest."

2. **If you're overtired, it will affect all areas of your life:** how well you concentrate in class, your ability to remember simple facts, your health—even your social life. "When we don't get enough sleep it affects our mood, making us prone to feeling depressed and less sociable," explains Wolfson. To combat this, make sure you sleep for at least nine hours and keep a regular sleep schedule by going to bed and waking up at roughly the same time each day.

3. Instead of pulling an all-nighter, you'd probably do better on the exam if you studied and slept. **"Memory is impaired when you don't get a good night's sleep,"** explains sleep researcher Mary Carskadon. Without sleep, it's likely that you'll forget some of what you learned the night before the test.

4. Common causes of sleeplessness in teens are anxiety, poor diet, and lack of exercise. **Learning to deal with stress and not overloading your schedule are keys to a better night's sleep.** Reducing your intake of caffeine and sweets and getting regular physical activity can also help you sleep at night. ◼

forth quickly. **REM sleep** usually begins about 90 minutes after falling asleep and occurs in bursts that total about two hours a night. This is the period when most dreams take place.

NONHUMAN primates, such as chimps, monkeys, and baboons, sleep about 10 hours a day. Brown bats sleep nearly 20 hours a day, while giraffes sleep less than two hours a day.

PEOPLE fall asleep more easily when body temperature drops, which is why it is often difficult to drop off during hot summer nights.

Sources: Dr. Eric Chudler, University of Washington; Australian Broadcasting Corp.; ThinkQuest; Stanford University

TIME TO THINK...

About Sleep Habits

For seven consecutive nights, record the number of hours you sleep. Compute the average number of hours you slept each night. Compare your average with those of your classmates. On days you sleep fewer hours than your average, do you notice any difference in the way you feel and in how you perform in school? Set a goal to get an adequate amount of sleep each night.

TRACKING DOWN THE FACTS

Model

Some teens take health risks without realizing it because they act on subjective, rather than objective, information.

Read this conversation between Eli and Samuel. The objective information is in green. The subjective information is in red.

Hey, Samuel. I didn't know you were going to try out for the wrestling team.

Yep! I've been working on my technique.

Me too. What have you been doing to get ready for tryouts?

Well, I've been eating lots of fruits, vegetables, and pasta. My health book says that athletes need complex carbohydrates. I've also been trying to get enough sleep. I read in the newspaper that most teens don't get enough sleep.

I'm thinking about using some pills to lose weight. I don't want to wrestle in the higher weight class. My brother says diet pills aren't dangerous and they help you lose weight fast. He says all the good wrestlers use them.

Are you doing anything to improve your strength and endurance?

Yeah. I got this workout idea in a wrestling magazine. I do aerobic exercises, like jogging, to increase my stamina. I do weight training to build strength. I'm also taking several vitamins every day. I'm convinced you can't get too many vitamins.

Hey, maybe we could work out one day soon.

Practice

Below are seven statements about health. Can you separate the subjective from the objective information? Use your textbook to find the facts. When you find a subjective statement, change it to an objective statement.

- Anger is a bad emotion.
- Regular shampooing prevents head lice.
- Almost half of the deaths of young people result from accidents.
- Snacking is bad for you.
- Most of your body is water.
- All stress is negative and should be avoided.
- Smokeless tobacco is a safe alternative to cigarettes.

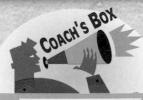

COACH'S BOX

Accessing Information

Ask yourself these questions about any source of information.

- Is it scientific?
- Does it give only one point of view?
- Is it trying to sell something?
- Does it agree with other sources?

Apply/Assess

Finding accurate information improves your ability to make healthful choices. It can also help you be a source of accurate information for your friends and family. Choose an area of health that interests you. You may use the Table of Contents in this book to review the different areas of health.

Use sources of objective information to find four health facts that teens should know. Report your facts to the class in the form of a chart. See the example below.

Self-√Check

- Does my chart include four health facts?
- Does my chart show where to find objective information?
- Does my chart explain why each source I found provides objective information?

Fact	Source(s)	Why I Believe This Source Is Objective
Eating chocolate does NOT cause acne.	www.familydoctor.org	uses the logo of the American Academy of Family Physicians
	www.aad.org	site of the American Academy of Dermatology

After You Read

Use your completed Foldable to review the information on the three aspects of health.

FOLDABLES™
Study Organizer

Reviewing Vocabulary and Concepts

On a sheet of paper, write the numbers 1–5. After each number, write the term from the list that best completes each statement.

- self-assessment
- physical
- wellness
- mental/emotional
- social

Lesson 1

1. Your _____ health involves the condition of your body.
2. Being patient with yourself when learning a new skill and taking responsibility for your actions are both examples of _____ health.
3. How well you get along with others is a key part of your _____ health.
4. Careful examination and judgment of your own patterns of behavior is _____.
5. One sign of a high level of _____ is a consistent feeling of well-being.

On a sheet of paper, write the numbers 6–18. Write *True* or *False* for each statement below. If the statement is false, change the underlined word or phrase to make it true.

Lesson 2

6. <u>Air pollution</u> is an environmental factor that can affect your health.

7. <u>Heredity</u> is one part of your health framework that does not change.
8. A friend who encourages you to smoke is an example of a <u>positive</u> influence.
9. The beliefs, customs, and traditions of a specific group of people is known as <u>culture</u>.
10. <u>Media</u> are the various methods for communicating information.
11. It is important to <u>accept</u> the information you learn from television programs, magazines, or any other media source.

Lesson 3

12. <u>Risks</u> are the possibility that something harmful may happen to your health and wellness.
13. A fallen tree in the middle of a bicycle path and a high level of dietary fat are both examples of <u>abstinence</u>.
14. Injuries and disabilities are two possible physical <u>consequences</u> of taking unnecessary risks.
15. If a statement is <u>objective</u>, it is based on a person's views and beliefs, not necessarily on facts.
16. If a statement is <u>subjective</u>, it is based on facts.
17. Going canoeing without wearing a life jacket when the current is strong and with someone who has no experience is an example of <u>cumulative risks</u>.
18. Not smoking is one example of <u>hazards</u>.

Thinking Critically

Using complete sentences, answer the following questions on a sheet of paper.

19. **Hypothesize** If your mental/emotional health improves, how might other aspects of your health be affected?
20. **Assess** How can you contribute to the strengthening of health-related policies at your school?

21. **Evaluate** In your opinion, which factor is a greater influence on your health: heredity or environment? Why?

22. **Apply** Imagine that you are getting to know a group of new friends. Tell how you would decide whether these friends were going to be a positive or negative influence on your health.

23. **Explain** Interpret critical issues related to solving problems: How can you resist peer pressure to try alcohol or other drugs?

Career Corner

Health Teacher Do you like learning about health? Do you think you have a talent for helping others learn new information? If so, a career as a health teacher might be for you. This career requires excellent communication skills and the ability to motivate others. You'll also need a four-year teaching degree with specialized courses in health education. One way to prepare for this career is by tutoring others. For more information, visit Career Corner at health.glencoe.com.

Standardized Test Practice

Reading & Writing

Read the paragraphs below and then answer the questions.

It is early morning and Mead Park Recreation Center is bustling with activity. A few joggers are making their way around the pond. Tennis partners are unpacking their racquets and balls for a morning match. Players and coaches are out on the softball field getting ready for another game.

More and more people are becoming physically active on a regular basis. Some engage in physical activity to improve their level of fitness or to achieve a healthful weight. Many people are physically active because they know how much better they feel after a game or a run. There are many reasons to be active, but one thing is clear: physical activity benefits physical, mental/emotional, and social health.

1. In the passage, the word "bustling" helps the reader see that the scene is

   (A) busy.

   (B) beautiful.

   (C) peaceful.

   (D) confused.

2. Which of the following best describes the organization of the second paragraph?

   (A) ranking reasons to be physically active in order of importance

   (B) explaining the pros and cons of physical activity

   (C) presenting events in the order in which they occur

   (D) presenting different reasons for being physically active

3. Write a paragraph giving the reasons why you think more people are engaging in regular physical activity.

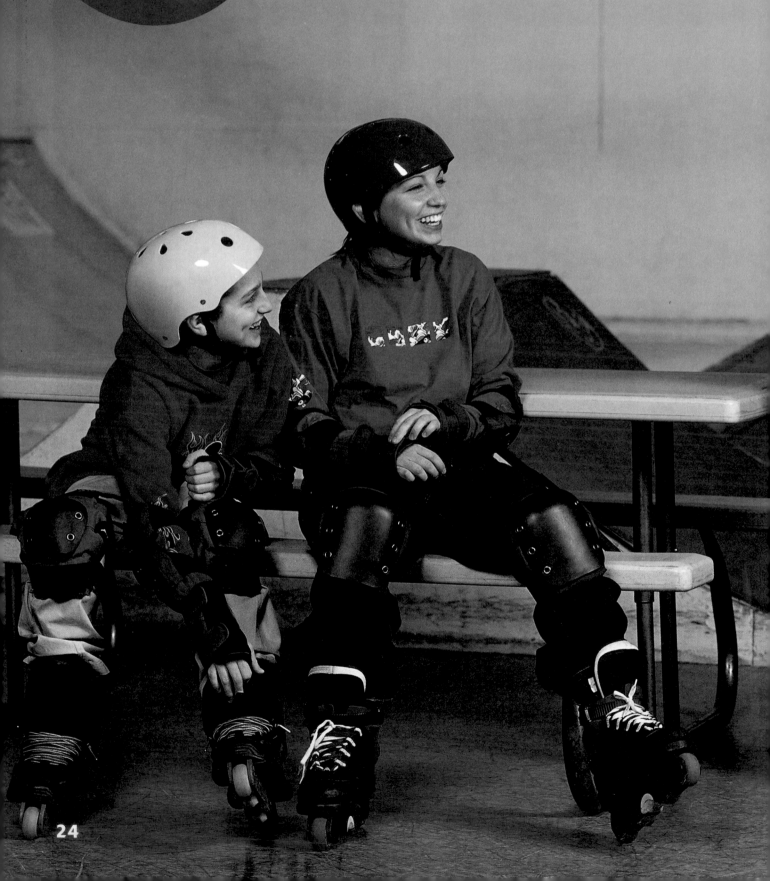

Taking Responsibility for Your Health

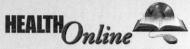

HEALTH *Online*

Do you take responsibility for your decisions? Take the Chapter 2 Health Inventory at health.glencoe.com to see how you rate.

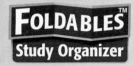

FOLDABLES™
Study Organizer

Before You Read

Make this Foldable to help you organize what you learn in Lesson 1 about building health skills. Begin with a plain sheet of 11″ × 17″ paper.

Step 1

Fold a sheet of paper in half along the long axis, then fold in half again. This makes four rows.

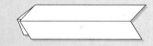

Step 2

Open and fold the short side on the left to make a 3″ column.

Step 3

Label the chart with the health skills shown.

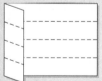

As You Read

Define and take notes on the health skills listed in the chart.

Building Health Skills

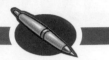

Skills for Balanced Health

Your health involves every aspect of your life—your body, your thoughts and emotions, and your relationships with others. There are many skills and practices that will help you achieve, maintain, and protect good health. If you develop these health skills and practices now, they will have a positive effect throughout your life. **Figure 2.1** provides an overview of the basic health skills.

FIGURE 2.1

THE HEALTH SKILLS

These skills are related to your physical, mental/emotional, and social health. *Give one or two examples of areas in which the development of these skills will benefit you as you grow older.*

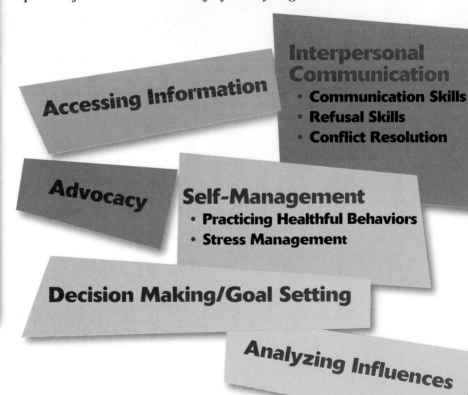

Accessing Information

Interpersonal Communication
- Communication Skills
- Refusal Skills
- Conflict Resolution

Advocacy

Self-Management
- Practicing Healthful Behaviors
- Stress Management

Decision Making/Goal Setting

Analyzing Influences

Accessing Information

From billboards to cereal boxes, you are exposed to information everywhere you look. You can develop good fact-finding skills so that you can gather the information you need to make healthful decisions. Your home, school, and community provide many valuable resources for finding reliable information.

Not all sources of information are equally valid. That's why it's important to verify your sources. For printed materials, check the credentials of the author and anyone the author quotes. Are they experts on the topic? Then check the author's sources and findings. Is the information based on reliable scientific studies?

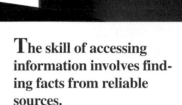

The skill of accessing information involves finding facts from reliable sources.

Self-Management

Developing self-management skills means that you act in specific ways to stay physically healthy and that you take responsibility for your mental and emotional wellness. Practicing healthful behaviors and managing stress are two key components in developing the skills of self-management.

HEALTH SKILLS ACTIVITY

ACCESSING INFORMATION

How to Find Reliable Information

Advances in technology allow you to access information 24 hours a day. Here are some tips to help you make wise choices among the available resources.

- **Parents, guardians, and other trusted adults** (such as teachers, counselors, and school nurses) should be your first source of reliable health information.
- **Library resources**—such as encyclopedias and nonfiction books on science, medicine, nutrition, and fitness—provide facts.
- **Reliable media sources** include newspaper and magazine articles by health professionals or experts, television and radio interviews with health professionals, and reports on current scientific studies related to health.

- **The Internet** contains up-to-the-minute information on health-related topics provided by government agencies, health care providers, universities, and scientific publications.
- **Community resources** are valuable sources of health information. Call or visit local chapters of organizations such as the American Heart Association and government offices such as the local department of health. Collect pamphlets about services and programs at hospitals, clinics, and universities in your area.

ON YOUR OWN
Select a health-related topic. Then develop evaluation criteria for health information and find reliable sources of information on your topic. Make a chart to evaluate at least five sources that you find.

Practicing Healthful Behaviors

When you practice healthful behaviors, you use skills that will not only protect you from immediate illness or injury but also increase your level of physical wellness over the long term. Drinking plenty of water, for example, helps your body function efficiently. Participating in regular physical activity strengthens your muscles and increases your energy. Getting regular medical and dental checkups maintains your health.

Stress Management

Your body reacts to everything that happens to you. Some of the events in your life may create **stress**, *your body's response to changes around you.* Stress can be positive or negative. Positive stress can help you work toward and reach goals. For example, you may spend more time studying so that you can avoid becoming too nervous before a big test. Negative stress can cause you discomfort and even keep you from doing things you need or want to do. For example, if you are worried that others will make fun of your lack of artistic ability, you may not enter your artwork in a school competition. Stress is a factor in everyone's life. It affects personal and family health. **Stress management** is *identifying sources of stress and learning how to handle them in ways that promote good mental and emotional health.*

Analyzing Influences

Being able to analyze influences means that you recognize the ways in which internal and external factors affect your health choices. Internal factors include your knowledge and feelings, interests, likes and dislikes, desires, and fears. External influences include relationships with people such as your family, friends, teachers, counselors, and role models. Media sources, such as books you read and advertisements you see and hear, also play a role in your health choices. Learn to tell the difference between influences that promote your health and those that harm your health.

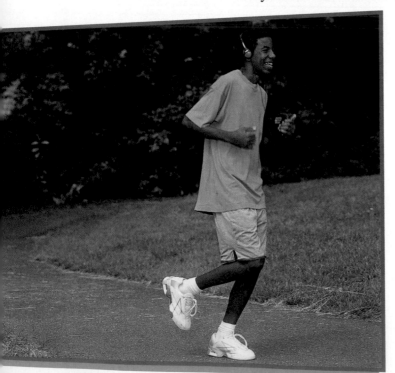

Participating in regular physical activity promotes good health and can help you manage stress. *What physical activities do you take part in on a regular basis?*

Interpersonal Communication

Developing your speaking and listening skills will help you express your ideas and feelings in healthful ways. It will also allow you to understand the messages that others send to you. Part of **interpersonal communication**, *the sharing of thoughts and feelings between two or more people,* is saying no to risk behaviors. These skills also enable you to handle difficult situations safely and fairly.

Communication Skills

Communication skills involve much more than being able to speak clearly. You can also get your message across by your facial expressions, tone of voice, choice of words, and body posture. You even communicate by the way you listen. Effective communication skills can help prevent misunderstandings. They will also allow you to give support to others when they need it.

Refusal Skills

Saying no can be a challenge. To stand up for your own decisions and beliefs, you need strong **refusal skills**, which are *ways to say no effectively.* When you say no to risk behaviors, you are showing respect for yourself. If a friend urges you to do something that you feel is not in your best interest, your beliefs will help you to refuse. A true friend will respect your decision. If you still feel pressured, you will need to examine your relationship with that person.

Reading Check

Investigate word meanings. *Managing* and *coping* are synonyms. List as many words as you can that mean the same, or nearly the same, as *stress, refuse,* and *communicate.*

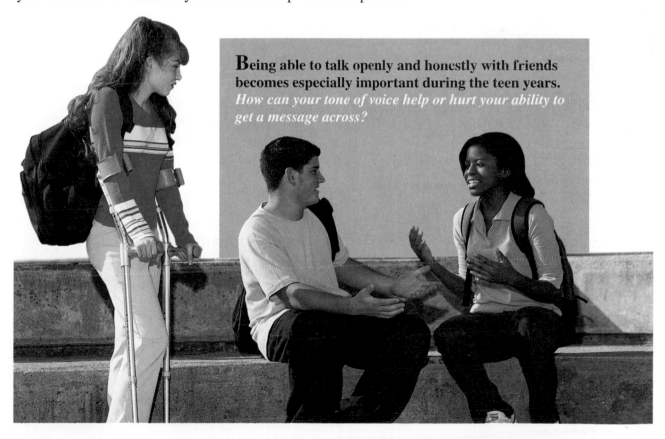

Being able to talk openly and honestly with friends becomes especially important during the teen years. *How can your tone of voice help or hurt your ability to get a message across?*

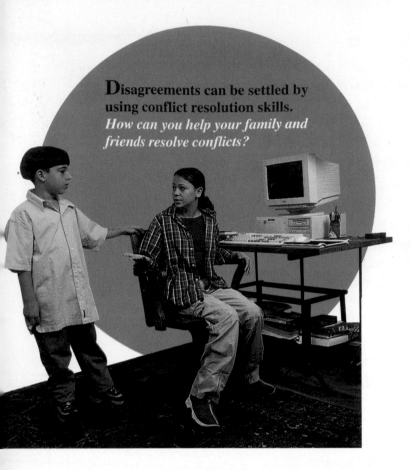

Disagreements can be settled by using conflict resolution skills. *How can you help your family and friends resolve conflicts?*

Conflict Resolution

Effective communication skills will be useful when you face **conflict**, *a disagreement between people with opposing viewpoints.* Conflicts are not good or bad. They indicate differences in opinion. Conflict is normal and can help bring about change. Many conflicts can be avoided, but you need to be prepared to face both small and large conflicts. **Conflict resolution** means *finding a solution to a disagreement or preventing it from becoming a larger conflict.* If you and a friend disagree about how to spend money that you have earned together, conflict-resolution skills can help you find an acceptable compromise. Begin by taking a time-out—at least 30 minutes. Allow each person to tell his or her side uninterrupted. Let each person ask questions. Keep brainstorming to find a good solution. Be committed to finding positive and constructive solutions to the conflict.

Lesson 1 Review

Using complete sentences, answer the following questions on a sheet of paper.

Reviewing Terms and Facts

1. **Identify** Name the basic health skills.
2. **Contrast** What is *stress*? Explain the difference between positive stress and negative stress.
3. **Vocabulary** Define the term *conflict*. Give an example of a conflict that you have faced recently.

Thinking Critically

4. **Judge** How can you tell the difference between a helpful influence and one that might lead you to try a risk behavior?

5. **Analyze** Suppose that two of your friends have stopped talking to each other because they had a fight about whom to invite to a party. Explain how communication skills and conflict resolution might help them reach a peaceful solution.

Applying Health Skills

6. **Refusal Skills** Think of a situation in which you were pressured to behave in a way that you felt was wrong. In a paragraph, explain the situation. Did you give in to the pressure? If you were able to stand up to it, explain how you used refusal skills to say no. If you gave in, explain how you could have handled the situation differently by using refusal skills.

Making Responsible Decisions

Responsibility for Your Health

As you grow up, you take on greater responsibility. This added responsibility involves making some important decisions. **Decision making** is *the process of making a choice or solving a problem.*

You make decisions about every area of your life—your health, family, friends, activities, and more. The choices you make show others what you think is important. Learning how to make positive decisions that show respect for your health and the health of others is part of becoming a responsible person.

When you make a decision, consider the critical issues and possible outcomes of that decision. Ask yourself:

- How will this decision affect my well-being?
- How will it affect the health of others?
- Is it harmful?
- Is it unlawful?
- How will my family feel about this decision?
- How might this decision affect my life goals?

Quick Write

Are you the type of person who makes decisions quickly, without giving them much thought, or do you weigh the pros and cons before taking action? Briefly describe the way you typically make decisions.

Learn About...

- the types of decisions that affect your health and the health of others.
- how values play a role in the decisions that you make.
- the steps of the decision-making process.

Vocabulary

- decision making
- values
- criteria

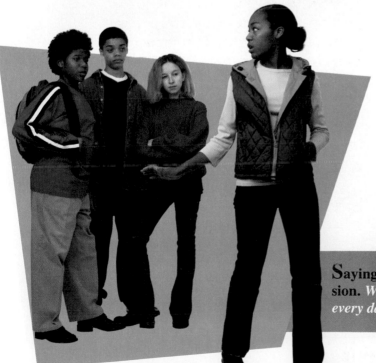

Saying no to harmful behavior is a responsible decision. *What other health-related decisions do you make every day?*

Values and the Decisions You Make

Responsible decisions should be based on values. **Values** are *the beliefs that guide the way a person lives, such as beliefs about what is right and wrong and what is most important.* In order for people to have healthy relationships, they must uphold core ethical values. Action that is ethical is considered right. People around the world place importance on values such as trust, respect, and citizenship.

Other values are completely individual. For example, you may believe that it is important to conserve natural resources. Values develop from many sources, as shown in **Figure 2.2**.

FIGURE 2.2

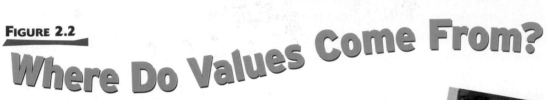

Basing your decisions on values will help ensure that these decisions are healthful. *How do values influence your decisions?*

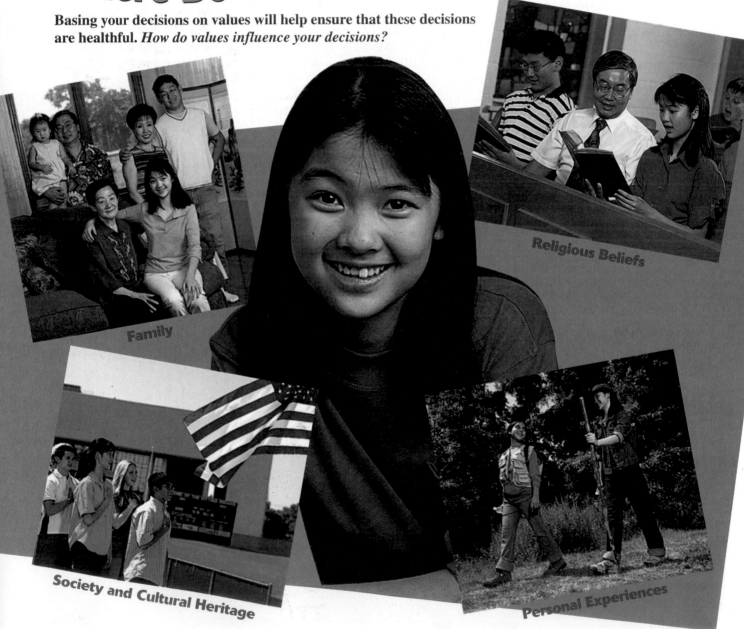

Family

Religious Beliefs

Society and Cultural Heritage

Personal Experiences

Evaluating Your Choices

Values provide you with **criteria** (kry·TIR·ee·uh), or *standards on which to base your decisions.* Criteria help you evaluate a situation. They can also help you evaluate the outcomes of your decisions.

Consider this situation. You place a high value on your health and safety. You also try to do what is right. A friend of yours has seen some athletes using smokeless tobacco and wants to try it with you. Your friend says that it won't be as dangerous as smoking cigarettes because you won't be inhaling the chemicals that are found in cigarettes. On the basis of your values and what you know about tobacco, you could evaluate the situation by applying the H.E.L.P. criteria:

- **H (Healthful)** Is your friend's claim correct? What are the actual health risks of using smokeless tobacco?
- **E (Ethical)** An action that is ethical is considered right, according to values. Is it right to use tobacco?
- **L (Legal)** Is it lawful for someone your age to use this product?
- **P (Parent Approval)** Would your parents approve of your choice?

In this case, using the above criteria to evaluate the situation would help you decide not to use smokeless tobacco. Your analysis will show that using this type of tobacco has many risks. You can explain your reasons and try to convince your friend to follow your lead.

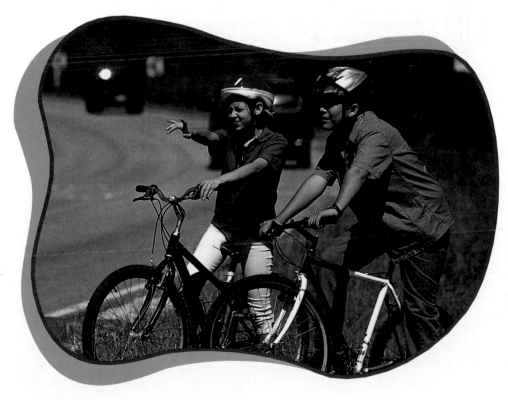

Taking a shortcut can be tempting, but you should think about the situation carefully before you decide. *How can these teens use the H.E.L.P. criteria to evaluate this situation?*

The Decision-Making Process

The decision-making process can be broken down into six steps. These steps are illustrated in **Figure 2.3**. Although you will usually use this skill to make important decisions, you can practice it with any decision.

FIGURE 2.3

THE STEPS OF THE DECISION-MAKING PROCESS

The decision-making process can help you to think through your choices. *Relate practices and steps necessary for making health decisions.*

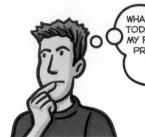

1. State the Situation
What is the decision I have to make? How much time do I have to make a decision?

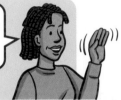

2. List the Options
What are my choices? Can a reliable source, such as my parent or guardian, help me think of other choices?

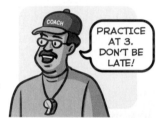

3. Weigh the Possible Outcomes
What are the consequences of each option? How will my choice affect me, both now and in the future? Will my choice affect anyone else, and if so, how?

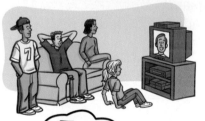

4. Consider Values
For some decisions I will need to ask myself, "How does each of my options fit in with my values? How will my values influence my decision?"

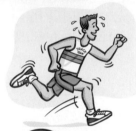

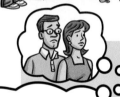

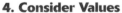

5. Make a Decision and Act
What choice shall I make? What do I need to do to follow through on my decision?

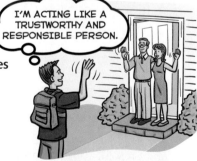

6. Evaluate the Decision
What were the consequences of my decision? Did the results turn out as I planned? Would I make the same choice if I had to do it again? What did I learn?

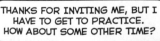

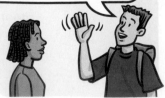

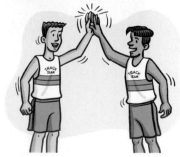

THE LINKS BETWEEN DECISIONS

Ms. Chen assigned a short essay on Friday. It is due on Tuesday. Sophia has to decide when she will write the essay. If she works on it on Saturday, she won't be able to go hiking. She was planning to practice for a gymnastics competition on Sunday. If she waits until Monday, she may have to stay up late to complete the essay.

WHAT YOU WILL NEED
- construction paper
- scissors and markers or pens
- tape, a stapler, or a glue stick

WHAT YOU WILL DO
1. Cut strips of construction paper. Write one of Sophia's possible decisions on a strip of paper.
2. Roll the strip into a loop. Staple, tape, or glue the loop together so that the writing appears on the outside of the loop.

3. On another strip write a decision that Sophia will have to make as a result of her first decision. Link it to the first loop.
4. Keep adding loops to show one chain of decisions that Sophia might make. Read your completed chain to the class.

IN CONCLUSION
1. In your opinion, which decisions created the most healthy decision chain? Why?
2. How did making a chain of decisions help you evaluate Sophia's situation?

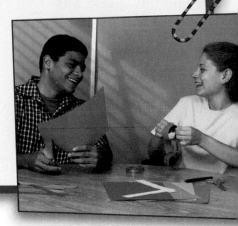

Lesson 2 Review

Using complete sentences, answer the following questions on a sheet of paper.

Reviewing Terms and Facts
1. **Vocabulary** Define the term *decision making*.
2. **Recall** Name three sources from which values develop.
3. **List** What are the four H.E.L.P. criteria?
4. **Summarize** Identify the six steps of the decision-making process.

Thinking Critically
5. **Explain** Why should you think about values before making a major decision?

6. **Analyze** Which of the six steps in the decision-making process do you think is the most important? Explain your answer.

Applying Health Skills
7. **Refusal Skills** When you make a decision that goes against what everyone else wants to do, you may need to use refusal skills. Imagine the following situation: A friend wants you to go swimming, but you don't want to go because there are no lifeguards on duty. With a classmate, role-play a scenario in which you use refusal skills to stand by your decision.

Setting Personal Health Goals

Quick Write

What does it mean if someone is "all talk and no action"? Write down a few ideas about how this approach to life could affect a person's health.

LEARN ABOUT...

- the benefits of setting goals.
- the types of goals you might set.
- how to create and follow a goal-setting plan to reach a goal.

VOCABULARY

- long-term goal
- short-term goal

Benefits of Setting Goals

You may wonder why it is important to have goals. Goals can give direction to your behavior and a pattern to your decisions. They allow you to develop a focus on the future. A goal is also one way to measure your success. You can look at goals as milestones on a journey. They help you evaluate how far you've traveled and how far you have left to go.

Some goals may be easy to achieve, while others are much more challenging. Suppose, for example, that your goal is to improve your grade in science class. Getting a high score on one quiz may not be a problem for you. Getting an A in science for the whole year, however, may be more difficult. In either case, achieving a goal that you have set for yourself is a rewarding experience.

It is important to recognize one's own strengths and limitations when setting goals. Although some of your goals may seem difficult to achieve, your best efforts will always be worthwhile. Striving to reach your goals will have a positive effect on your self-confidence. The knowledge that you have reached some goals in the past will give you the confidence you need to reach new goals. Meeting the goals you have set for yourself is an appropriate way to gain attention and recognition. Your success can also inspire others to work toward their own goals.

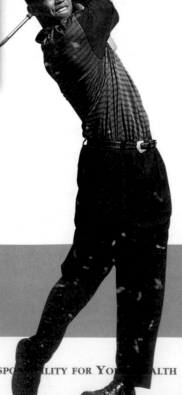

Athletes must set and reach many goals to succeed in their sports. *Think of an example of a health-related goal that an athlete might set.*

Long-Term and Short-Term Goals

Time is an important element in the process of setting goals. Some goals will take much longer to achieve than others. A **long-term goal** is *a goal that you plan to reach over an extended length of time.* Examples of long-term goals include learning to play an instrument, becoming class president, making the soccer team, and working in a specific profession. These goals could take months or years to achieve. Each step you take toward your long-term goal brings you closer to it.

You will be able to accomplish some goals quickly. A **short-term goal** is *a goal that you can reach in a short length of time.* Examples of short-term goals include cleaning your room and finishing your homework. Setting and meeting a series of short-term goals can help you achieve a long-term goal. **Figure 2.4** shows how one teen works to reach a challenging long-term goal.

Developing Good Character

Perseverance

To *persevere* means to continue even when the going gets tough. Think about a health-related goal that you have achieved recently. Did you ever feel like you wanted to give up on your goal? Write a paragraph describing how you got past that moment and kept on trying.

FIGURE 2.4

Achieving a Personal Health Goal

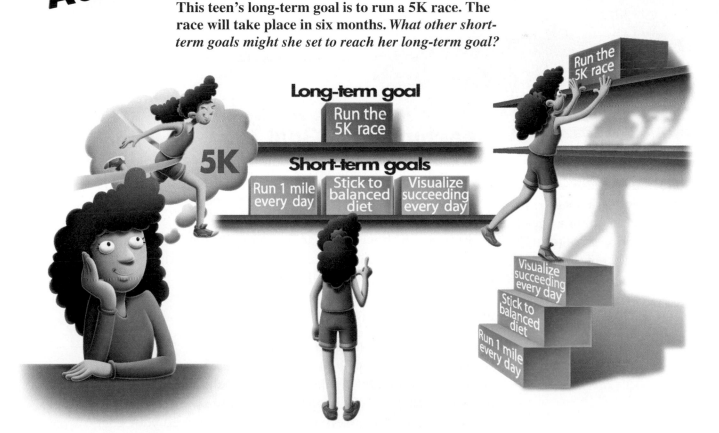

This teen's long-term goal is to run a 5K race. The race will take place in six months. *What other short-term goals might she set to reach her long-term goal?*

Long-term goal
Run the 5K race

Short-term goals
Run 1 mile every day | Stick to balanced diet | Visualize succeeding every day

Run the 5K race

Visualize succeeding every day
Stick to balanced diet
Run 1 mile every day

GOAL SETTING

Managing Your Habits

A habit is a pattern of behavior that you repeat often enough so that you come to do it almost without thinking. Habits can be difficult to change because you are often unaware of them. The first step in managing your habits is to think about the positive and negative behaviors that are part of your everyday life.

Some habits have lifelong benefits. For example, getting enough sleep each night will improve your energy and alertness. Others may be harmful or unsafe. For example, leaving your clothes or books on the floor can lead to an injury if you or someone else trips and falls.

Habits become stronger with repetition. To acquire a positive habit, repeat the action regularly. Soon you will practice the healthful behavior almost automatically. To eliminate a harmful habit, set specific goals toward stopping it and stick to them.

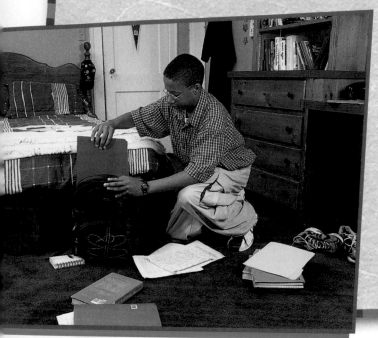

ON YOUR OWN

Identify and analyze a harmful or unsafe habit that you have. How long have you had this habit? Why do you act this way? When? After you complete your evaluation, create a goal-setting plan to change the habit.

Reading Check

Understand cause and effect. For each goal-setting step, state a specific activity, or cause, which will produce a desired result, or effect.

Reaching Your Goal

After you decide on a goal, you'll need to create and follow a goal-setting plan to help you stay on track. A goal-setting plan is a series of steps you'll take to reach your goal.

Figure 2.5 shows the plan one teen outlined to reach his goal of going to baseball camp. Notice how his goal-setting plan helps him organize his efforts and manage his time so that he can achieve the results he wants. You can follow these steps to build an effective goal-setting plan:

Step 1: Set a specific goal and write it down.
Step 2: List the steps you will take to reach your goal.
Step 3: Get help from others who can help and support you.
Step 4: Evaluate your progress by setting checkpoints.
Step 5: Reward yourself after you have achieved your goal.

FIGURE 2.5

CREATING A GOAL-SETTING PLAN

This teen's outline includes all five steps of an effective goal-setting plan. *How could you use these steps to achieve your own long-term goal?*

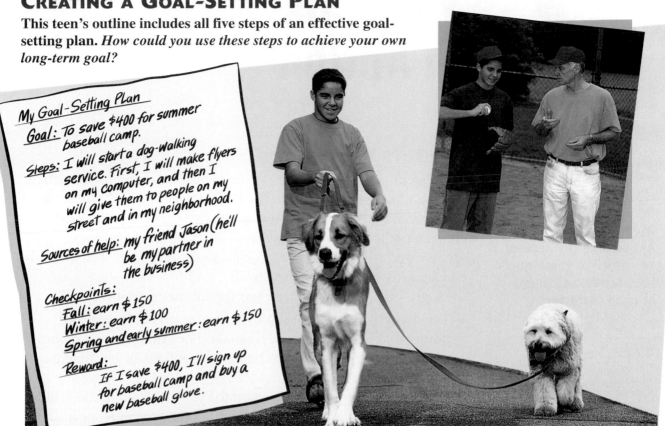

My Goal-Setting Plan

Goal: To save $400 for summer baseball camp.

Steps: I will start a dog-walking service. First, I will make flyers on my computer, and then I will give them to people on my street and in my neighborhood.

Sources of help: my friend Jason (he'll be my partner in the business)

Checkpoints:
Fall: earn $150
Winter: earn $100
Spring and early summer: earn $150

Reward: If I save $400, I'll sign up for baseball camp and buy a new baseball glove.

Lesson 3 Review

Using complete sentences, answer the following questions on a sheet of paper.

Reviewing Terms and Facts

1. **Vocabulary** Define the term *short-term goal.* Then use it in an original sentence.
2. **Describe** Give two examples of short-term goals and two of long-term goals.
3. **Restate** Describe the five steps of an effective goal-setting plan.

Thinking Critically

4. **Analyze** How can short-term goals help you achieve a long-term goal?
5. **Apply** Develop three strategies for setting long-term personal and vocational goals.

Applying Health Skills

6. **Advocacy** Create a comic strip, or write a short story that will encourage young readers to develop a specific healthful habit. Choose a habit that you want to encourage young people to practice. Then create characters and a plot that show how this habit can improve health. Also, give readers hints about ways to develop this habit. For example, if you want to emphasize the health benefits of eating vegetables, you might create a tale about a character who learns to enjoy vegetables. Keep your audience in mind as you write.

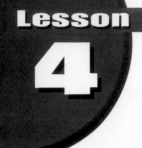

Your Character in Action

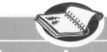

Quick Write

List some of the qualities that you value most in friends and other people. As you read this lesson, see which of these qualities are also elements of good character.

LEARN ABOUT...

○ the elements of good character.
○ how you can develop good character.

VOCABULARY

○ character
○ advocacy
○ role model

What Is Character?

What kind of person are you? Are you honest and trustworthy? Do you treat everyone with respect? *The way in which you think, feel, and act* is your **character**. A person is said to have good character when she or he has the qualities of trustworthiness, respect, responsibility, fairness, caring, and citizenship. These qualities are illustrated in **Figure 2.6**.

A person of good character has the following traits:

- **Trustworthiness.** A trustworthy person is reliable and honest—someone you can count on. For example, a trustworthy teen can be depended on to be honest with his or her parents and teachers.
- **Respect.** When you show regard for your health and the health of other people, you are demonstrating the trait of respect. Respectful listening and speaking are important communication skills. A respectful person also realizes that others have a right to see situations and ideas differently.
- **Responsibility.** Being accountable for your actions is a large part of responsibility. Responsible people are willing to step forward

FIGURE 2.6

BUILDING GOOD CHARACTER

Good character is built from a combination of attitudes, behaviors, and values. *What types of behavior might be connected to fairness?*

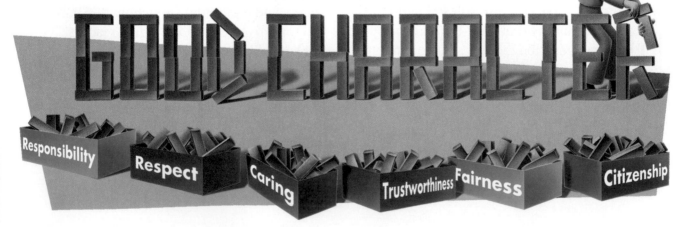

and say, "It's up to me to do this task. I'll take the credit if I handle it wisely or accept the consequences if I don't." If you have a test coming up, it's your responsibility to study for it. How well you do is up to you.

- **Fairness.** Fairness means treating everyone equally and honestly. Someone who is fair is open-minded and does not favor one person over another.
- **Caring.** Caring means showing understanding and compassion toward others. A caring person treats people with kindness and generosity, listening to them and trying to help when possible. For instance, a caring person offers support and encouragement to a classmate who is upset.
- **Citizenship.** Citizenship consists of all the responsibilities and privileges of being a citizen. Good citizenship means obeying rules and laws. It also means doing what you can to help your school, community, and country, and encouraging others to get involved as well. Part of good citizenship is protecting the environment. Citizenship is also related to the skill of advocacy. **Advocacy** is *taking action in support of a cause.* When you find an issue you really care about, such as preventing violence in your school, contribute your talents to help build a safer community.

The teen years are a good time to develop many positive character traits. People with good character are able to be a positive influence on their families, friends, and communities.

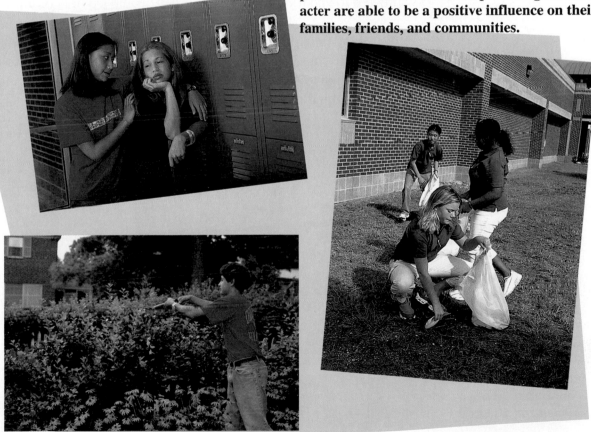

Reading Check

Create your own chart to present and explain each element of good character.

Developing Your Character

Unlike curly hair or brown eyes, the qualities of good character aren't present at birth. Character must be learned when you're young and developed throughout your life. You learn about character from parents, teachers, religious leaders, and others.

Life experiences with other people can teach you about the qualities of good character. For example, children learn about fairness by playing games and sports. Think of the first time you heard someone say, "Hey, no fair! That's cheating!" You learned that fair play and honesty are valued traits.

You also learn about the qualities of good character by watching people around you. Some of these people may become models for you to imitate. A **role model** is *a person who inspires you to act or think in a certain way.* Parents or guardians are important role models for their children.

Know Yourself

To develop good character, become aware of your words and actions. Are you an honest person? Are you kind? Do you stand up for what you believe in? Do you help people who are in trouble? Do you listen to and try to understand other people's points of view?

You can learn about your character by thinking about such questions. If you discover some behavior or attitude in yourself that you'd like to change or improve, start today. Take action to become the kind of person you want to be.

Dr. Ben Carson, the director of brain surgery for children at Johns Hopkins University, encourages teens to excel. The Carson Scholars Fund rewards students who, through their performance in school and their efforts in the community, serve as role models for others.

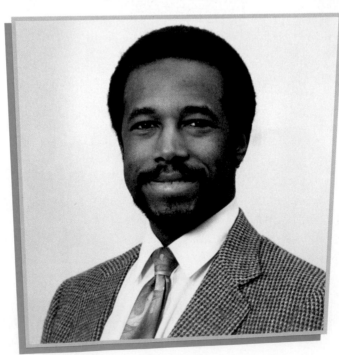

PRACTICING HEALTHFUL BEHAVIORS

Maintaining Parents' Trust

Your relationship with your parents or guardians is particularly important, so you need to follow their guidelines regarding behavior that is healthy and safe for you. Here are some ways to maintain your parents' or guardians' trust.

- Do what you say you are going to do.
- Accept responsibility for your mistakes.

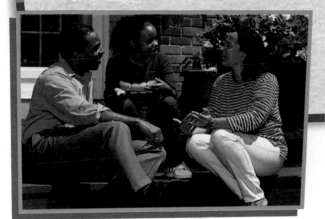

- Talk openly and honestly with your parents or guardians. Tell the truth about what you're thinking and feeling.
- Listen carefully to your parents' or guardians' advice. Ask questions to make sure that you really understand what they are telling you.
- Think before you speak. Don't let emotions control you. Explain your opinions and ideas respectfully and clearly. Look for solutions.

ON YOUR OWN

Write a short story in which a teen gains his or her parents' or guardians' trust. Show how the main character chooses a course of action that supports this trust.

Lesson 4 Review

Using complete sentences, answer the following questions on a sheet of paper.

Reviewing Terms and Facts

1. **Recall** What is *character*? What six traits contribute to a person's character?
2. **Compare and Contrast** What is the difference between respect and responsibility?
3. **Vocabulary** Define the term *advocacy*. Describe one way that advocacy can improve your physical health.
4. **Explain** Give an example of how life experiences can teach you about good character.

Thinking Critically

5. **Analyze** How might working to develop good character be an acceptable way for someone to gain attention and recognition?
6. **Infer** Explain how good character can have a positive effect on community health.

Applying Health Skills

7. **Communication Skills** Invent a situation in which a parent makes a new rule, such as an earlier curfew or a limit on television viewing, that a teen thinks is unfair. Write a dialogue between the teen and the parent in which the teen's response reflects the qualities of good character.

3 Teens Making A Difference

Armed with character and creativity, these goal-driven teens are out to make a positive difference.

Triathlete
Rudy Garcia-Tolson, 14, *Bloomington, CA*

AMAZING RACE: "I've been doing triathlons since I was 10 years old, even though when I was five, both my legs were amputated below the knee. With prosthetic legs, I can run a six-minute mile, and I'm a few seconds shy of the American record among disabled athletes in the swimming individual medley."

THE BEGINNING: "I was born with pterygium (teh-RIJ-ee-um) syndrome, a disease that bound my legs together and left me unable to walk. I wanted to be active, and the doctors said I'd spend the rest of my life in a wheelchair unless I had my legs amputated, so I had them cut off."

GETTING THE WORD OUT: "As a Challenged Athletes Foundation spokesperson, I talk about being a disabled athlete at schools nationwide."

HOW HE'LL MAKE A DIFFERENCE: "When I first started running, there were no races for double amputees because people didn't think that we could do it. I'm proving them wrong. I want to show other disabled kids that it's worth coming out and competing."

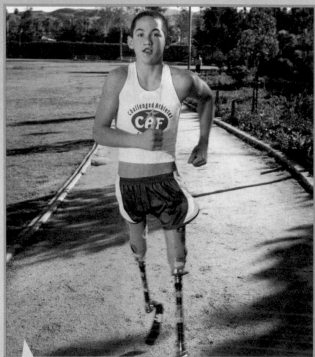

"I was tired of being in my room sitting down," says disabled athlete Rudy Garcia-Tolson.

Literacy Advocate
Lauren Echstenkamper, 16, *Sarasota, FL*

READ ALERT: "Less fortunate children in my area didn't have books to read at home, so in September 2000, I started the Bookworm Project. I asked kids at my school to donate children's books, and we collected more than 2,000 in just two weeks and gave them to Alta Vista, a local elementary school. Now the Zonta Club of Sarasota, a women's service organization, is helping me expand the program in Florida and beyond."

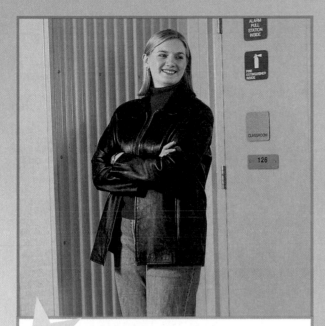

Lauren returns to her alma mater, Pine View School, in Osprey, Florida.

GREAT EXPECTATIONS: "When I first brought the books to Alta Vista, the kids were waiting outside. They immediately plopped down on the sidewalk and started reading. I've since started Bookworms on Tape. I got teachers and friends to read books aloud, and I'd tape them."

THE FINAL CHAPTER: "I threw a party for the Alta Vista kids. One child wrote me a card: 'Because of you, I can read.' I knew then that my hard work had really paid off."

HOW SHE'LL MAKE A DIFFERENCE: "I grew up in a house full of books. I want other kids to have the same opportunities I had. I hope that I can help children gain a love for reading, because it leads to success later in life."

Activist, Teen Connect
Alfred Ciffo III, 16, *Hallandale, FL*

CALL TO ACTION: "I founded Teen Connect, an organization that fosters friendships between teens and senior citizens through regular phone calls. It started with a few kids in my hometown. Now we've got hundreds of teens and seniors throughout Florida involved; there are local chapters across the country."

THE LEGACY: "While I was growing up, my grandmother and my great-aunt were like second parents and friends [to me]. After they died, I wanted to help others gain from intergenerational relationships the way I had."

THE REWARDS: "Seniors love sharing the experiences of today's youth. At a meeting [I once had], this 101-year-old man stood up and read a poem he'd written about how much Teen Connect meant to him. Most teens in the program say they've found new and dear friends."

HOW HE'LL MAKE A DIFFERENCE: "We all need to get back to basics and be good to each other by starting with a phone call, a conversation, or an act of kindness. I hope to bring that idea to people everywhere." ■

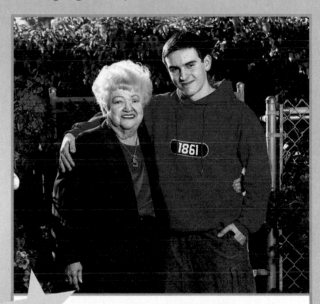

Alfred pals around with Selma Kahan, a senior friend he has been phoning since Teen Connect began.

TIME TO THINK...

About Character in Action
As a class, discuss how each teen in the article demonstrates a positive character trait. Then, think of someone in your life who also shows good character. Write a definition of good character and describe how the person you've chosen fits that definition. Add a paragraph detailing what actions you might perform to show that you are a person of good character.

SAYING NO AND FEELING GOOD ABOUT IT IT

Model

S.T.O.P. is an easy way to remember how to use refusal skills. S.T.O.P. stands for **S**ay no in a firm voice, **T**ell why not, **O**ffer another idea, and **P**romptly leave. See how Megan uses S.T.O.P. to show that she is responsible.

BEN: How about another game? You've got to give me the chance to even the score.

MEGAN: No, I can't. [**S**ay no in a firm voice.] I wish I could, but I've got to get home to watch my little brother. [**T**ell why not.]

BEN: You can be a little late. Your dad is cool. He'll understand.

MEGAN: I can't this afternoon. Maybe we can play again tomorrow. [**O**ffer another idea.]

BEN: I can't believe you're going to ditch me for your little brother.

MEGAN: (walking away) I'm sorry, but I've gotta go now. [**P**romptly leave.]

Practice

As Cody and Bailey leave a store, Bailey pulls a new CD out of his pocket. Read the dialogue below between the two friends. List each of Cody's refusals on a sheet of paper, and identify which part of S.T.O.P. is being used. Which character trait does Cody demonstrate?

BAILEY: What do you think of my new CD? It was free!
CODY: What do you mean free?
BAILEY: I mean you can just take what you want if you know what you're doing. C'mon, I'll show you.
CODY: No. I don't want to steal CDs.
BAILEY: What's the problem? These stores make tons of money.
CODY: That's shoplifting. We could get in real trouble.
BAILEY: I've done it a million times and haven't gotten caught.
CODY: Getting away with it doesn't make it right. I'm leaving.

Apply/Assess

Using S.T.O.P., write a script for one of the following scenarios. With a partner, role-play your script for the class, and explain the character trait it demonstrates.

You are at a sleepover with a group of friends. One of your friends offers to pierce everyone's ears. You don't like the idea, but others seem to want to do it.

You are at a Halloween party. One of your friends brings toilet paper to T.P. his neighbor's house and yard. Your friend wants you to help "get even." You don't want to participate.

Refusal Skills

S.T.O.P. is an easy way to remember how to use refusal skills.
S Say no in a firm voice.
T Tell why not.
O Offer another idea.
P Promptly leave.

Self-√Check

- Does my script contain each part of S.T.O.P.?
- Does my script demonstrate a character trait?

CHAPTER 2 ASSESSMENT

After You Read

Use your completed Foldable to review the information on building health skills.

FOLDABLES™
Study Organizer

Reviewing Vocabulary and Concepts

On a sheet of paper, write the numbers 1–5. After each number, write the term from the list that best completes each sentence.

> - conflict resolution
> - refusal skills
> - interpersonal communication
> - accessing information
> - stress management

Lesson 1

1. When _____, it is important to check the accuracy of the content.
2. Learning how to handle stress in healthful ways is known as _____.
3. By developing effective speaking and listening skills, you will improve your _____.
4. Strong _____ will help you say no effectively.
5. You can use _____ skills to find a solution to disagreements.

Lesson 2

On a sheet of paper, write the numbers 6–8. Write *True* or *False* for each statement below. If the statement is false, change the underlined word or phrase to make it true.

6. The process of making a choice or finding a solution is <u>accessing information.</u>
7. Every decision you make should <u>oppose</u> values.

8. The standards on which you base a decision are called <u>influences</u>.

Lesson 3

On a sheet of paper, write the numbers 9–12. After each number, write the letter of the answer that best completes each of the following.

9. Striving to reach your goals will have a positive effect on your
   a. empathy.
   b. fairness.
   c. self-confidence.
   d. loyalty.
10. Which is an example of a long-term goal?
    a. Eating a balanced breakfast
    b. Becoming a pediatrician
    c. Getting a good score on a quiz
    d. Writing a book report
11. Which of the following elements is *not* part of an effective goal-setting plan?
    a. A description of your goal
    b. A list of reasons you can't reach a goal.
    c. The steps you will take to reach the goal
    d. A set of checkpoints to monitor progress
12. Which strategy will help you develop healthful habits?
    a. Focus only on your short-term goals.
    b. Focus only on your long-term goals.
    c. Repeat positive behaviors.
    d. Avoid setting goals.

Lesson 4

On a sheet of paper, write the numbers 13–16. Write *True* or *False* for each statement below. If the statement is false, change the underlined word or phrase to make it true.

13. When you recognize that others are free to have perspectives that differ from yours, you show <u>influences.</u>
14. The key to practicing <u>responsibility</u> is to be accountable for your actions.
15. <u>Advocacy</u> means showing compassion toward others.

16. A <u>role model</u> inspires you to act or think in a certain way.

Thinking Critically

Using complete sentences, answer the following questions on a sheet of paper.

17. Apply Write a short story about a student who makes a healthful choice.

18. Assess Evaluate a recent decision you made. How well did you follow the decision-making steps?

19. Hypothesize Explain why it isn't good to set too many or too few goals.

20. Interpret Suppose your school is launching a Good Character Award. How might winners be selected?

Career Corner

Exercise and Aerobics Instructor Do you like exercising and staying physically fit? Do you like music and dancing? If so, you could turn your interests into a career as an exercise and aerobics instructor. These professionals help people reach their fitness goals by teaching aerobics or other types of exercise. The American Council on Exercise certifies many exercise and aerobics instructors. Visit Career Corner at health.glencoe.com to find out more about this and other health careers.

Standardized Test Practice

Reading & Writing

Read the paragraphs below and then answer the questions.

Sunburn is the most preventable risk factor for skin cancer. This means you can keep yourself safe from skin cancer by taking advantage of the protection you get from using a sunscreen. You can take control over your own health.

Sunscreens are chemical compounds that either absorb ultraviolet (UV) rays or reflect them. The type that absorbs rays is more popular with consumers, probably because they are invisible when applied to the skin. Experts advise using a sunscreen with a SPF (sun protection factor) of 30 or greater.

Sunscreens may fail when people use just a single application when a second one is needed, or when users overestimate the effectiveness of the sunscreen and stay out in the sun for too long.

1. Which phrase helps readers understand the meaning of the word "preventable"?
   A keep yourself safe
   B using a sunscreen
   C control over your own health
   D take advantage of the protection

2. What is the main purpose of this passage?
   A to express emotions
   B to inform
   C to entertain
   D to persuade

3. Write a paragraph describing a decision or action that shows how you can take control over your own health and well-being.

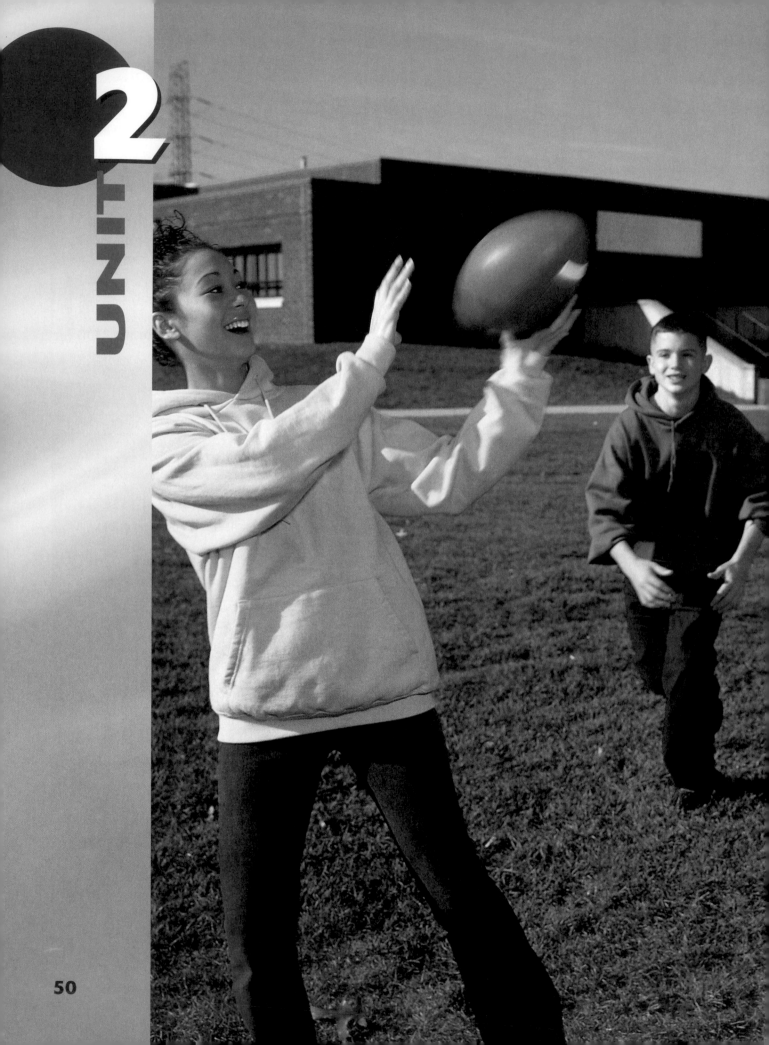

UNIT

2

50

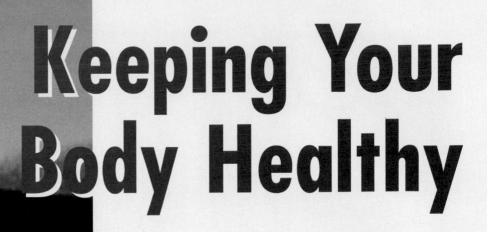

Keeping Your Body Healthy

HEALTH in Action

How can eating an apple help you catch a football?

Proper nutrition has a major effect on the way your body performs. Eating healthful foods can help you grow stronger, give you energy, and improve your vision and reaction time—all of which can enhance your performance, whether you're playing a sport, riding a bike, or studying for a test. So, while the decision you make about what to have for breakfast might not seem like a big deal, it goes a long way toward determining how well you'll do for the rest of the day!

51

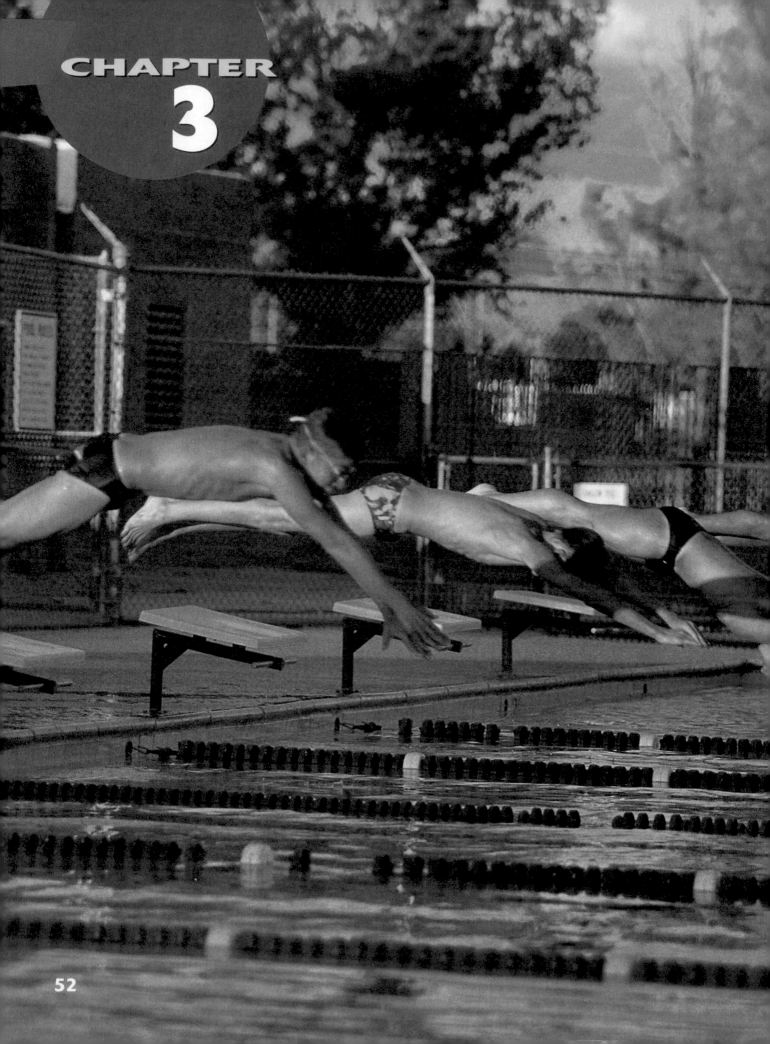

Physical Activity and Fitness

HEALTH *Online*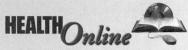

Rate your physical activity and fitness habits. Take the Health Inventory for Chapter 3 at health.glencoe.com.

FOLDABLES™ Study Organizer

Before You Read

Make this Foldable to record the information presented in Lesson 1 about the three elements of fitness. Begin with a plain sheet of 11″ × 17″ paper.

Step 1

Fold a sheet of paper into thirds along the short axis.

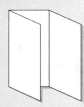

Step 2

Open and fold the bottom edge up to form a pocket. Glue the edges.

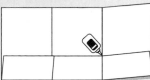

Step 3

Label each pocket as shown. Place an index card or quarter sheet of notebook paper into each pocket.

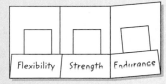

Flexibility   Strength   Endurance

As You Read

Write down key points on each element of fitness on index cards or sheets of notebook paper cut into quarter sections. Store the cards in the appropriate pocket of your Foldable.

Physical Activity and Health

Quick Write

List as many physical activities as you can. Which do you think are the most beneficial to health, and why?

LEARN ABOUT...

- the benefits of physical activity.
- how to increase your strength, endurance, and flexibility.

VOCABULARY

- physical activity
- fitness
- exercise
- strength
- endurance
- heart and lung endurance
- muscle endurance
- aerobic exercise
- anaerobic exercise
- flexibility

Physical Activity and You

You do many types of physical activity every day: running to catch the school bus, walking up a flight of stairs, doing chores. **Physical activity** is *any kind of movement that causes your body to use energy.* Participating in regular physical activity

- helps build and maintain healthy bones, muscles, and joints.
- helps control weight and reduce fat.
- helps keep blood pressure within a healthy range.

The ability to handle the physical work and play of everyday life without becoming tired is known as **fitness.** You can become more fit by exercising. **Exercise** is *physical activity that is planned, structured, and repetitive and that improves or maintains personal fitness.* Exercising regularly increases your energy level, allowing you to be more active during the day. Also, if you want to play a sport, exercising regularly can help you develop the skills you will need.

The Benefits of Physical Activity

Do you ever feel calmer about a situation after you've gone for a bike ride? Not only does physical activity improve your physical well-being, it can enhance mental/emotional and social health, too. **Figure 3.1** lists the benefits of physical activity.

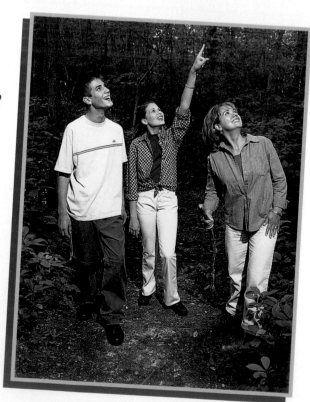

Physical activity is a way for people of all ages to stay fit and enjoy one another's company. *What activities do you think you will enjoy throughout your life?*

FIGURE 3.1

PHYSICAL ACTIVITY AND YOUR TOTAL HEALTH

Being physically active enhances all aspects of your health.

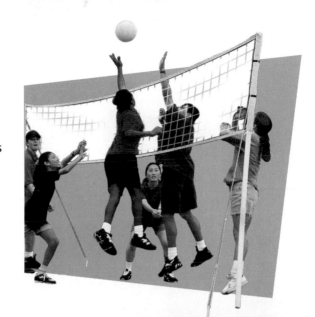

Benefits to Physical Health
• Maintenance of a healthy weight
• Improved strength and flexibility
• Better performance of heart and lungs
• Higher energy level
• Decreased risk of certain diseases
• Stronger bones
• Greater freedom of movement
• Better coordination
• Better sleep

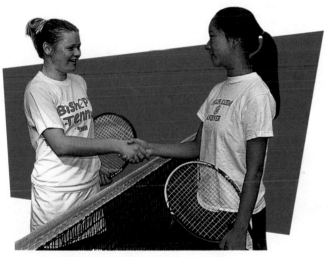

Benefits to Social Health
• Additional chances to meet new people
• Opportunities to share common goals with others
• Increased ability to interact and cooperate with others
• Opportunities to use talents to help others

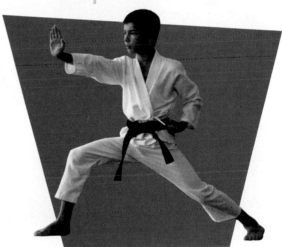

Benefits to Mental/Emotional Health
• Enhanced self-confidence
• Sharpened mental alertness
• Reduced stress
• More relaxed attitude
• More enjoyment of free time

Strength

The first element of fitness is **strength**, *the ability of your muscles to exert a force.* Strength is measured according to the most work your muscles can do at a given time. Building strength through physical activity enables you to lift heavy objects more easily with less chance of injury. It also makes it easier for you to develop skills for sports and other activities. **Figure 3.2** on page 56 shows three types of strength-building exercises.

FIGURE 3.2

STRENGTH-BUILDING EXERCISES

To build your strength, gradually increase the number of repetitions you do during each exercise session. *Which muscles do you strengthen when you do push-ups?*

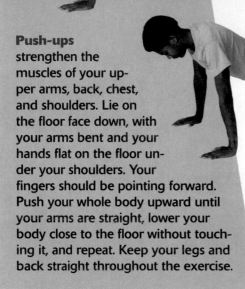

Push-ups strengthen the muscles of your upper arms, back, chest, and shoulders. Lie on the floor face down, with your arms bent and your hands flat on the floor under your shoulders. Your fingers should be pointing forward. Push your whole body upward until your arms are straight, lower your body close to the floor without touching it, and repeat. Keep your legs and back straight throughout the exercise.

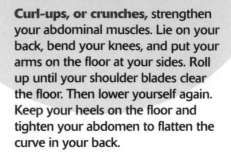

Curl-ups, or crunches, strengthen your abdominal muscles. Lie on your back, bend your knees, and put your arms on the floor at your sides. Roll up until your shoulder blades clear the floor. Then lower yourself again. Keep your heels on the floor and tighten your abdomen to flatten the curve in your back.

Step-ups strengthen your leg muscles. Step up onto a step with your left foot, and then bring up the right foot. Step down with the left foot first, then the right. Repeat, alternating legs.

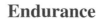

Endurance

The second element of fitness is **endurance** (in·DUR·uhnts), *the ability to perform vigorous physical activity without getting overly tired.* There are two basic types of endurance. **Heart and lung endurance** is *the measure of how effectively your heart and lungs work during moderate-to-vigorous physical activity or exercise.* It is also a measure of how quickly your heartbeat and breathing return to normal when you stop exercising. **Muscle endurance** is *the ability of a muscle to repeatedly exert a force over a prolonged period of time.*

Two types of exercise can help build endurance: aerobic and anaerobic. **Aerobic** (ehr·OH·bik) **exercise** is *rhythmic, nonstop, moderate-to-vigorous activity that requires large amounts of oxygen and works the heart*. Aerobic exercises include walking, jogging, bicycling, swimming laps, and cross-country skiing. Doing aerobic exercises for a minimum of 20 minutes at least three times a week is the best way to build heart and lung endurance. **Anaerobic** (AN·ehr·oh·bik) **exercise** is *intense physical activity that requires little oxygen but involves short bursts of energy*. Weight lifting and sprinting are examples of anaerobic exercises. Such activities help build and maintain strength and muscle endurance.

Flexibility

Flexibility, the third element of fitness, is *the ability to move joints fully and easily*. Some people are naturally more flexible than others are. Nevertheless, you can increase your flexibility by doing regular, gentle stretching of muscles and joints. Improving your flexibility will help you feel more comfortable and reduce your risk of injury during strength or endurance training. **Figure 3.3** shows two exercises that you can do to improve your flexibility.

FIGURE 3.3

STRETCHING EXERCISES

These exercises will stretch the muscles of your upper body and your legs.

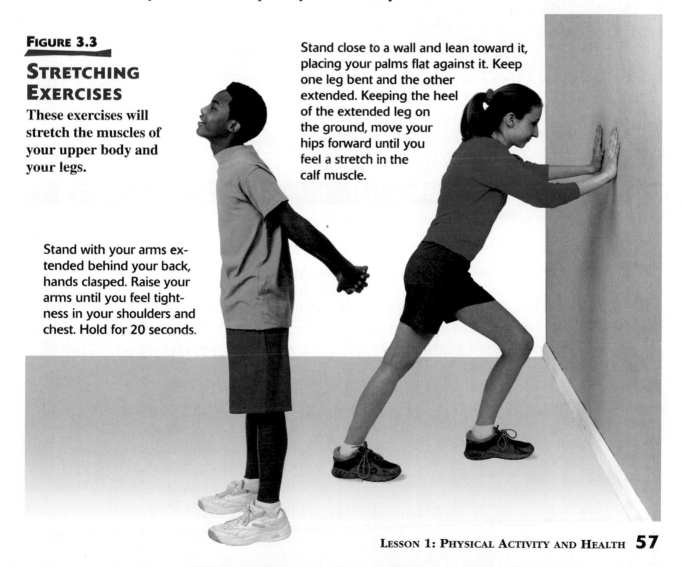

Stand close to a wall and lean toward it, placing your palms flat against it. Keep one leg bent and the other extended. Keeping the heel of the extended leg on the ground, move your hips forward until you feel a stretch in the calf muscle.

Stand with your arms extended behind your back, hands clasped. Raise your arms until you feel tightness in your shoulders and chest. Hold for 20 seconds.

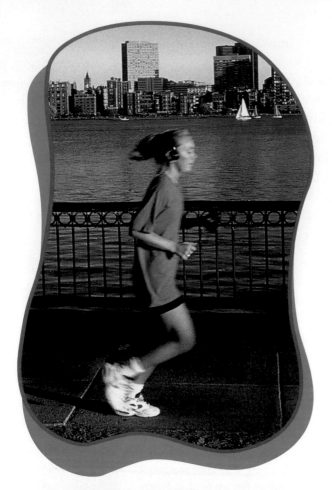

Jogging is a form of aerobic exercise. *What other out-of-school fitness activities promote fitness and health?*

Selecting the Right Exercises

To reach your fitness goals, plan a program that is convenient, affordable, and enjoyable. Think about the type of exercises that you would like to do, the equipment you will need, and when and where you will exercise. Your workouts should include a variety of physical activities to promote balanced fitness. Here are some ways to add physical activity to your life.

- Do a variety of aerobic exercises and/or active sports and recreational activities for at least 20 minutes, three to five times a week.
- Aim to do strength and flexibility exercises two or three times a week.
- Try not to spend more than half an hour at a time watching television or playing computer games. Staying active is important to good health.

Lesson 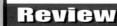 Review

Using complete sentences, answer the following questions on a sheet of paper.

Reviewing Terms and Facts

1. **Vocabulary** Define the term *physical activity*. Write a sentence explaining why it is important to your health.
2. **List** What are the three elements of fitness? Define each element.
3. **Distinguish** What is the difference between heart and lung endurance and muscle endurance?

Thinking Critically

4. **Analyze** Explain how the three parts of the health triangle may be linked through physical activity.
5. **Explain** Why should a good exercise program include several kinds of activities?

Applying Health Skills

6. **Practicing Healthful Behaviors** Ask a physical education teacher or another exercise professional to demonstrate a strength, endurance, or flexibility exercise. Demonstrate this exercise for your class, and explain its benefits.

The Skeletal and Muscular Systems

Bones for Support, Muscles for Movement

You depend on your skelctal and muscular systems to support you and help you move. The **skeletal system** is *the framework of bones and other tissues that supports the body.* It is made up of 206 bones as well as many joints and connecting tissues. Your skeletal system gives your body structure and protects your internal organs.

Your muscles supply the power to move your body. The **muscular system** consists of *tissues that move parts of the body and operate internal organs.* The human body has more than 600 muscles.

The Skeletal System

Besides supporting and protecting your body, your bones also store calcium and other minerals and make blood cells. The *places where two or more bones meet* are called **joints**. Some joints are immovable, such as those in the skull. Others allow a wide range of movement.

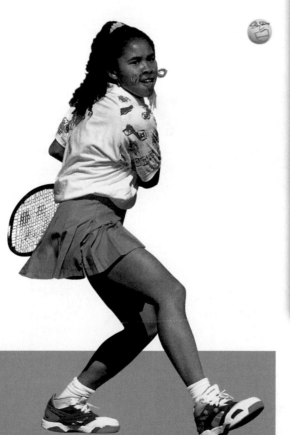

Any physical activity requires that bones and muscles work smoothly together. *How many bones and muscles does the human body have?*

Quick Write

Have you ever felt sore the day after you tried a new physical activity? Explain in a few sentences why you think this occurred.

LEARN ABOUT...

- the functions of the skeletal and muscular systems.
- how bones and muscles work together to allow movement.
- how to keep your bones and muscles healthy.

VOCABULARY

- skeletal system
- muscular system
- joint
- cartilage
- ligament
- tendon

Figure 3.4 identifies some of the major bones in the skeletal system and describes several types of joints. Connecting tissues link bones to muscles so that the two can work together to move parts of the body. Each type of connecting tissue has a specific function. **Cartilage** *allows joints to move easily, cushions bones, and supports soft tissues, such as those in the nose and ear.* **Ligaments** *hold bones in place at the joints;* for example, in the knee and ankle. **Tendons** *join muscle to muscle or muscle to bone.* An example is the Achilles tendon, which attaches the calf muscle to the heel bone.

FIGURE 3.4

THE SKELETAL SYSTEM

Here are some of the major bones and joints of the skeletal system. *The shoulder is what type of joint?*

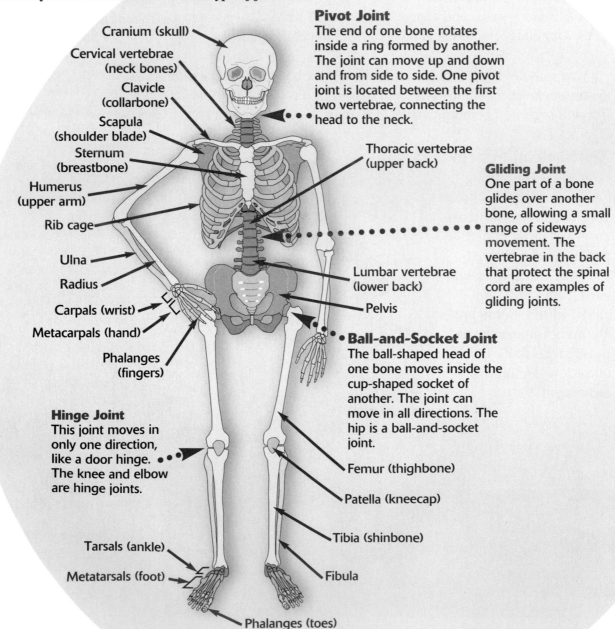

Pivot Joint
The end of one bone rotates inside a ring formed by another. The joint can move up and down and from side to side. One pivot joint is located between the first two vertebrae, connecting the head to the neck.

Gliding Joint
One part of a bone glides over another bone, allowing a small range of sideways movement. The vertebrae in the back that protect the spinal cord are examples of gliding joints.

Ball-and-Socket Joint
The ball-shaped head of one bone moves inside the cup-shaped socket of another. The joint can move in all directions. The hip is a ball-and-socket joint.

Hinge Joint
This joint moves in only one direction, like a door hinge. The knee and elbow are hinge joints.

Cranium (skull)
Cervical vertebrae (neck bones)
Clavicle (collarbone)
Scapula (shoulder blade)
Sternum (breastbone)
Humerus (upper arm)
Rib cage
Ulna
Radius
Carpals (wrist)
Metacarpals (hand)
Phalanges (fingers)

Thoracic vertebrae (upper back)
Lumbar vertebrae (lower back)
Pelvis
Femur (thighbone)
Patella (kneecap)
Tibia (shinbone)
Fibula

Tarsals (ankle)
Metatarsals (foot)
Phalanges (toes)

The Muscular System

Muscle tissue responds to messages from the brain and contracts, or shortens, to cause movement. Smooth muscles, which include the muscles of internal organs and blood vessels, are involuntary; they move without your being aware of it. Cardiac muscle, found only in the heart, is also involuntary. Skeletal muscles, shown in **Figure 3.5**, are voluntary, or under your control.

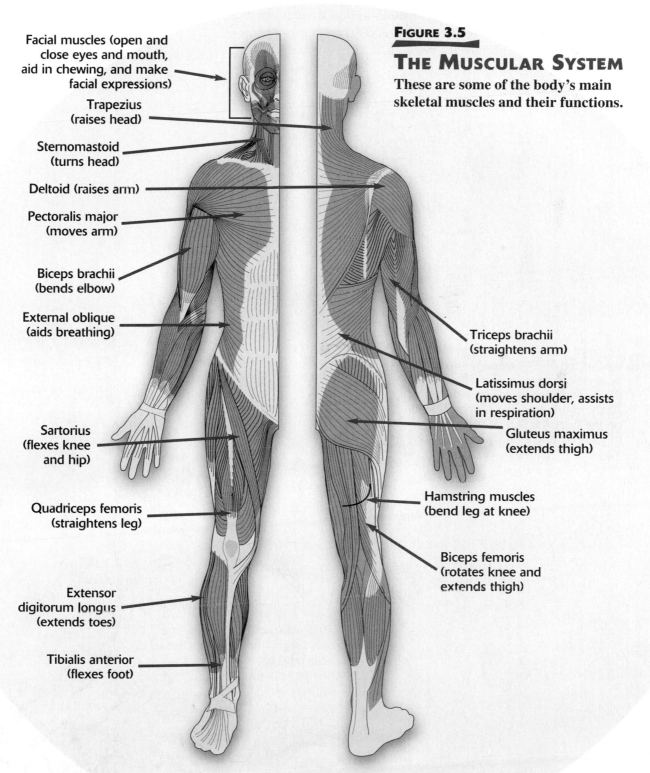

FIGURE 3.5

THE MUSCULAR SYSTEM

These are some of the body's main skeletal muscles and their functions.

Facial muscles (open and close eyes and mouth, aid in chewing, and make facial expressions)

Trapezius (raises head)

Sternomastoid (turns head)

Deltoid (raises arm)

Pectoralis major (moves arm)

Biceps brachii (bends elbow)

External oblique (aids breathing)

Sartorius (flexes knee and hip)

Quadriceps femoris (straightens leg)

Extensor digitorum longus (extends toes)

Tibialis anterior (flexes foot)

Triceps brachii (straightens arm)

Latissimus dorsi (moves shoulder, assists in respiration)

Gluteus maximus (extends thigh)

Hamstring muscles (bend leg at knee)

Biceps femoris (rotates knee and extends thigh)

Skeletal muscles work in pairs to move bones, as shown in **Figure 3.6**. Each member of the pair is connected to the bone that is to be moved. When one muscle contracts, the opposite muscle extends, or lengthens.

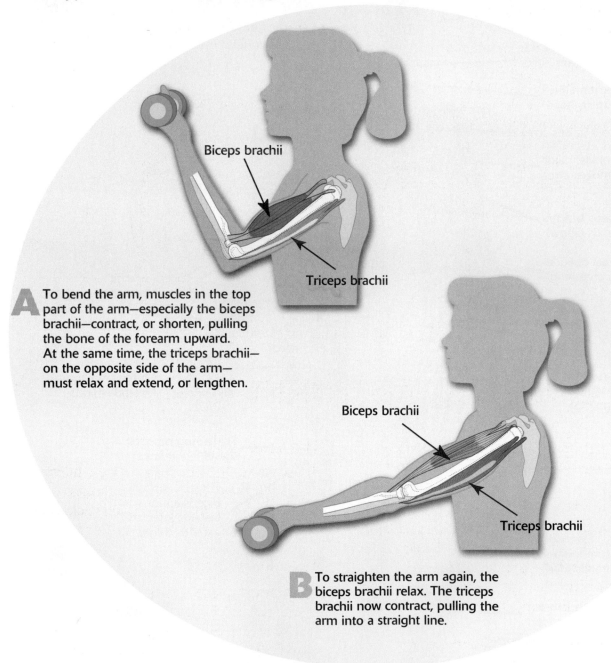

FIGURE 3.6

MUSCLE PAIRS

Muscle pairs are said to work in opposition—to create movement, two muscles must perform opposite actions. *Try bending your arm and see if you can feel the muscles working.*

Biceps brachii

Triceps brachii

A To bend the arm, muscles in the top part of the arm—especially the biceps brachii—contract, or shorten, pulling the bone of the forearm upward. At the same time, the triceps brachii— on the opposite side of the arm— must relax and extend, or lengthen.

Biceps brachii

Triceps brachii

B To straighten the arm again, the biceps brachii relax. The triceps brachii now contract, pulling the arm into a straight line.

Caring for Your Skeletal and Muscular Systems

Keep your skeletal and muscular systems healthy by following these tips.

- **Participate in regular physical activity.** Exercises that build strength will make your bones and muscles stronger. Activities that build heart and lung endurance will strengthen the muscles in your heart and lungs. Exercises that increase flexibility will make it easier for you to move and can prevent some types of injuries.
- **Follow a nutritious eating plan.** Foods that are rich in calcium and vitamin D promote bone growth and strength. Carbohydrates will give your muscles energy, and foods high in protein will build muscle tissue.
- **Practice good posture.** Sit and stand in a correct but relaxed manner so that bones, joints, and muscles maintain proper alignment.
- **Lift objects carefully.** When lifting something heavy, keep your back straight and your knees bent.
- **Treat injuries quickly.** If you are injured, see a physician. Avoid putting stress on an injured body part.

To prevent backaches, make sure that your backpack is not overloaded and that you are using all the straps available for support.

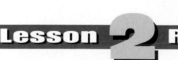

Lesson 2 Review

Using complete sentences, answer the following questions on a sheet of paper.

Reviewing Terms and Facts

1. **Vocabulary** Define the terms *skeletal system* and *muscular system,* and explain how these systems work together.
2. **Explain** What are the three types of connecting tissue? What is the function of each type?
3. **Identify** Name the four types of joints, and describe the movement allowed by each.

Thinking Critically

4. **Analyze** Why do you think the human body has more muscles than bones?
5. **Interpret** Why do you think backaches may be caused by poor posture?

Applying Health Skills

6. **Accessing Information** At birth everyone has 350 bones, but adults have 206. Use resources at home and in your library to find out how bones develop and change as people grow. Write a paragraph explaining this change.

The Circulatory System

Quick Write

Have you ever felt that your heart was "pounding" or that it "skipped a beat"? What do you think caused that sensation?

LEARN ABOUT...

- the functions of the circulatory system.
- how blood circulates through the body.
- how to keep your circulatory system healthy.

VOCABULARY

- circulatory system
- artery
- vein
- capillary
- pulmonary circulation
- systemic circulation
- plasma
- blood pressure

Your Heart and Blood Vessels

A healthy circulatory system is important to a lifetime of good health. The **circulatory system** is *the group of organs and tissues that transport essential materials to body cells and remove their waste products.* This system consists of the heart, the blood vessels, and the blood itself. Another name for the circulatory system is the cardiovascular system. *Cardio-* refers to the heart and *-vascular* means having to do with vessels.

An organ composed of cardiac muscle, the heart pumps blood throughout the network of blood vessels. The blood flows through three types of vessels—arteries, veins, and capillaries. The heart pumps blood into the **arteries**, *the blood vessels that carry blood away from the heart to all parts of the body.* The **veins** are *the blood vessels that carry blood back to the heart from all parts of the body.* **Capillaries**, the smallest blood vessels, *provide body cells with blood and connect arteries with veins.*

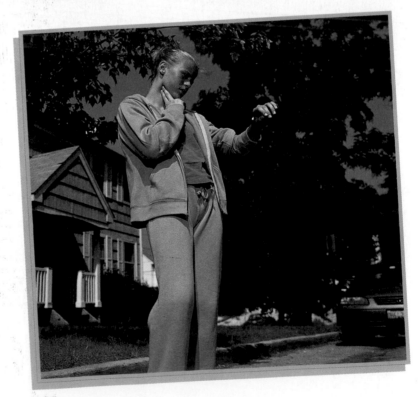

A pulse is produced by the regular contractions of the heart as it pumps blood throughout the body.

How Circulation Works

Two types of circulation are always at work in your body. **Pulmonary** (PUL·muh·nehr·ee) **circulation** *carries the blood from the heart, through the lungs, and back to the heart.* This stage of circulation allows the blood to become enriched with oxygen before it is sent throughout the body. **Systemic** (sis·TE·mik) **circulation** *sends oxygen-rich blood to all the body tissues except the lungs.* **Figure 3.7** shows you how these two types of circulation work together to keep your body cells supplied with nutrients and free of waste products.

Reading Check
Understand word parts. Investigate the words *circulatory* and *pulmonary*. What are their roots and suffixes? What does each mean?

FIGURE 3.7

PULMONARY AND SYSTEMIC CIRCULATION

Oxygen-rich blood coming from the lungs is circulated through the heart and pumped to body tissues. This blood returns to the heart depleted of oxygen and is pumped to the lungs.

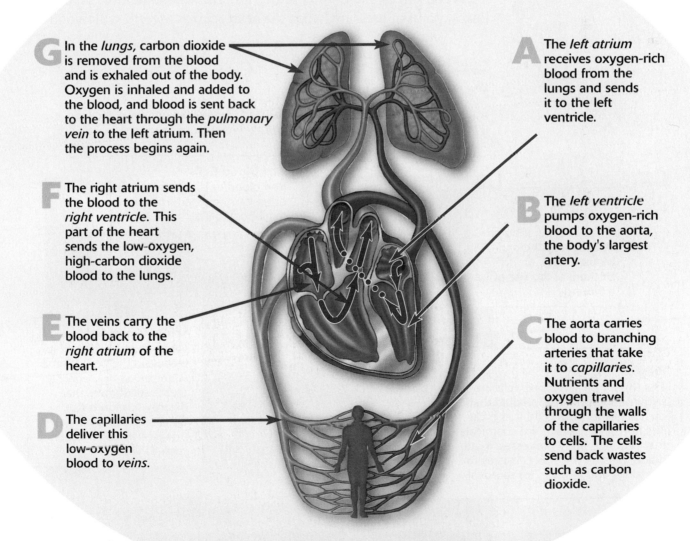

G In the *lungs*, carbon dioxide is removed from the blood and is exhaled out of the body. Oxygen is inhaled and added to the blood, and blood is sent back to the heart through the *pulmonary vein* to the left atrium. Then the process begins again.

F The right atrium sends the blood to the *right ventricle*. This part of the heart sends the low-oxygen, high-carbon dioxide blood to the lungs.

E The veins carry the blood back to the *right atrium* of the heart.

D The capillaries deliver this low-oxygen blood to *veins*.

A The *left atrium* receives oxygen-rich blood from the lungs and sends it to the left ventricle.

B The *left ventricle* pumps oxygen-rich blood to the aorta, the body's largest artery.

C The aorta carries blood to branching arteries that take it to *capillaries*. Nutrients and oxygen travel through the walls of the capillaries to cells. The cells send back wastes such as carbon dioxide.

Blood has to flow upward, against gravity, in some parts of your body. Try the following experiment. Stretch one arm high above your head. Let the other arm hang down by your side. Hold this position for a minute. What differences do you find between your hands?

What's in Your Blood

The different parts of blood carry out several important functions in the body. Many of these functions involve transporting various substances through the body and protecting the body from harm. Over half of the volume of blood is **plasma** (PLAZ·muh), *a yellowish fluid, the watery portion of blood.* The rest of the volume of blood is made up of three kinds of cells: red blood cells, white blood cells, and cell fragments called platelets (PLAYT·luhts). The parts of the blood and their functions are described in **Figure 3.8.**

Blood Pressure

When you have a medical checkup, the nurse or doctor may take your blood pressure. **Blood pressure** is *the force of blood pushing against the walls of the blood vessels.* A blood pressure reading consists of two numbers, usually written in this way: 110/70. The first number is the pressure at its highest point, when the heart contracts and forces blood into the arteries. The second number is the lowest point of pressure, when the heart relaxes to refill with blood.

Figure 3.8

Parts of the Blood

Each element of the blood helps the body in a different way. *How do white blood cells help you stay healthy?*

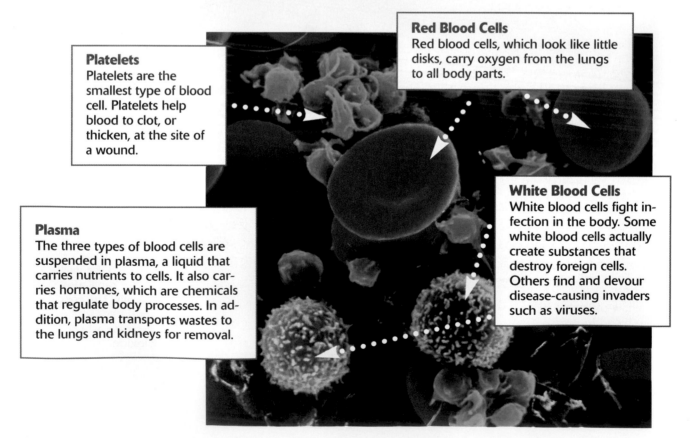

Platelets
Platelets are the smallest type of blood cell. Platelets help blood to clot, or thicken, at the site of a wound.

Red Blood Cells
Red blood cells, which look like little disks, carry oxygen from the lungs to all body parts.

White Blood Cells
White blood cells fight infection in the body. Some white blood cells actually create substances that destroy foreign cells. Others find and devour disease-causing invaders such as viruses.

Plasma
The three types of blood cells are suspended in plasma, a liquid that carries nutrients to cells. It also carries hormones, which are chemicals that regulate body processes. In addition, plasma transports wastes to the lungs and kidneys for removal.

FIGURE 3.9

COMPATIBLE BLOOD TYPES

Hospital workers determine a person's blood type before allowing him or her to receive blood from someone else. In most cases the donor's blood should be the same type as the recipient's blood. A person can, however, receive a different, compatible blood type in an emergency.

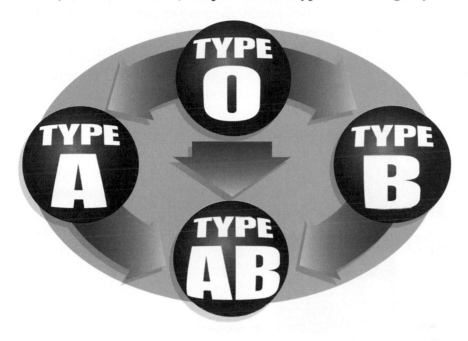

Blood Types

All blood is not the same. The four types—A, B, AB, and O—are classified according to the type of red blood cells they contain. Some blood types are compatible, or able to coexist in one person's body. Compatible blood types can be mixed safely. If blood types that are not compatible are combined, the red blood cells in one type of blood clump together and block the blood vessels. **Figure 3.9** shows which blood types are compatible.

Blood may also contain a substance called an Rh factor. Most people are Rh-positive, meaning that their blood has this substance. Rh-negative blood does not contain this substance. People with Rh-positive blood can receive blood from people who are either Rh-positive or Rh-negative. People who are Rh-negative, however, can accept blood only from others who are Rh-negative.

Caring for Your Circulatory System

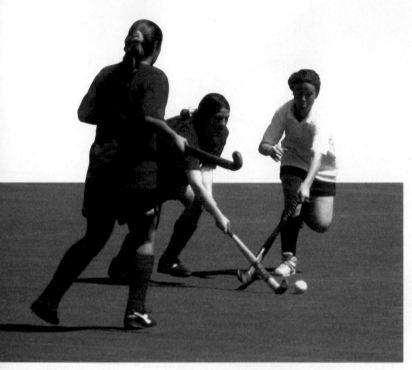

These teens are keeping their circulatory systems healthy by enjoying a fast-paced sport. What other physical activities would benefit the circulatory system?

You can take action now to care for your circulatory system throughout your life. First, eat a balanced diet that is low in fats. Learn to manage stress—it can put a strain on your heart and blood vessels. Avoid smoking. The nicotine in tobacco narrows the blood vessels and prevents your blood from carrying oxygen effectively. Activities that build heart and lung endurance also benefit your circulatory system in the following ways:

- When you engage in aerobic activity, your heart, blood vessels, and blood become more efficient at delivering oxygen and nutrients to your muscles and other organs. After several weeks of regular aerobic activity, your heart can pump more blood each minute, and your muscle cells can use more oxygen.
- Moderate and vigorous physical activity may lower the levels of fatty materials in your blood and help keep your arteries free of fatty deposits.
- Regular participation in moderate and vigorous physical activities and exercise will help you maintain a healthy weight, allowing your heart to work efficiently.

Lesson 3 Review

Using complete sentences, answer the following questions on a sheet of paper.

Reviewing Terms and Facts

1. **Vocabulary** Define the term *circulatory system*.
2. **Distinguish** How do arteries, veins, and capillaries differ?
3. **Discuss** Name the two types of circulation. Why is each type important?
4. **Summarize** List the components of blood, and explain what each one does.

Thinking Critically

5. **Explain** Why do you think a blood pressure reading is taken during a medical checkup?
6. **Conclude** Why is it necessary for hospital workers to know patients' blood types?

Applying Health Skills

7. **Analyzing Influences** Advertisers often emphasize the fact that certain types of food are good for your heart. Find print ads for two such products. Then decide whether each product really enhances the health of your heart, and explain how you came to that conclusion.

Developing a Personal Fitness Program

Fitness and Body Composition

You've learned that fitness is the ability to handle the physical work and play of everyday life without becoming tired. One factor that affects your overall fitness is your body composition. **Body composition** is *the proportions of fat, bones, muscle, and fluid that make up body weight.* Participation in regular physical activity increases the amount of muscle and decreases the amount of fat in your body, allowing you to become fit and stay healthy.

Achieving Your Fitness Goals

Now that you know how fitness can benefit your skeletal, muscular, and circulatory systems, you may want to start a fitness program. To do this, first think about your goals. Perhaps you want to increase your heart and lung endurance or develop specific skills for a sport. You may just want to feel healthier. If you set a specific goal, you'll be more inspired to stick with your fitness program, and you'll feel a sense of accomplishment when you reach that goal.

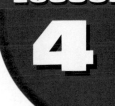

Quick Write

Do you feel that there is enough physical activity in your daily life? If so, list three reasons you think this is so. If not, list three ways to increase your physical activity.

LEARN ABOUT...

- factors to consider when planning a fitness program.
- how to plan your workouts.
- how to calculate your target heart rate range.
- how to assess your progress in meeting your fitness goals.

VOCABULARY

- body composition
- warm-up
- cool-down
- frequency
- intensity
- target heart rate

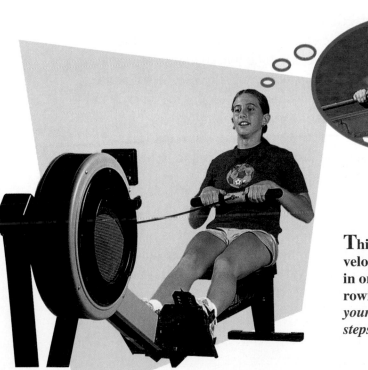

This teen is working to develop the skills she will need in order to meet her goal of rowing a boat well. *What is your fitness goal, and what steps can you take to reach it?*

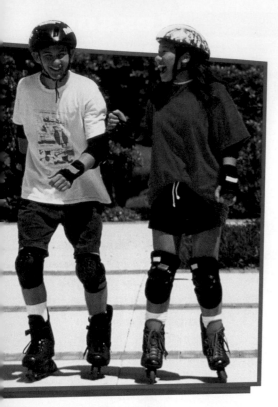

Some activities require protective gear. *What are these teens wearing, and why?*

Working Out Safely

As you plan your fitness program, it is important to think about safety and know what precautions to take. First, dress appropriately for your workout. Loose-fitting clothing is usually best. If your workout takes you outdoors at night, wear light colors and reflective coverings so that others can see you better. For cold-weather workouts, dress in several thin layers of clothing. In hot weather, shorten your workouts and drink plenty of fluids. Always wear sunscreen to protect your skin.

Consider the best location and equipment for your workout. For example, soft, even surfaces are easier on your bones and muscles. Be careful when working out alone outdoors, especially at night or in a deserted place. If possible, work out with a friend. Consider your equipment carefully, too. Make sure that your shoes or skates provide good support and are comfortable. Always wear the protective gear that is appropriate for your activity.

If you get injured, treat the injury according to the R.I.C.E. formula: **R**est, **I**ce, **C**ompression, and **E**levation. Stop your activity immediately and rest. Then use ice to keep swelling down and to ease any pain. Compression means putting pressure on the injured area to reduce swelling, as with an elastic bandage. Elevation involves raising the injured part, also to reduce swelling.

Making a Schedule

A written schedule can help you stick to your fitness program. Write out a weekly plan that includes your school physical education classes and your activities before and after school. Then make a chart or calendar to remind yourself of what activities you've planned and when you'll work out each day. Keep track of how often you work out and how long each session lasts. It's satisfying to look back and see how much you've accomplished!

Be flexible when you make your schedule. Your goals and needs may change as your level of fitness increases. You may want to try new activities or take advantage of seasonal sports. In fact, varying your workouts will keep you interested in your program.

Elements of a Good Workout

A good workout consists of 20 to 30 minutes of moderate-to-vigorous physical activity. It should include a warm-up, the workout activity, and a cool-down. You may choose aerobic activities, strength-building activities, or both. If you are including both types of physical activity, work on strength training after the aerobic activity because your muscles will function more smoothly then.

Warm-Up and Cool-Down

Before you start your workout, you need to warm up your muscles. A **warm-up** routine is *gentle exercise you do to prepare your muscles for moderate to vigorous activity.* Include some stretching activities after your warm-up. When you have completed your workout, it is important to allow time for a cooling-down stage. The **cool-down** involves *gentle exercises that let your body adjust to ending a workout.* **Figure 3.10** illustrates the warming-up and cooling-down processes.

HEALTH *Online*

Topic: Fitness goals

For a link to more information on setting and reaching your fitness goals, go to **health.glencoe.com**.

Activity: Using the information provided at this link, create a written plan to improve your fitness level.

FIGURE 3.10

WARMING UP AND COOLING DOWN

By warming up and cooling down, you help to ensure a safe workout. *What else can you do to make your workouts safer?*

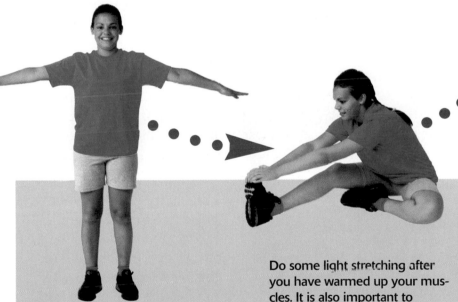

Your warm-up should take about ten minutes and consist of easy aerobic exercise. When you warm up, blood flows into your muscles so that they are more flexible. In addition, your heart rate increases gradually and safely.

Do some light stretching after you have warmed up your muscles. It is also important to stretch after your cool-down to maintain or increase your flexibility. Stretch only to a point where you feel a gentle pull and hold the stretch for a count of 15 to 20 seconds. To prevent injury, avoid bouncing or jerking.

Cool down after your workout so that your muscles don't tighten. Cooling down also brings your circulation back to normal and lowers your body temperature. To cool down, continue the movements of your workout at a slower pace for about five to ten minutes. Follow this with about five minutes of stretching. Remember to drink plenty of fluids after exercising.

The F.I.T. Formula

Using the F.I.T. formula will help you meet your fitness goals. F.I.T. stands for the **F**requency, **I**ntensity, and length of **T**ime of your workout sessions. Increase all of these factors over time.

- **Frequency** is *the number of days you work out each week.* At first, work out two or three days a week. Gradually increase your workouts to five days a week. Remember that you will probably want to vary your routine from day to day.
- **Intensity** means *how much energy you use when you work out.* There is an easy way to determine if the intensity of your workout is appropriate. If you are able to talk, you're probably moving at the right pace. If you find you are out of breath and can't talk, slow down. If you are able to sing while engaged in your activity, you may not be working hard enough.
- **Time** is how long each workout lasts. Begin by working out for about 20 minutes. Then gradually increase your physical activity to 30 to 45 minutes at each session.

Target Heart Rate

You can monitor the intensity of your workout by taking your pulse to see if you are in your target heart rate zone. Your **target heart rate** is the *number of heartbeats per minute that you should aim for during moderate to vigorous activity to benefit your circulatory system the most.* **Figure 3.11** explains how to calculate the range of your target heart rate.

To see whether you are exercising within your target heart rate range during a workout, take your pulse for 6 seconds and multiply this number by 10 to get your pulse rate for one minute. (To take your pulse, place the first two fingers of one hand on the inside of the other wrist, or on either side of the neck, right below the jaw line. Don't use your thumb, which has its own pulse.) Where does the number fall within your range?

FIGURE 3.11

CALCULATING YOUR TARGET HEART RATE

Knowing the range of your target heart rate can help you assess the intensity of a workout.

$$\begin{array}{r} 220 \\ -12 \\ \hline 208 \end{array}$$

Step 1
Subtract your age from 220. The resulting number is your maximum heart rate—an estimate of how fast your heart is capable of beating.

$$\begin{array}{r} 208 \\ \times\ 0.6 \\ \hline 124.8 \end{array}$$

Step 2
Multiply your maximum heart rate by 0.6 to find the low end of your target heart rate range. When you first begin an exercise plan, you should aim for this heart rate.

$$\begin{array}{r} 208 \\ \times\ 0.8 \\ \hline 166.4 \end{array}$$

Step 3
Multiply your maximum heart rate by 0.8 to find the high end of your target heart rate range. As you become more fit, you can work up to this level. Do not exceed this heart rate while exercising.

Checking Your Progress

Once you've established your fitness program and started to follow your weekly schedule, take some time to think about what you've accomplished and where you are going. Is your program working for you? Do you need to make adjustments? Are you close to reaching your goals? The following tips can help you assess your program and monitor your progress.

If you've been working out for four to eight weeks, you should see some results. You may feel better, be more flexible, and have more heart and lung endurance and muscular endurance. Keeping a fitness log as you go will help you see how far you've come.

If you feel that you're not any closer to your goal, think about whether you've been keeping to your schedule. If not, how can you make sure that you do? If you have kept to your schedule, you may need to reevaluate your goal. Is it realistic? Maybe you need more time than you thought.

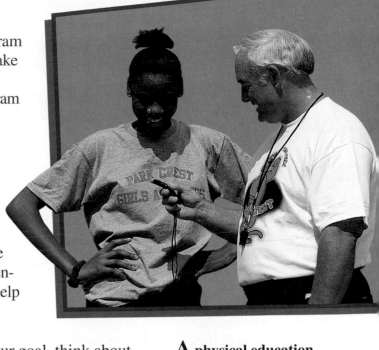

A physical education teacher is a source of advice about how to set fitness goals. Talk to your physical education teacher about the goals you'd like to achieve.

Lesson 4 Review

Using complete sentences, answer the following questions on a sheet of paper.

Reviewing Terms and Facts

1. **Vocabulary** Define the term *body composition.*
2. **Identify** What are some safety issues you need to consider when you work out?
3. **Explain** What is the purpose of warm-up and cool-down periods?
4. **Describe** Explain the F.I.T. formula.
5. **Discuss** How is target heart rate related to the intensity of a workout?

Thinking Critically

6. **Describe** What would you advise a friend to do if he or she became injured while working out?

7. **Justify** Why is it important to be flexible when you plan a workout schedule?

Applying Health Skills

8. **Advocacy** Demonstrate ways to use health information to help others: Imagine that your friend starts a fitness program but loses interest after a week. What health information could you give to this friend to help him or her stick to the program?
9. **Goal Setting** List some ways you can engage in physical activities outside of school. From this list, choose an activity that you think you would enjoy and set a goal to participate in this activity regularly. Use the goal-setting steps to help you reach your goal.

Sports and Physical Wellness

LEARN ABOUT...

- the advantages of both individual and team sports.
- how to avoid sports injuries.
- how eating habits can affect the level of performance.
- why it is harmful to take drugs to improve sports performance.

VOCABULARY

- individual sports
- team sports
- dehydration
- conditioning
- overtraining
- anabolic steroids

Sports for Health

Starting and following a well thought-out program is a good way to achieve fitness. One way to remain fit is by playing sports. Some people play sports for fun. Others make a serious commitment to a sport, working hard to develop their skills.

What do you like about sports? Do you like the excitement of competing against another person or team? Do you enjoy mastering a new skill? Do you prefer one-on-one competition or the support of teammates? Do you enjoy competing at all? Think about these questions. Choose sports that you think will be fun. You'll be more likely to get the greatest benefit out of a sport if you have a good time doing it.

Health behaviors and knowledge, including those related to fitness and sports, vary with age. Older adults may engage in low-impact activities and sports to prevent injuries. Younger generations may participate in more vigorous sports and activities.

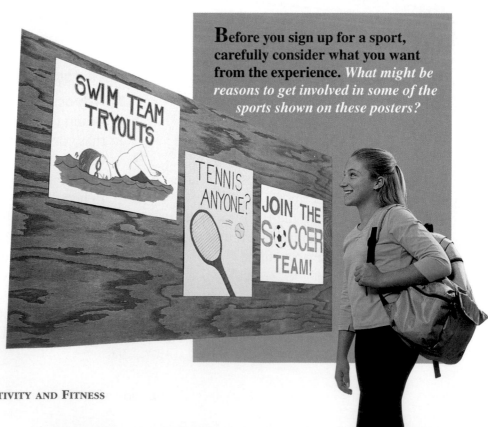

Before you sign up for a sport, carefully consider what you want from the experience. *What might be reasons to get involved in some of the sports shown on these posters?*

Individual and Team Sports

Individual sports are *physical activities you can take part in by yourself or with another person, without being part of a team.* Biking, hiking, swimming, running, surfing, skating, and horseback riding are all individual sports. You can set your own schedule and determine your own level of commitment in individual sports. You don't have to be compared to anyone else, and you can establish the pace of the activity. However, you miss some of the mental/emotional, and social health benefits of playing on a team.

Team sports are *organized physical activities with specific rules, played by opposing groups of people.* Baseball, basketball, football, soccer, and volleyball are popular team sports. In team sports you have the companionship and encouragement of teammates and coaches. Playing against another team may push you to excel. Having to attend regularly scheduled practices can help you to become more responsible. However, some people may find that playing a team sport is too time-consuming.

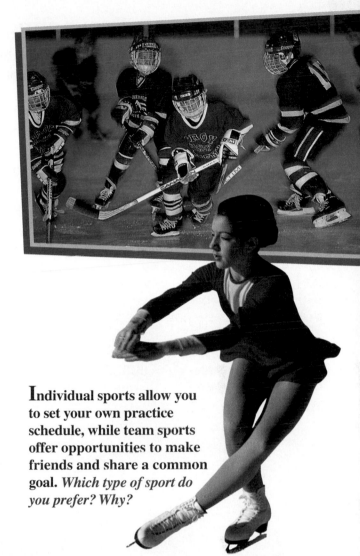

Individual sports allow you to set your own practice schedule, while team sports offer opportunities to make friends and share a common goal. *Which type of sport do you prefer? Why?*

HEALTH SKILLS ACTIVITY

DECISION MAKING

Balancing Your Activities

Kate loves ballet, and she's a good ice-skater. In seventh grade Kate discovered that she liked basketball too. She made the school team.

Now she has a problem, however. Seventh grade demands more homework time than Kate expected. Her grades are starting to slip. Also, because Kate is at basketball practice most afternoons and ballet class on the weekends, her sister feels as if she is doing more than her share of chores at home.

How can Kate solve her problem?

WHAT WOULD YOU DO?

With a small group, role-play a family discussion of Kate's situation. Then work through the steps of the decision-making process.

1. **STATE THE SITUATION.**
2. **LIST THE OPTIONS.**
3. **WEIGH THE POSSIBLE OUTCOMES.**
4. **CONSIDER VALUES.**
5. **MAKE A DECISION AND ACT.**
6. **EVALUATE YOUR DECISION.**

Preventing Injuries

The following tips can help you avoid sports-related injuries.

- See a doctor for a physical exam before you participate in a sport.
- Warm up, stretch adequately, and cool down.
- Learn the proper techniques for your sport.
- Use the correct safety and protective equipment properly. See **Figure 3.12** for a description of some of the gear that can help protect you.
- Observe safety rules during sports and other physical activities.
- Report any injury to your coach or teacher and to your parents.
- Don't return to the sport until a health care professional says that you are well enough to play.

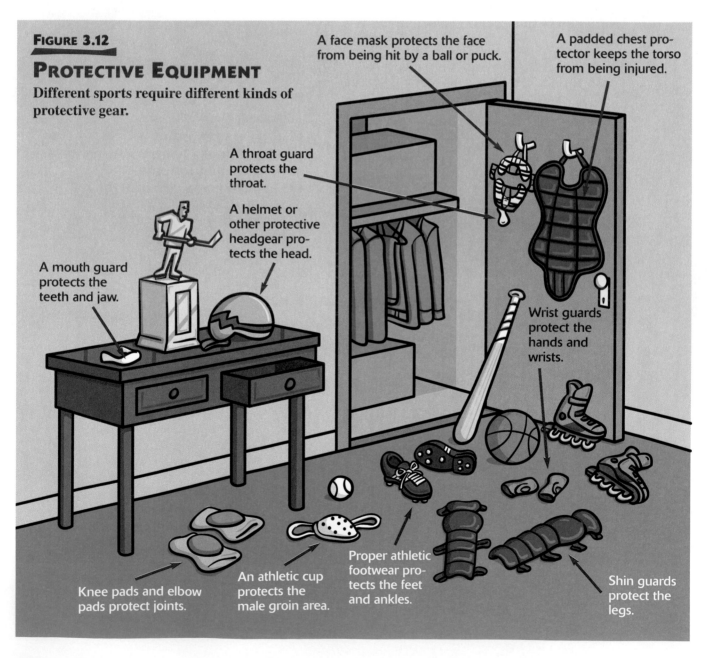

FIGURE 3.12

PROTECTIVE EQUIPMENT

Different sports require different kinds of protective gear.

A face mask protects the face from being hit by a ball or puck.

A padded chest protector keeps the torso from being injured.

A throat guard protects the throat.

A helmet or other protective headgear protects the head.

A mouth guard protects the teeth and jaw.

Wrist guards protect the hands and wrists.

Knee pads and elbow pads protect joints.

An athletic cup protects the male groin area.

Proper athletic footwear protects the feet and ankles.

Shin guards protect the legs.

Sports Nutrition

If you play a sport, remember that you will need to keep your body supplied with additional energy. This need may require some changes in what you eat as well as when you eat.

What to Eat

When you play a sport, you may need more food to provide your body with the fuel it requires. **Figure 3.13** identifies a variety of activities in terms of the calories they burn. If you play a more vigorous sport for a longer period of time, you may need to eat more. This added intake helps give you the energy you will need while you play. A good approach to providing your body with enough fuel is to choose a variety of foods from the five major food groups every day. A balanced diet will supply your body with what it needs for you to perform at your best.

You also need to make sure that you drink enough water when you play sports. If you don't replace the water you lose by sweating, dehydration can occur. **Dehydration** is the *excessive loss of water from the body.* It can result in muscle cramps, heatstroke, and harm to some body systems. Don't wait until you're thirsty before you drink.

Reading Check
Make your own judgments. Which sports or activities in your own life burn the most calories?

FIGURE 3.13

SPORTS AND ENERGY USE

If you do the activities shown here for the amount of time stated, you will burn about 150 calories. You can burn roughly the same number of calories by playing a less vigorous sport for a longer time or by playing a more intense sport for a shorter time.

Less Vigorous, More Time

More Vigorous, Less Time

Activity	Minutes
Volleyball	45
Touch football	30–45
Shooting baskets	30
Cycling 5 miles	30
Swimming laps	20
Wheelchair basketball	20
Cycling 4 miles	15
Running 1½ miles	15

Source: Centers for Disease Control and Prevention

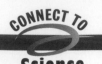
When to Eat

When you first take up a sport, you will have to consider how much energy you will need, when you will need it, and how your sport will affect your digestion. It is also important to make sure that you always have water available and drink it all day long. Here are a few more tips.

- Eat a light snack one to two hours before a sporting event. Foods like bananas, bagels, and fruit juices are good choices.
- Drink plenty of fluids before a game. A good guideline is 2 cups (16 ounces) of water about two hours before the event, followed by 1 cup of water every 15 minutes.
- Continue to drink water during the game. This helps to control your body temperature and cool working muscles. Sports drinks can restore fluids and minerals to your body if you are involved in an activity that lasts for more than one hour.
- Refuel your body with a hearty, balanced meal after the game. Also, keep track of your weight before and after a game. For every pound that you have lost during the event, drink 3 cups of water.

Shaping Up Safely

If you want to play a sport regularly, you'll need to get into shape for it. *Training to get into shape* is called **conditioning**. Different sports demand different levels of strength, endurance, and flexibility. For example, a gymnast needs strength, flexibility, muscle endurance, and balance to perform a variety of routines. Talk to a physical education teacher, a coach, or an athletic trainer to help you establish a conditioning routine.

Athletes should drink fluids before, during, and after sporting events.

You can get into shape for your sport with regular conditioning and good nutrition. However, too much exercise without enough rest can be harmful. **Overtraining** is *exercising too hard or too often, without enough rest in between sessions.* Signs of overtraining include an elevated resting heart rate, frequent illness, disturbed sleeping habits, and frequent muscle strain or injury. To avoid overtraining, take a day off from exercise every week. Alternate intense workout days with light ones. Every two months reduce your exercise frequency, intensity, and time for a week.

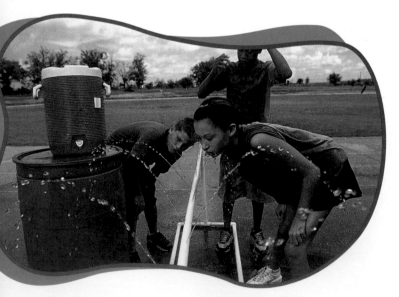

Avoiding Harmful Substances

Anabolic steroids (a·nuh·BAH·lik STIR·oydz) are *synthetic compounds that cause muscle tissue to develop at an abnormally high rate.* Anabolic steroids, often referred to simply as *steroids,* have legitimate medical uses, such as in the treatment of some types of cancer. However, it is not only unfair but also illegal to use them to improve athletic performance. Anabolic steroids can also have many different side effects, including

- weakening of tendons, possibly leading to joint or tendon injury.
- damage to the cardiovascular system, affecting heart rate and blood pressure and increasing the risk of a heart attack.
- bone damage because the bones can become more brittle.
- brain and liver cancer.
- harmful changes in sexual characteristics, including the growth of facial hair in females and breast development in males.
- the development of acne.
- increased irritability, anxiety, suspicion, or sudden rage.

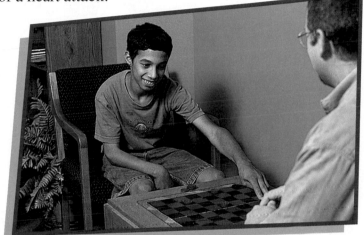

To avoid overtraining, take one day a week off from working out. *What are some signs of overtraining?*

Lesson 5 Review

Using complete sentences, answer the following questions on a sheet of paper.

Reviewing Terms and Facts

1. **Vocabulary** Define the terms *individual sports* and *team sports.*
2. **Recall** What are three ways to avoid sports injuries?
3. **Describe** How much water should an athlete drink before a game?
4. **Vocabulary** Define the term *dehydration,* and discuss its effects.
5. **Apply** What is *overtraining?* What advice would you give to someone who is showing signs of overtraining?

Thinking Critically

6. **Evaluate** Describe your own thoughts and feelings about the benefits of individual sports compared to those of team sports.
7. **Predict** How might playing a sport throughout your life benefit your health?

Applying Health Skills

8. **Refusal Skills** With a classmate, write a skit in which an athlete is persistently pressured by a teammate to take anabolic steroids. Incorporate facts about steroid use into the athlete's refusal.

The New Gym

The emphasis is on lifelong fitness habits, not competition.

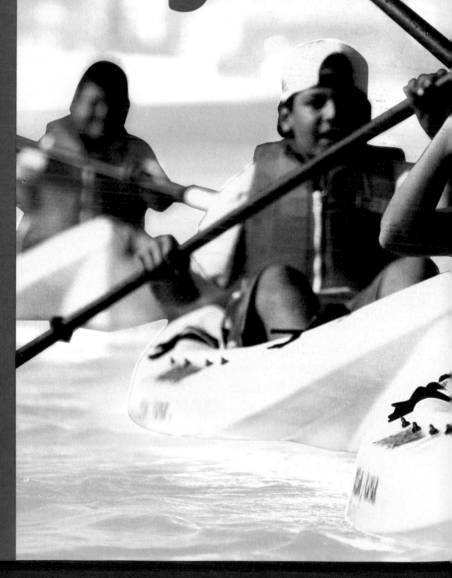

Fitness Tips

Want to feel good, have fun, and stay healthy? Here are some tips from Judy Young, executive director of the National Association for Sport and Physical Education.

Get moving: Be physically active for at least an hour every day. Kick a soccer ball, take a walk with your family, go dancing with friends—whatever! Try new and varied activities so you work different muscles in your body.

Stick with it: Perform one of your daily physical activities for at least 10 minutes at a time. Increase the time as you get stronger.

Set limits: Don't spend more than two hours a day playing computer games or watching TV.

Fuel up: Eat a nutritious, balanced diet that includes whole grains; fruits and vegetables; low-fat dairy products; and protein-rich foods such as lean meats or beans. Drink at least eight glasses of water every day.

Have fun: Exercise is more fun with a partner. Invite a friend or family member the next time you're ready to get active.

It's a sunny day, and 12-year-old Liza Parisaca is on the banks of Biscayne Bay in Miami, Florida. She pulls on a life vest over her T-shirt and cautiously climbs into the sailboat bobbing in the clear blue water. Today, the first-time sailor will learn how to tack, or change course, on the boat. "Ready?" asks the instructor. Liza nods her head. She steers the boat through the wind, and it changes direction smoothly. "I wasn't really scared," she says with a big grin.

This isn't an end-of-summer sailing trip. It's gym class at Riverside Elementary School. Riverside is one of many schools around the country that have begun adding fun new activities to gym classes.

In schools like Riverside, gym class is no longer about lining up and choosing teams. A new physical education (P.E.) movement is helping kids find activities they'll enjoy so much that they'll stay active for the rest of their lives. The activities include cycling, martial arts, dance, kickboxing, in-line skating, using treadmills, and even sailing and kayaking. The goal is to teach children sports and workouts that they can enjoy outside of school.

Time to Shape Up

The movement comes in response to studies that show that young people are less active than ever before. According to a report released by the Institute of Medicine, American children and adults need much more physical activity. The report calls for at least an hour a day of some type of physical activity.

Unfortunately, most children do not even come close to meeting that standard. Fewer than one in four children gets even 20 minutes of vigorous activity on a daily basis. One in four young people receives no physical education in school, according to P.E. 4 Life, a group that promotes fitness for kids.

Young peoples' general activity level peaks in 10th grade, then slowly declines all the way into adulthood. "We want them to find something they can enjoy doing for a lifetime," says Dr. Jayne Greenberg, director of P.E. programs for the Miami-Dade County Schools in Florida.

Greenberg says the key to the new P.E. programs is that they work for all kids regardless of skill level. "Traditional P.E. programs tended to focus on competitive team sports and appeal mainly to the strongest athletes in the class," she says. In the sailing unit at Riverside, even disabled children take a turn as skippers of the boat. Says Greenberg: "Kids should never have to feel like they aren't good enough in their gym classes." ◢

TIME TO THINK...

About Fitness

Turn the "Fitness Tips" into a personal checklist. Create a chart with the seven days of the week listed on the left and the five tips—or goals—listed on the bottom. For one week, check off the goals that you accomplish each day. Use this information to determine what physical activity goals you need to work on.

STAYING ON THE PATH TO FITNESS

Model

During the summer Hayley decided that she wanted to be more active. She planned out what activities she would do and when. She went swimming at the community pool. She also went in-line skating and bicycling, and she asked her friends to play tennis. She was pleased with her progress at the end of the summer.

However, Hayley realized that the pool would close soon and that she would be unable to do a lot of her activities once it started getting dark earlier. After thinking and talking with her family and friends, Hayley decided to continue working toward her goal of adding physical activity to her life by working out to exercise videos after school.

Practice

When you set a goal, it is important to set up checkpoints so that you can evaluate your progress. This step will help you make adjustments for any obstacles that may arise. Read the situation below and write a paragraph explaining what you think Jared can do to meet his fitness goals. How might revisiting his checkpoints help him meet his goals?

After finding himself out of breath from running a mile in gym class, Jared has decided that he'd like to work to become more fit. He created a plan to reach this goal. The problem is that between homework, studying, and watching his younger brother in the afternoon, he hasn't been able to find the time to work out.

Apply/Assess

Use the goal-setting steps to design a fitness program for yourself. When you set up your checkpoints, consider any issues that could prevent you from meeting your goal. For example, you might want to go jogging but live in an area where high or low temperatures discourage you from engaging in outdoor activities for part of the year. Brainstorm other ways to meet your goal. Exchange fitness programs with a classmate. Make suggestions for how your classmate can meet his or her goal when obstacles come up.

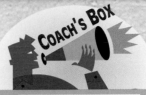

COACH'S BOX

Goal Setting

1. Set a specific goal.
2. List the steps to reach your goal.
3. Get help from others.
4. Evaluate your progress.
5. Reward yourself.

Self-√ Check

- Did I use the goal-setting steps to design a fitness program?
- Did I come up with other ways to meet my goal when obstacles arose?

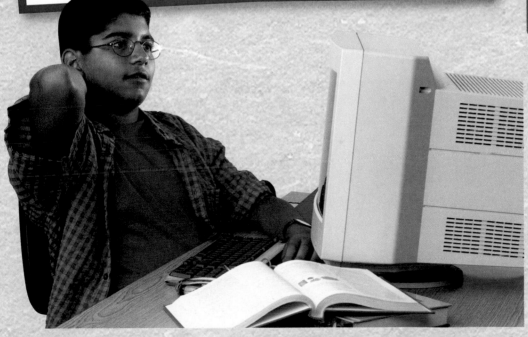

Reviewing Vocabulary and Concepts

On a sheet of paper, write the numbers 1–7. After each number, write the term from the list that best completes each statement.

- tendon
- fitness
- exercise
- involuntary
- strength
- aerobic
- skeletal

Lesson 1

1. The ability to handle the physical work and play of everyday life without becoming tired is known as _____.

2. Physical activity that is planned, structured, and repetitive is called _____.

3. The ability of muscles to exert a force is called _____.

4. Rhythmic, nonstop, moderate-to-vigorous activity that requires large amounts of oxygen and works the heart is _____ exercise.

Lesson 2

5. The tissue that attaches muscle to bone or muscle to muscle is called a(n) _____.

6. _____ muscles are found in the heart and other internal organs.

7. Pairs of _____ muscles work in opposition.

On a sheet of paper, write the numbers 8–13. Write *True* or *False* for each statement below. If the statement is false, change the underlined word or phrase to make it true.

Lesson 3

8. The group of organs that transports essential materials to body cells and removes waste is the <u>nervous</u> system.

9. The watery part of the blood is <u>plasma</u>.

10. Oxygen is carried from the lungs to other parts of the body by <u>platelets</u>.

Lesson 4

11. Gentle exercise that prepares your body for moderate to vigorous activity is a <u>warm-up</u>.

12. Gentle exercise that lets your body adjust to ending a workout is a <u>target heart rate</u>.

13. <u>Intensity</u> refers to the number of days you work out each week.

Lesson 5

On a sheet of paper, write the numbers 14–16. After each number, write the letter of the answer that best completes each statement.

14. Training to get into shape is called
  a. sports nutrition.
  b. conditioning.
  c. overtraining.
  d. dehydration.

15. If you have an elevated resting heart rate, are frequently ill, and experience disturbed sleeping patterns, you may be
  a. overtraining.
  b. dehydrated.
  c. malnourished.
  d. overconfident.

16. Anabolic steroids cause muscle tissue to
  a. maintain its flexibility.
  b. stop developing.
  c. develop at an abnormally high rate.
  d. perform at its best.

Thinking Critically

Using complete sentences, answer the following questions on a sheet of paper.

17. Explain How might staying fit help you cope with stress?

18. Integrate Describe how a program of regular exercise designed to improve strength, endurance, and flexibility can help the skeletal and muscular systems.

19. Apply Explain why you agree or disagree with this statement: "I have no control over the health of my circulatory system."

20. Analyze If you play a sport, why might you want to continue a conditioning program even in the off-season?

Career Corner

Sports Medicine Are you interested in sports? Do you also have an interest in helping people get well? Put both interests together, and become a doctor who specializes in sports medicine. These professionals treat people with sports- or exercise-related injuries.

To enter this career, you'll need a four-year college degree, four years of medical school, and one to seven years of residency training. Learn more about this and other health careers by clicking on Career Corner at health.glencoe.com.

Standardized Test Practice

Reading & Writing

Read the paragraphs below and then answer the questions.

My dad and I went white-water rafting this summer and it was an experience I will never forget.

The first mile or so of the trip was easy since we just started in a slow-moving current to get used to paddling and to listen to the guide give us instructions. Then we approached the rapids and everything changed. I can't explain the feeling of moving so fast down the rapids, with water rushing all around us while we tried to navigate. At one point our guide had to help me navigate through the "eye of the needle," a difficult stretch of the rapids. I just missed hitting a rock, but I lost my balance for a moment and almost fell overboard. It was scary, but great, and the trip seemed to be over too soon.

1. The mood of the letter writer can best be described as

   A relieved.

   B excited.

   C nervous.

   D mysterious.

2. From the information in the second paragraph, the reader can conclude that the writer found white-water rafting to be

   A difficult.

   B easy.

   C boring.

   D not for young people.

3. Write a paragraph describing how you feel when you participate in a sport or other physical activity that you enjoy.

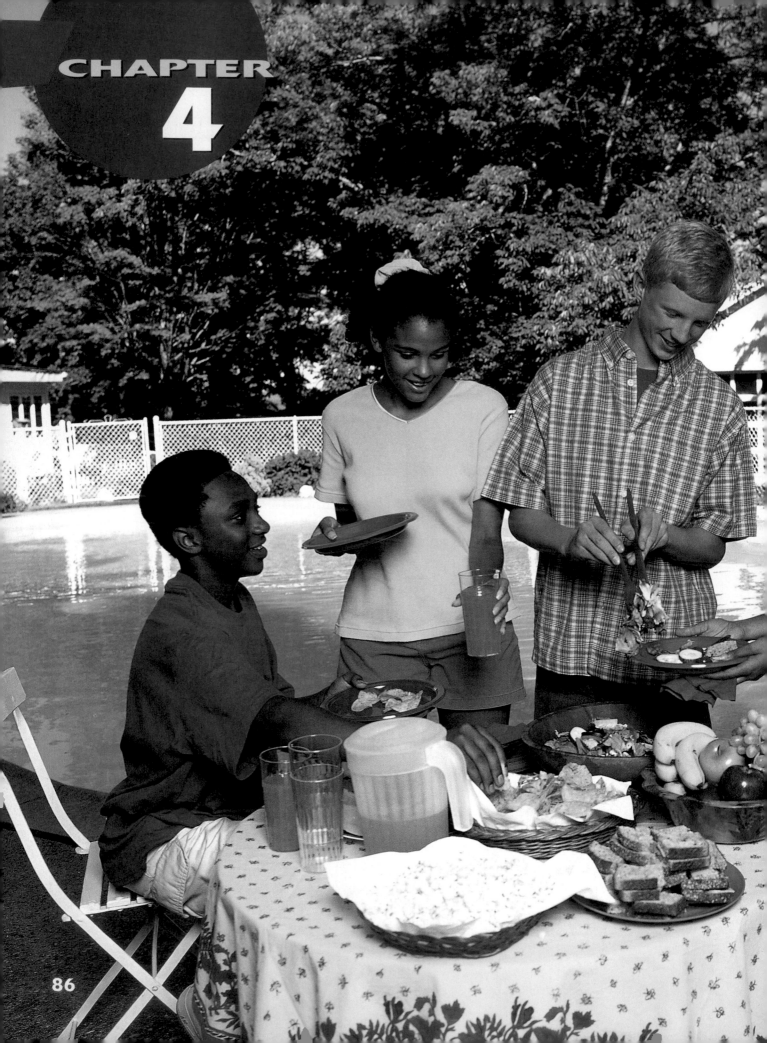

4

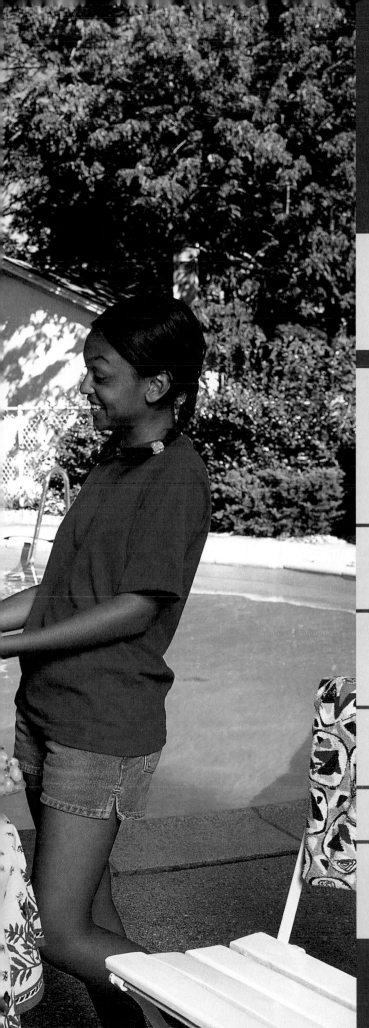

Food and Nutrition

HEALTH *Online*

Do you practice healthful nutrition habits? Go to health.glencoe.com and take the Health Inventory for Chapter 4 to find out how you rate.

FOLDABLES™
Study Organizer

Before You Read

Make this Foldable to help you organize what you learn in Lesson 1 about the six types of nutrients. Begin with four plain sheets of 8½″ × 11″ paper.

Step 1

Collect four sheets of paper, and place them ½″ apart.

Step 2

Roll up the bottom edges, stopping them ½″ from the top edges. This makes all tabs the same size.

Step 3

Crease the paper to hold the tabs in place and staple along the fold.

Step 4

Label the tabs as shown.

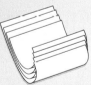

Six Major Nutrients
Carbohydrates
Proteins
Fats
Vitamins
Minerals
Water
Vocabulary

As You Read

Record information on each type of nutrient and define key vocabulary terms under the appropriate tab.

87

Nutrients for Health

The Six Major Nutrients

Eating healthful food helps you feel good and do your best. **Nutrients** (NOO·tree·ents) are *substances in foods that your body needs in order to grow, have energy, and stay healthy.* The six categories of nutrients are described below.

Carbohydrates, Proteins, and Fats

Carbohydrates (kar·boh·HY·drayts) are *the starches and sugars that provide energy.* Starches are complex carbohydrates. They are found in foods such as rice, pasta, breads, potatoes, beans, and corn. Sugars are simple carbohydrates. They occur naturally in milk, fruit, and honey. Sugar is also added to many foods.

Proteins (PROH·teenz) are *nutrients used to repair body cells and tissues.* Proteins are made up of amino (uh·MEE·noh) acids. Complete proteins contain all the essential amino acids. They are found in foods from animal sources, such as meat, dairy products, and eggs. Plant foods lack one or more essential amino acids, so they're incomplete proteins. However, eating a variety of plant foods, such as beans, nuts, and grains, can provide all the essential amino acids.

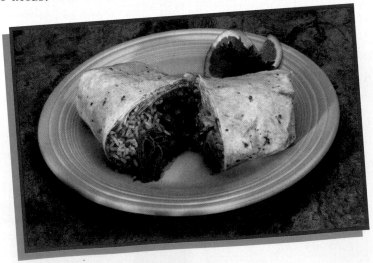

Burritos are a good source of several different nutrients, including proteins and carbohydrates.

Fats are *nutrients that supply energy, keep the skin healthy, and promote normal growth.* They also transport certain vitamins through the body and help build cell membranes. **Saturated fats** are *fats that are solid at room temperature.* Examples include butter; stick margarine; and the fats in meat, poultry, and dairy products. Eating large amounts of foods that are high in saturated fats increases the risk of heart disease. **Unsaturated fats**, *fats that are liquid at room temperature,* come mainly from plant sources. Foods with mostly unsaturated fats include vegetable oils, nuts, olives, and avocados. *Trans fats* are unsaturated fats that have been chemically altered to make them solid. These fats are linked to heart disease.

Vitamins, Minerals, and Water

Vitamins are *substances that help to regulate the body's functions.* Your body needs vitamins to produce energy, to fight infections, and to help with other tasks. Water-soluble vitamins, including vitamin C and the B vitamins, dissolve in water. Only small amounts of water-soluble vitamins are stored in the body, so these vitamins must be replaced every day. Fat-soluble vitamins, including vitamins A, D, E, and K, dissolve in fat. The body can store these vitamins until they are needed. Fruits and vegetables are the best sources of vitamins A and C. Whole-grain and enriched breads and cereals supply B vitamins. Milk is a good source of vitamin D and the B vitamin riboflavin.

Minerals are *nutrients that strengthen bones and teeth, help keep blood healthy, and keep the heart and other organs working properly.* Calcium, phosphorus, and magnesium are minerals that help build and renew your bones. Iron is needed for making red blood cells. Potassium, sodium, and chloride help maintain the body's balance of fluids. Milk is a rich source of calcium and phosphorus. Meat, spinach and other leafy green vegetables, fruits, and dry beans supply iron. Sodium comes from salt and is found in many packaged foods.

Water is a nutrient, too! Without water your body would not be able to function. Water helps with digestion, carries nutrients throughout the body, removes wastes from the body, and regulates body temperature. Drink eight to ten glasses of water each day.

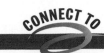

Science

CALCIUM FROM FOOD
During the teen years, your bones are still growing. If you do not eat enough calcium-rich foods, over time your bones will weaken, leading to osteoporosis (ahs·tee·oh·puh·ROH·suhs). This disabling disease causes bones to fracture easily. *List three ways to add calcium-rich foods to your diet.*

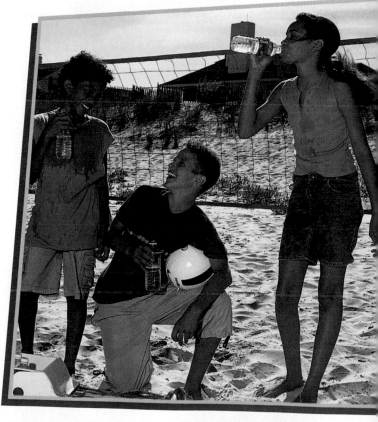

When you're thirsty, reach for water. This nutrient helps the body function properly.

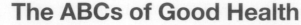
The ABCs of Good Health

Getting enough physical activity and eating a variety of foods will help you stay healthy. The U.S. Department of Agriculture (USDA) has developed the Dietary Guidelines for Americans. The guidelines focus on the ABCs of good health: **A**im for fitness, **B**uild a healthy base, and **C**hoose sensibly.

Aim for Fitness

Being physically active every day and maintaining a healthy weight are important for fitness. You can easily get the recommended 60 minutes of daily physical activity by walking, running, skating, or making other activities part of your daily routine.

Build a Healthy Base

You can help your body stay healthy and function well by eating a variety of foods. Make grains, fruits, and vegetables the foundation of your meals. Grains (especially enriched and whole grains), fruits, and vegetables supply the vitamins and minerals your body needs for healthy eyes, skin, bones, and blood. They're your best energy source, too. Many of these foods are also good sources of **fiber**, *the part of grains, fruits, and vegetables that the body cannot break down.*

Fiber helps move wastes out of your system, and may also help prevent some diseases, such as heart disease. One way to increase the fiber in your diet is to eat at least five servings of fruits and vegetables daily. Another way is to choose whole-grain cereals, whole-grain breads, and brown rice whenever you can.

A healthy base also involves making sure that food is safe to eat. Handle and prepare foods properly at home and take care when eating out to avoid food-borne illnesses. Harmful bacteria, viruses, and parasites can cause food to spoil and may make you sick.

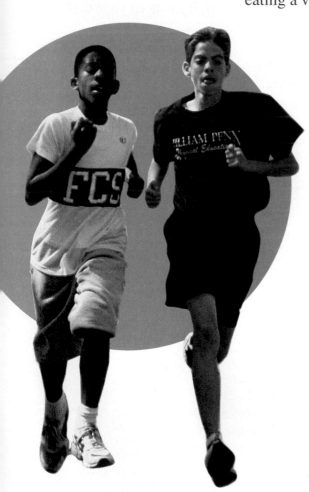

Staying physically active is an important part of good health. *How can you fit physical activity into your daily*

Choose Sensibly

Avoid consuming too much fat. Good nutrition depends on an eating plan that is low in cholesterol and saturated fat. **Cholesterol** (kuh·LES·tuh·rawl) is *a waxy substance used by the body to build cells and make other substances.* Saturated fats tend to raise the body's level of cholesterol, which increases the risk of heart disease and stroke. Choose foods low in saturated fats and keep your overall fat intake to no more than 30 percent of daily calories.

Avoid consuming too much sugar. Many foods contain sugars. Foods that have large amounts of added sugar include soft drinks, fruit punch, cakes and cookies, candy, and ice cream. Remember that foods containing sugars and starches promote tooth decay. Be sure to check canned and processed foods for hidden sugars. If a product's ingredient list includes words such as *corn syrup, sucrose,* or *dextrose,* the food is likely to be high in added sugars.

Avoid consuming too much salt. Sodium, a mineral in salt, helps the body regulate fluids and blood pressure. Your body needs only a small amount of sodium (less than 1/4 teaspoon of salt daily). Too much sodium may increase your risk of high blood pressure and can decrease the amount of calcium in your body, weakening your bones. To cut down on salt, choose low-sodium foods; use herbs and spices to season foods; and go easy on salty snacks.

✓ Reading Check

Understand how text is organized. The introduction presents a handy tip for remembering the Dietary Guidelines. Locate this tip on these two pages.

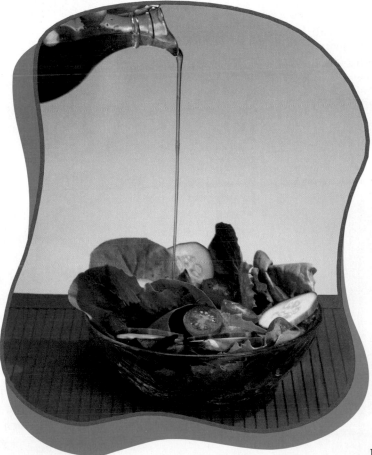

Fats perform many important functions in the body, but consuming too much fat is not healthful. *List three ways of adding flavor to salads without adding a lot of fat.*

Reading a Nutrition Facts Panel

Most packaged foods come with a food label that includes a Nutrition Facts panel. The panel lists the product's nutritional value. This information can help you make smart food choices. **Figure 4.1** on page 93 shows how to read the various sections of a Nutrition Facts panel.

The Nutrition Facts panel tells you how large one serving is and the number of calories and amounts of nutrients in a serving. Studying the % Daily Value column will tell you if a food is high or low in certain nutrients. Look for foods that have low daily value percentages (below 5 percent) for fats, cholesterol, and sodium. Choose foods whose labels show high percentages (20 percent or above) of fiber, vitamins, and minerals.

HEALTH SKILLS ACTIVITY

PRACTICING HEALTHFUL BEHAVIORS

Keeping Food Safe

Have you ever felt sick to your stomach and thought to yourself, "It must have been something I ate"? If you handle and prepare foods properly, you will greatly decrease your risk of getting a foodborne illness. To keep food safe, follow these steps:

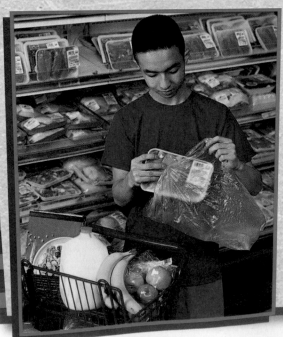

- **CLEAN.** Before you handle food or utensils, wash your hands with warm, soapy water. Wash your hands after handling raw meats, poultry, eggs, and fish as well as everything that comes into contact with these foods. Clean kitchen surfaces as you work.
- **SEPARATE.** Separate raw, cooked, and ready-to-eat foods while buying, preparing, and storing them.
- **COOK.** Make sure that you cook foods to the proper temperature by using a food thermometer. Reheat leftovers thoroughly.
- **CHILL.** Keep perishable foods refrigerated. Thaw frozen foods in the refrigerator.
- **FOLLOW THE LABEL.** Read labels and follow directions such as "Refrigerate after opening."
- **SERVE SAFELY.** Keep hot foods hot and cold foods cold.
- **WHEN IN DOUBT, THROW IT OUT.** Do not eat any food that you think has not been handled or stored properly.

ON YOUR OWN

On a sheet of paper, describe how you would prepare or store each of the following foods to keep it safe:

- Tuna sandwich
- Raw ground beef
- Raw spinach

FIGURE 4.1

GETTING THE NUTRITION FACTS

Reading Nutrition Facts panels will help you choose healthful food products. *Do you look at the serving size when deciding how much of a food to eat?*

What is the total amount of fat in the product? How much of that fat is saturated?

The % Daily Value column helps you judge the amounts of the listed nutrients in one serving of the product. The general guideline is that 20 percent or more is a lot and 5 percent or less isn't very much.

This section shows the suggested amounts of nutrients and food substances the average person should aim for each day. Your individual needs may be higher or lower.

The serving size is the portion most people eat. The amounts listed for calories, nutrients, and food substances are based on one serving of the package's contents.

How many calories does one serving contain? How many of those calories come from fat?

This shows the percentage of Daily Values for selected vitamins and minerals in one serving of the food.

Nutrition Facts

Serving Size: 2 bars (42g)
Servings Per Package: 1

Calories 180
Calories from Fat 60

Amount Per Serving: % Daily Value*

Total Fat 6g — 10%
Saturated Fat 0.5g — 3%
Cholesterol 0mg — 0%
Sodium 160mg — 7%
Total Carbohydrate 29g — 10%
Dietary Fiber 2g — 9%
Sugars 11g
Protein 4g

Vitamin A 40% • Vitamin C 0%
Calcium 0% • Iron 6%

*Percent Daily Values are based on a 2,000 calorie diet. Your daily values may be higher or lower depending on your calorie needs:

	Calories:	2,000	2,500
Total Fat	Less than	65g	80g
Saturated Fat	Less than	20g	25g
Cholesterol	Less than	300mg	300mg
Sodium	Less than	2,400mg	2,400mg
Total Carbohydrate		300g	375g
Dietary Fiber		25g	30g

Lesson 1 Review

Using complete sentences, answer the following questions on a sheet of paper.

Reviewing Terms and Facts

1. **Recall** Identify the six categories of nutrients.
2. **Vocabulary** What are *carbohydrates*?
3. **Discuss** What are *proteins,* and how do they help the body?
4. **Distinguish** Explain the difference between *saturated* and *unsaturated fats*. What food sources contain each of these types of fats?
5. **List** Name three minerals, and explain how each one helps your body.

Thinking Critically

6. **Evaluate** How do the ABCs of good health work together to help you achieve a healthful lifestyle?
7. **Suggest** What would you tell someone who isn't sure how old the leftovers in the refrigerator are? Why?

Applying Health Skills

8. **Accessing Information** Study the Nutrition Facts panel on a package or can of food. Would this food help you fulfill the Dietary Guidelines? Write a short report in which you list your findings and explain the product's nutritional value.

The Food Guide Pyramid

Quick Write
List three reasons variety is important in your meals and snacks.

LEARN ABOUT...

- what influences a person's food choices.
- how to use the Food Guide Pyramid to make healthful food choices.

VOCABULARY

- nutrition
- Food Guide Pyramid
- calorie

The Foods You Choose

The foods you eat enable your body to grow and function properly. **Nutrition** (noo·TRI·shuhn) is *the process of taking in food and using it for energy, growth, and good health.* Eating fulfills the body's physical needs. It can also satisfy emotional and social needs.

Influences on Food Choices

Many factors influence food choices:

- **Personal taste.** The way foods look, smell, feel, and taste influences what you choose to eat.
- **Geography.** The land, climate, and agricultural products where you live affect food availability and influence your food choices.
- **Family, friends, and cultural background.** Your family's traditions or ethnic background may influence your food choices. You may also select certain foods because of your friends.
- **Advertising.** Food ads may influence you to choose one food over others.
- **Cost.** If you don't have much money to spend, you may choose certain foods because they cost less than others.
- **Convenience.** Sometimes you may select foods that you can prepare quickly and easily.

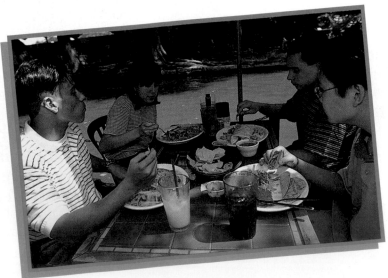

Seeing what foods your friends choose to eat may inspire you to eat some foods you've never tried before. *Name at least two ways in which your friends influence you to make positive food choices. What might influence the food choices of adults?*

The Food Guide Pyramid

You can combine many foods in different ways to create a wholesome and delicious eating plan. To help you decide what foods to eat, the USDA developed the **Food Guide Pyramid**, *a guide for making healthful daily food choices.* **Figure 4.2** shows how foods are grouped on the Pyramid according to the nutrients they provide to the body.

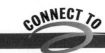

CONNECT TO
Science

VITAMIN AND MINERAL SUPPLEMENTS
Vitamin and mineral deficiencies can result from a poor diet. Symptoms may include fatigue and frequent bruising. Consult with a doctor to determine when it's appropriate to take a vitamin or mineral supplement to correct a deficiency.

FIGURE 4.2

THE FOOD GUIDE PYRAMID

The Food Guide Pyramid is an excellent tool to help you build a healthy base. Eat plenty of foods from the widest part of the Pyramid and limited amounts of food from the Pyramid tip. *How many servings did you eat from the fruit group yesterday?*

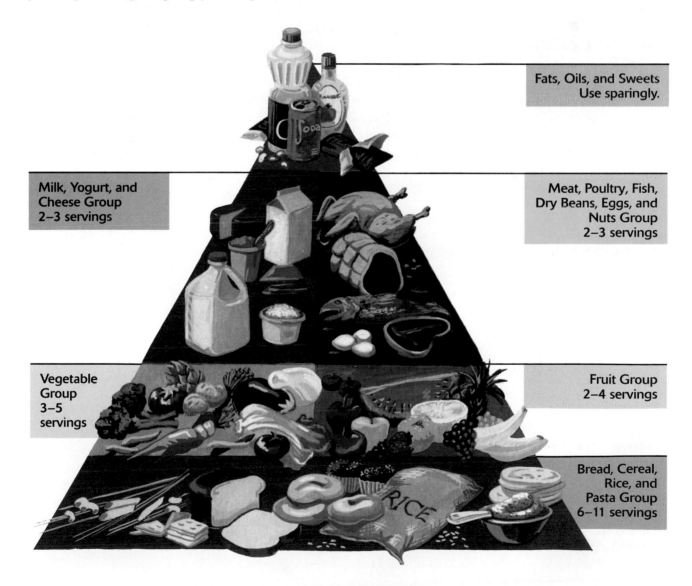

Fats, Oils, and Sweets
Use sparingly.

Milk, Yogurt, and Cheese Group
2–3 servings

Meat, Poultry, Fish, Dry Beans, Eggs, and Nuts Group
2–3 servings

Vegetable Group
3–5 servings

Fruit Group
2–4 servings

Bread, Cereal, Rice, and Pasta Group
6–11 servings

Reading Check

Build your vocabulary.
The word *calorie* comes from a Latin word meaning "heat." How does this meaning relate to calories in food?

Using the Pyramid to Meet Your Needs

The Food Guide Pyramid shows the suggested range of daily servings from each of the five major food groups. The number of servings that is right for you will depend on the amount of energy that you need each day. Various factors, including your age, your gender, and how active you are, affect your energy needs. **Figure 4.3** shows the recommended daily servings in each food group for teen girls and teen boys.

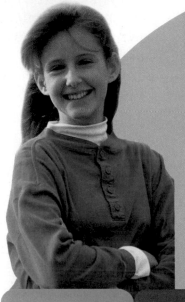

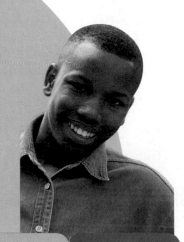

FIGURE 4.3

Recommended Daily Servings for Teens

Teen boys usually require larger amounts of food from most food groups than teen girls do. Look at this table. *Do you think that you might need to increase or decrease servings from any of the food groups? If so, which ones?*

Food Group		Sample Serving Sizes	Teen Girls	Teen Boys
Bread, Cereal, Rice, and Pasta Group		• 1 slice of bread • 1 ounce ready-to-eat cereal • 1/2 cup cooked cereal, rice, or pasta	▢▢▢▢▢▢▢▢▢	▢▢▢▢▢▢▢▢▢▢▢
Vegetable Group		• 1/2 cup cooked or raw chopped vegetables • 1 cup raw leafy vegetables • 3/4 cup vegetable juice	🥕🥕🥕🥕	🥕🥕🥕🥕🥕
Fruit Group		• 1 medium apple, banana, or orange • 1/2 cup chopped, cooked, or canned fruit • 3/4 cup fruit juice	🍎🍎🍎	🍎🍎🍎🍎
Milk, Yogurt, and Cheese Group		• 1 cup milk or yogurt • 1 1/2 ounces natural cheese • 2 ounces processed cheese	🥛🥛🥛	🥛🥛🥛
Meat, Poultry, Fish, Dry Beans, Eggs, and Nuts Group		• 2 to 3 ounces cooked lean meat, poultry, or fish. The following are equal to 1 ounce of meat: ▲ 1 egg ▲ 1/2 cup cooked dry beans ▲ 2 tablespoons peanut butter ▲ 1/3 cup nuts	🍗🍗	🍗🍗🍗

Eating a Variety of Foods

Using the Food Guide Pyramid can help you get enough nutrients each day. Many of the foods you eat have ingredients from two or more food groups. A slice of pizza, for example, combines bread, cheese, tomato sauce, and possibly vegetables and meat. Because no single food or food group supplies all the nutrients your body needs, it's a good idea to eat a variety of foods from every group over time.

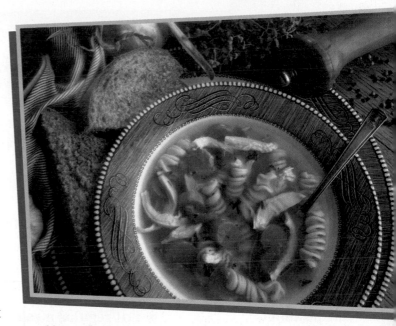

Foods that are high in sugars and fats—represented by the tip of the Food Guide Pyramid—are generally low in nutrients but high in calories. A **calorie** (KA·luh·ree) is *a unit of heat that measures the energy available in foods.* An eating plan that has more calories than your body can use results in weight gain. A high-fat diet is often high in calories, too. Most teens need about 2,200 to 2,800 calories per day, depending on their activity level. Try to get most of your calories from the lower levels of the Food Guide Pyramid to maintain your health.

Many foods contain ingredients from several different food groups. *What food groups are represented in this meal?*

Lesson 2 Review

Using complete sentences, answer the following questions on a sheet of paper.

Reviewing Terms and Facts

1. **Vocabulary** Define the term *Food Guide Pyramid,* and explain how the Pyramid can be used to make healthful food choices.
2. **List** Identify the five major food groups shown in the Food Guide Pyramid.
3. **Recall** What is the range of recommended daily servings for each of the five major food groups?

Thinking Critically

4. **Hypothesize** How are food choices behavioral factors that can put you at risk for contracting specific diseases?

5. **Distinguish** List some advertising claims you've seen and heard about the nutrients in foods and food supplements. How can you distinguish which are true and which are false?

Applying Health Skills

6. **Decision Making** Imagine that you are at the supermarket. You need to purchase foods to prepare dinner for a family of four, and you have a food budget of $20.00. What foods will you choose for a healthful meal that will not cost more than you have budgeted? On the same budget, what foods would you buy at the food court in the mall to provide a healthful lunch for a group of six friends? Share your budgets with the rest of the class.

Healthful Meals and Snacks

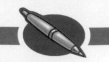

Planning Healthful Meals

The Dietary Guidelines and the Food Guide Pyramid can help you plan healthful meals and snacks. Here are a few suggestions to help you get the nutrients you need and still enjoy your food:

- **Eat regular meals.** Avoid skipping meals. People who skip meals tend to overeat at other times.
- **Watch portion sizes.** Suggested portion sizes may be smaller than you think. For example, one serving of meat is only 2 to 3 ounces. A cup of pasta may not seem like much, but it is two servings from the Bread, Cereal, Rice, and Pasta Group.
- **Eat small amounts of foods from the Pyramid tip.** You don't need to cut out fats and sugars entirely. An occasional candy bar or soft drink won't undo an otherwise healthful eating plan.
- **Aim to achieve balance over time.** Eat a variety of foods from all of the food groups over several days to get the right amounts and types of nutrients. If you eat a big lunch that is high in fats, balance it by making sure that your next few meals are lower in fats.

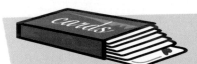

3 oz. (84 g) cooked meat, poultry, or fish = deck of cards

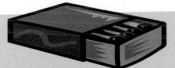

2 tbsp. (30 mL) peanut butter = matchbox

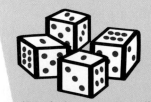

1 oz (28 g) cheese = four dice

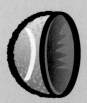

$\frac{1}{2}$ cup (125 mL) cooked vegetables = half a tennis ball

Some common items can help you visualize Pyramid serving sizes.

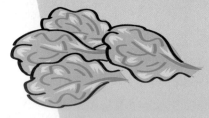

1 cup (250 mL) raw leafy greens = four lettuce leaves

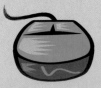

1 medium potato = computer mouse

Breakfast Starts Your Day

When you wake up in the morning, 10 or 12 hours may have passed since you last ate. Your body needs a fresh supply of energy. Start each morning with a healthful breakfast. Students who eat breakfast concentrate better at school and have a more positive attitude.

Breakfasts that include complex carbohydrates and some protein will give you the energy you need to start the day. You might eat oatmeal with milk along with a piece of fruit or combine whole-wheat toast and eggs. Even a bean burrito or a hamburger on a bun counts as breakfast. Adding Vitamin C-rich foods such as grapefruit or orange juice, or a calcium-rich dairy food such as milk will help you to fit in all the vitamins and minerals you need to stay healthy. If you're short on time, grab a cup of yogurt or a bowl of ready-to-eat cereal. Choose cereals that are made from whole grains or that have added vitamins and minerals. If you don't have time to eat at home, take something with you. A muffin, string cheese, and raisins plus a drink such as fruit or vegetable juice will give you the fuel you need for a great start.

Wake up your taste buds! Try leftover pizza for breakfast. It may not be a traditional breakfast food, but it is healthful and can provide the energy you need to start the day. *How can you improve your breakfast eating habits?*

HEALTH SKILLS ACTIVITY

PRACTICING HEALTHFUL BEHAVIORS

Breakfast on the Go

If you don't have a lot of time in the morning, try some of these healthful and quick-to-prepare breakfasts:

- Toaster waffle with blueberries, instant hot cocoa made with low-fat milk
- Low-fat ham and cheese on an English muffin, carrot sticks, grapefruit juice
- Bagel, yogurt drink
- Leftover pizza, cranberry juice
- Smoothie (blender shake made with milk and sliced fruit), whole-wheat toast
- Cereal with yogurt or milk, orange juice
- Celery sticks stuffed with peanut butter, apple juice

ON YOUR OWN

Make a list of some healthful breakfasts you could prepare when you are in a hurry. Include some items that can be eaten "on the go." Refer to your list when you need a quick breakfast.

Reading Check

Make your own word group. Of the three words listed below, leave out one, and add another that goes with them to make a group. Give the group a name. *grapes, carrot sticks, crackers*

Choosing foods that provide a variety of nutrients and textures will make your lunch nutritious and fun to eat. *How can you keep your lunch cold and safe to eat?*

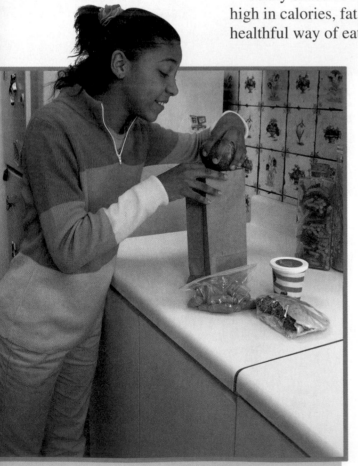

Packing a School Lunch

If you pack your own lunch, be sure to include a variety of nutritious foods. Vary your selections to avoid eating the same foods every day. Brainstorm ways to make your lunches more healthful. For example, using whole-grain bread instead of white bread for sandwiches will give you more fiber. Adding raw spinach leaves and tomatoes to tuna on rye bread boosts the meal's vitamin and mineral content. If you like deli meats, try lean roast beef, turkey, or ham for protein. Lean meats have less fat.

A packed lunch doesn't always have to include sandwiches. Many foods are available in individual servings. Look for single-serving containers of low-fat or fat-free salad dressings. Then you can pack a salad for lunch. Add low-fat yogurt, cheese sticks, applesauce, or granola bars. Instead of potato chips, pack carrot sticks or pepper slices for something crunchy. A crisp apple, a banana, or grapes make a great dessert, and these fruits are easy to transport. Instead of soft drinks or fruit drinks that contain added sugar, pack bottled water or plan to buy milk at school.

Nutritious Snacks

Many snack foods—such as potato chips and candy bars—are high in calories, fat, salt, and/or sugar, but low in nutrients. A more healthful way of eating is to choose snack foods that are **nutrient dense**, meaning that they *have a high amount of nutrients relative to the number of calories.* **Figure 4.4** shows examples of nutrient-dense snacks.

The snacks you eat give you energy and a chance to fit in the nutrients you may miss at other times during the day. Satisfy your hunger by choosing snack foods that combine grain products, fruits, vegetables, and dairy foods. Try some of these nutritious snacks:

- Baked tortilla chips with salsa
- Fruit smoothie made with milk or yogurt
- A peanut butter and banana sandwich on whole wheat bread
- Raw veggies with yogurt dip
- Apple and cheese slices with graham crackers
- Popcorn topped with chili powder or cinnamon
- Tomato or vegetable juice

FIGURE 4.4

COMPARING SNACKS

Snacks can be good for you if you choose wisely. *Why are nutrient-dense foods more healthful?*

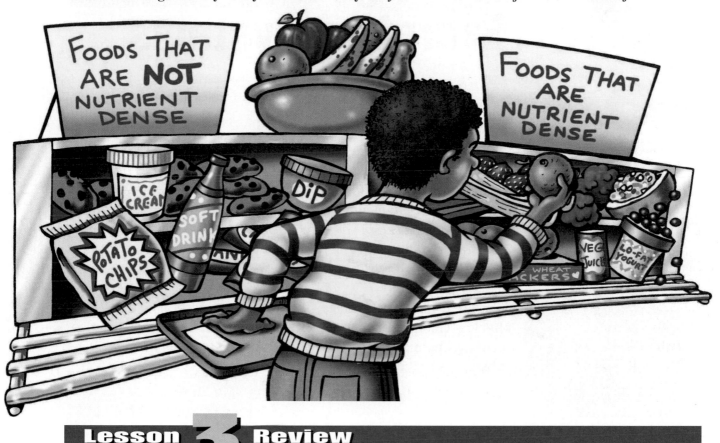

FOODS THAT ARE **NOT** NUTRIENT DENSE

FOODS THAT ARE NUTRIENT DENSE

Lesson 3 Review

Using complete sentences, answer the following questions on a sheet of paper.

Reviewing Terms and Facts

1. **List** Name two ways to make sure you get the nutrients you need.
2. **Recall** Explain why it is important to eat breakfast.
3. **Describe** Give two examples of nutritious lunches you could pack.
4. **Vocabulary** Define the term *nutrient dense.* List four nutrient-dense foods.

Thinking Critically

5. **Judge** How can you make sure that you eat portions of reasonable sizes at a restaurant?
6. **Evaluate** Analyze the nutritional value of each of the following breakfast menus.

Then suggest several foods that might be substituted to make each menu more nutritious and lower in fat.
Breakfast #1: orange juice, two fried eggs with bacon, whole wheat toast
Breakfast #2: whole-grain cereal with whole milk and sliced peaches, white toast with butter and jelly, glass of water

Applying Health Skills

7. **Advocacy** Using what you have learned from this chapter so far, write an advertisement for a healthful breakfast or snack. Combine words and pictures to persuade readers that the foods you suggest are healthful, easy to prepare, and delicious.

The Digestive and Excretory Systems

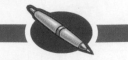

Quick Write

Jot down at least two or three parts of the body that help you digest the food you eat.

Learn About...

- how your body digests food.
- how your body removes waste products.

Vocabulary

- digestion
- digestive system
- saliva
- small intestine
- liver
- pancreas
- excretion
- excretory system
- colon
- kidneys

Turning Food into Fuel

When you eat, your body breaks the food down into smaller parts so that it can use the nutrients in the food for fuel. **Digestion** (dy·JES·chuhn) is *the process by which the body breaks down food into smaller components that can be absorbed by the bloodstream and sent to each cell in your body.* Your **digestive system** is *a group of organs that work together to break down foods into substances that your cells can use.*

Figure 4.5 shows the steps in digestion. Digestion involves physical changes, such as the crushing of food by the teeth. It also involves chemical changes, such as the transforming of food by substances in the body called enzymes.

Figure 4.5

Steps in Digestion

It takes 24 to 48 hours for your body to break down food into energy and get rid of wastes.

| **Mouth** | **Stomach** | **Small Intestine** | **Colon** |
| Crushing and Grinding | Chemical Breakdown | Useful Material Extracted | Water Removal |

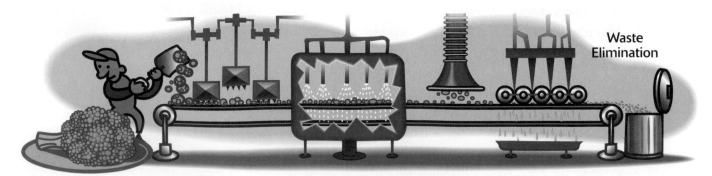

Waste Elimination

FIGURE 4.6

CHEWING AND SWALLOWING

Digestion begins in the mouth. *What roles do the epiglottis and uvula play in the digestive process?*

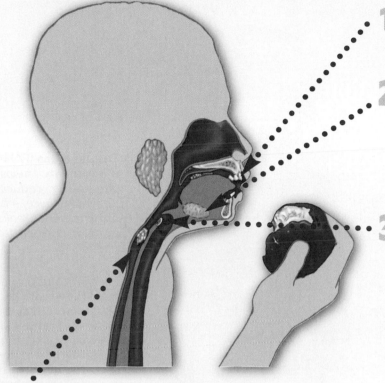

1 The teeth tear and grind the food into small shreds or chunks.

2 The salivary glands produce saliva. Enzymes in the saliva begin the chemical breakdown of carbohydrates, converting the starches to sugar. The saliva also moistens and softens the food for its transport.

3 Before you swallow, your air passages are open. Getting food into these passages could cause you to choke. Therefore, when you swallow, a flap of skin called the epiglottis (e•puh•GLAH•tuhs) closes off the trachea to keep food from entering it. The trachea (TRAY•kee•uh), or windpipe, is the passageway through which air gets to your lungs. At the same time, the uvula (YOO•vyuh•luh) closes off the airway to the nose.

4 Once the food is swallowed, it enters the esophagus (i•SAH•fuh•guhs), a long muscular tube that connects the mouth to the stomach.

How Digestion Begins

Does your mouth start to water when you sit down to eat a meal or smell something good cooking? That "water" is saliva. **Saliva** (suh·LY·vuh) is *a digestive juice produced by the salivary glands in your mouth.* Saliva starts to flow as a physical signal from your body that it is ready to begin the digestive process. When you chew food and then swallow it, the food begins a long journey through your body. **Figure 4.6** shows the first steps in the digestive process.

Organs of the Digestive System

Figure 4.7 on page 104 shows the path food takes during the next part of the digestive process. The esophagus pushes the food along until it reaches the stomach. The stomach's strong, muscular walls churn the food to break it into smaller pieces and mix them with gastric juice, a mixture of acid and enzymes. This process can take up to four hours.

FIGURE 4.7

THE DIGESTIVE SYSTEM

Food provides nutrients that the body needs in order to grow, develop, move, and stay healthy.

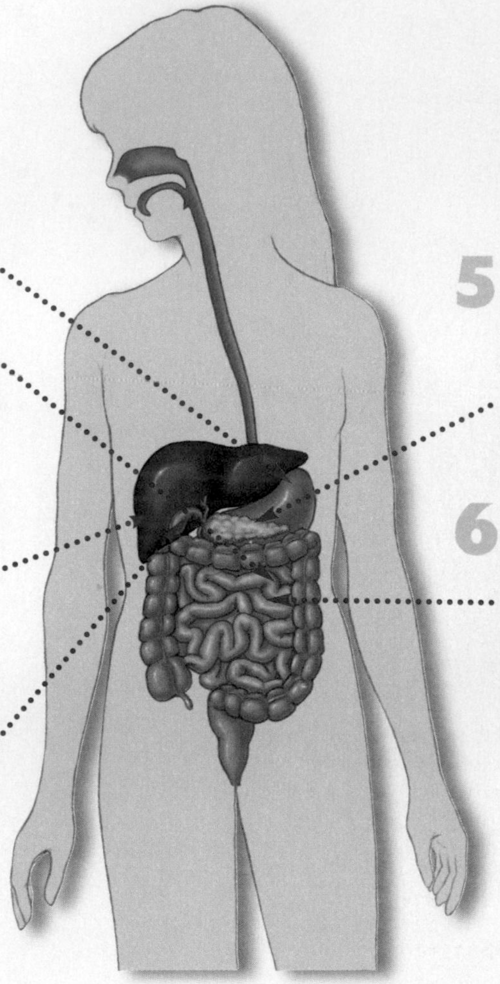

1 Acid and enzymes in the stomach break the food down until it resembles a thin soup called chyme (KYM).

2 Next the food moves to the **small intestine**, *a coiled tube, about 20 feet long, where most of the digestive process takes place.*

3 The **liver**, *the body's largest gland, secretes a liquid called bile that helps to digest fats.* In addition, the liver helps regulate the level of sugar in the blood, breaks down harmful substances such as alcohol, and stores some vitamins.

4 After the liver produces bile, it sends it to the gallbladder (GAWL•bla•duhr). The gallbladder stores the bile until it is needed.

5 The **pancreas** (PAN•kree•uhs) *is a gland that helps the small intestine by producing pancreatic juice, a blend of enzymes that breaks down proteins, carbohydrates, and fats.*

6 The walls of the small intestine are covered with fingerlike projections called villi (VI•ly). Nutrients from the digested material pass through the villi. This allows the nutrients to enter the bloodstream and eventually reach body cells.

Removing Wastes from the Body

Some foods that you eat contain materials that the body cannot use. During the digestive process, these substances—commonly called wastes—are separated out. These wastes must be removed from the body. **Excretion** (ek·SKREE·shuhn) *is the process by which the body gets rid of waste materials.*

The body produces three kinds of wastes: solids, liquids, and gases. Your **excretory** (EK·skruh·tohr·ee) **system** is *the system that removes wastes from your body and controls water balance.* Although your lungs get rid of carbon dioxide gas when you exhale, and your skin gets rid of some wastes when you sweat, the major organs of the excretory system are the kidneys, bladder, and colon.

Liquid Wastes

Liquid wastes are produced by cell activity. Approximately 50 to 80 percent of your body is water, and most waste materials are dissolved in it. **Figure 4.8** shows how the organs involved in excreting liquid wastes filter, store, and finally remove these wastes from your body.

Solid Wastes

Solid wastes are made up of foods that your body cannot break down, including fiber. After digestion, the body sends a mixture of water and undigested solid wastes into the **colon** (KOH·luhn), *a storage tube for solid wastes.* The colon is also called the large intestine. Most of the water is absorbed by the colon and returned to the body. The remaining solid wastes become material called feces. When the colon becomes full, strong muscles in its walls contract. This movement pushes the feces out of the body through an opening called the anus.

FIGURE 4.8

ELIMINATING LIQUID WASTES

Your kidneys and bladder get rid of liquid wastes.
How do you think drinking plenty of fluids helps you take care of your kidneys and bladder?

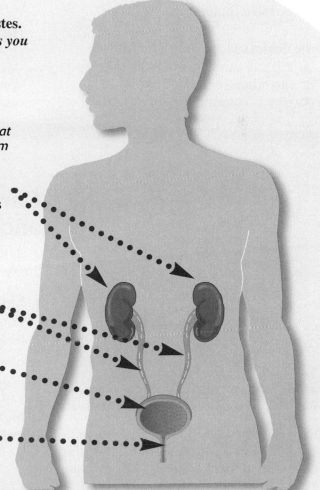

1 The **kidneys** are a pair of *organs that filter water and waste materials from the blood.* The kidneys also help to regulate the amounts of water and salts in the body. Urine is made up of the fluid and dissolved substances secreted by the kidneys.

2 The kidneys send the urine to the bladder through two tubes called ureters (YUR·uh·terz).

3 The bladder is a pouch in which urine is stored.

4 A signal from the nervous system lets the person know when the bladder is full. Urine passes out of the body through a tube called the urethra (yu·REE·thruh).

How Foods Break Down

PART I

Digestion begins when your teeth tear and crush large pieces of food into small chunks. The following activity will help demonstrate how chewing aids digestion.

WHAT YOU WILL NEED
- Two hard candies
- Two bowls filled with lukewarm water

WHAT YOU WILL DO
1. With a partner, crush one piece of candy into small pieces. Drop the whole candy into one bowl and the crushed candy into a second bowl at the same time.
2. Record the time each candy takes to dissolve completely.

IN CONCLUSION
1. Did one candy dissolve faster than the other?
2. Why is chewing part of digestion?

PART II

Bile, secreted by the liver, helps to digest fats. The following activity will demonstrate bile's role in the digestive process.

WHAT YOU WILL NEED
- A bowl of water
- Vegetable oil
- Dishwashing liquid

WHAT YOU WILL DO
1. Put several drops of vegetable oil into the water.
2. Put several drops of dishwashing liquid onto the oily surface of the water and observe what happens.

IN CONCLUSION
Suppose that the vegetable oil was fat and the dishwashing liquid was bile. From your observation, how do you think bile works to digest fat?

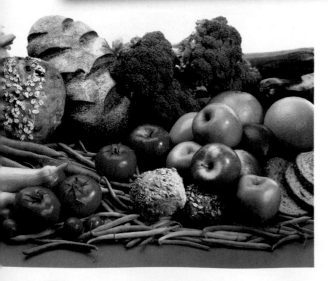

Whole grains and many fruits and vegetables contain fiber, a substance that helps your digestive system work properly. *How can you add more fiber to your eating plan?*

Caring for Your Digestive and Excretory Systems

Follow these guidelines to help keep the digestive and excretory systems working well.

- **Eat a balanced diet that is based on the Food Guide Pyramid.** Eating a variety of foods while taking care not to eat too many foods from the tip of the Pyramid promotes healthy digestion.
- **Eat plenty of foods that are low in fat and high in fiber.** Dietary fiber helps move wastes through the digestive system.

- **Eat at regular times each day.** This habit will help keep foods moving through your body at a steady pace.
- **Drink eight to ten glasses of water every day.** Your digestive and excretory systems need plenty of water in order to function. Foods that contain large amounts of water, such as fruit, soup, and juice, also count.
- **Take care of your teeth.** Your teeth are important to the digestive process. Brush them at least twice a day with a fluoride toothpaste, and floss daily. Remember to have regular dental checkups.
- **Stay active.** Regular physical activity aids digestion. Participate in moderate to vigorous physical activity on most, if not all, days of the week. Wait a while after eating before you engage in physical activity, however, to give your body time to digest some of the food you have eaten.

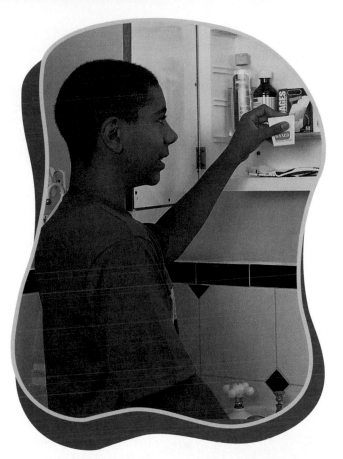

Take care of your teeth and have regular dental checkups. *What role do teeth play in the digestive process?*

Lesson 4 Review

Using complete sentences, answer the following questions on a sheet of paper.

Reviewing Terms and Facts

1. **Vocabulary** Define the term *digestion,* and explain why food has to be digested.
2. **Recall** How do the liver and the pancreas aid in the digestive process?
3. **Vocabulary** Define the term *excretory system.*
4. **List** Identify the major organs of the excretory system.
5. **Restate** What does the colon do?

Thinking Critically

6. **Predict** Describe possible consequences for the rest of the body if the digestive system is not working properly.

7. **Plan** Choose two of the tips in this lesson for caring for your digestive and excretory systems, and explain how you might make them part of your life.

Applying Health Skills

8. **Stress Management** Stress and anxiety can cause or worsen disorders of the digestive system such as indigestion. This particular disorder may cause pain in the upper abdomen and nausea. List at least three ways that you can reduce stressful situations to keep your digestive system healthy.

Managing Your Weight

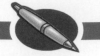

LEARN ABOUT...

- how to determine what weight is healthy for you.
- the dangers of eating disorders.
- healthful ways to manage your weight.

VOCABULARY

- Body Mass Index (BMI)
- eating disorder
- anorexia nervosa
- bulimia nervosa
- binge eating disorder

A Healthy Weight

What do you consider to be your healthy weight? External factors, such as the way models look in ads, may influence your idea of what you think you should weigh. However, the weight that you think is appropriate for you may not be healthy.

Your height, age, gender, inherited body type, and growth pattern determine your healthy weight. Maintaining a healthy weight is important for wellness. A healthy weight is not just one number but a range. To see if your weight falls within a healthy range, use the Body Mass Index chart for teens **(Figure 4.9)**. **Body Mass Index (BMI)** is *a way to assess your body size, taking your height and weight into account.* By using the BMI chart from year to year, you can look at your growth pattern to see if your weight is appropriate for your age.

FIGURE 4.9

BODY MASS INDEX RANGE

Calculate your BMI (See "Connect to Math" on page 109.) Then find your age on the bottom of the graph and trace an imaginary line straight up from your age to your BMI to see what range your BMI falls into.

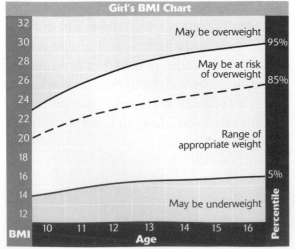

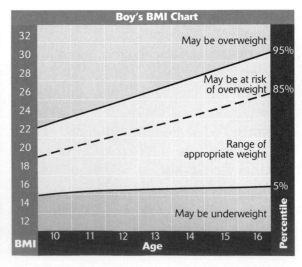

Benefits of a Healthy Weight

Being overweight or underweight may increase your risk of developing serious health problems. Staying in your healthy weight range will help you enjoy a long, healthy life.

Being seriously overweight strains the muscles and bones and makes the heart work harder. It increases the risk of heart disease, stroke, and diabetes (dy·uh·BEE·teez), a disease that prevents the body from converting food into energy. Being seriously underweight can cause fatigue, sleeplessness, and irritability.

Nutrition and Physical Activity

Your body runs on energy from food. You need to eat in order to move, to grow, to build and repair tissues, and to keep your body systems working. When you eat, your body converts the calories in the food to a type of energy that your cells can use.

To stay at a healthy weight, you must take in the same number of calories each day that you use for energy. If you eat too much, your body converts the extra calories into body fat. If you take in fewer calories than you need, your body converts its stored body fat to energy, causing you to lose weight. **Figure 4.10** shows how many calories are burned during some common activities. Choosing nutritious foods according to calculated energy expenditure will help you achieve a healthy body composition.

CONNECT TO
Math

CALCULATE YOUR BMI
Use this formula to calculate your BMI.
1. **Multiply your weight in pounds by 0.45.**
2. **Then multiply your height in inches by 0.025. Square the result.**
3. **Divide your answer in step 1 by the answer in step 2.**
Calculate the BMI of someone who is 5'2" (62 inches) tall and weighs 110 pounds.

FIGURE 4.10

ACTIVITY AND CALORIE USE

This chart shows the calculated energy expenditure of a 100-pound person performing each activity for one hour. *What happens when you use more calories than you take in?*

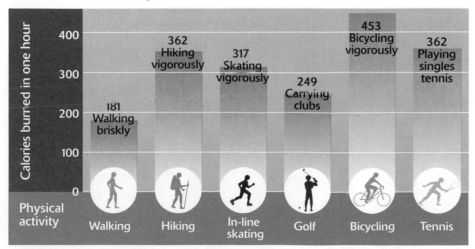

Eating Disorders

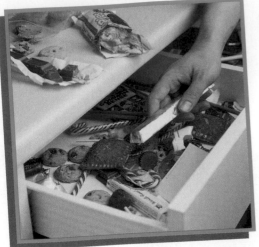

Eating disorders are *extreme eating behaviors that can lead to serious illness or even death.* These disorders are often related to other problems, such as an unrealistic body image, low self-esteem, depression, and other emotional pain. **Anorexia nervosa** (a·nuh·REK·see·uh ner·VOH·suh) is *an eating disorder in which a person has an intense fear of weight gain and starves herself or himself.* People who have anorexia nervosa risk heart problems, kidney failure, loss of bone minerals, and even death.

Bulimia (boo·LEE·mee·uh) **nervosa** is *an eating disorder in which a person repeatedly eats large amounts of food and then purges.* That is, the excess food is forced from the body through vomiting or using laxatives to speed up the excretory system. Although a bulimic person's weight may be within the normal range, medical problems such as dehydration, irregular heartbeat, and damage to the colon, liver, and kidneys can develop. **Binge eating disorder**, or compulsive overeating, is *an eating disorder in which a person repeatedly eats large amounts of food at one time.* Binge eaters do not purge but may frequently fast or diet. Over time, they may develop high blood pressure, diabetes, or certain types of cancer.

If you think that someone you know might have an eating disorder, encourage her or him to tell a trusted adult and to get professional help. *Look in a phone book to find groups that help people with eating disorders.*

HEALTH SKILLS ACTIVITY

ADVOCACY

Positive Body Image

Poor body image affects teens and adults alike. Often, people think that they are too fat, too thin, or just not muscular or shapely enough. A person with an unrealistic body image is in danger of developing an eating disorder. If you have negative feelings about the way you look, the following can help you develop a more realistic body image.

- **RECOGNIZE THAT THERE IS NO ONE BODY TYPE THAT IS RIGHT FOR EVERYONE.** Your body type depends on your height, weight, gender, and family characteristics.
- **BE HAPPY WITH WHO YOU ARE.** Accept the way you look now.

- **GET ADVICE FROM YOUR DOCTOR.** Remember that you need nutrients and food energy for your growing, active body.
- **SET REASONABLE GOALS.** Avoid drastic diets. Aim to lose or gain a few pounds slowly and get into better shape.
- **ADD PHYSICAL ACTIVITY TO YOUR DAILY ROUTINE.** Physical activity will help keep your body in a healthy weight range and will build muscle.

WITH A GROUP
Create a public service announcement that promotes having a realistic body image. You may create a poster, a radio ad, or a television commercial. Share your announcement with your class.

Tips for Managing Your Weight

To safely reach and maintain a healthy weight for you, eat moderate amounts of nutritious foods and be physically active each day. Avoid fad diets—those that are popular for only a short time. Many fad diets limit food variety, which is unhealthy. Also, any weight lost on these diets is usually regained.

Choose lean meats, low-fat dairy foods, and foods that are steamed or baked instead of fried. Watch portion sizes. Eat slowly, and chew your food well; this can help you eat less. It takes about 20 minutes for your brain to get the signal that your stomach is feeling full.

If you need to lose weight, do it gradually—aim for no more than 1/2 to 1 pound a week. Eat smaller servings, which supply fewer calories. Try to eat at regular times each day and drink plenty of water. If you need to gain weight, eat larger servings of nutritious foods. You may also want to drink more milk or juice.

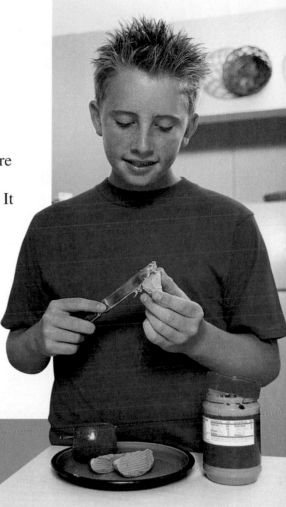

Healthful weight management depends on eating regular meals and choosing snacks wisely. *Why isn't it a good idea to skip meals as a way to lose weight?*

Lesson 5 Review

Using complete sentences, answer the following questions on a sheet of paper.

Reviewing Terms and Facts

1. **Vocabulary** What is *Body Mass Index*?
2. **Explain** Describe the possible health risks of being underweight.
3. **Restate** Identify and describe types of eating disorders, such as bulimia, anorexia, and binge eating disorder.
4. **List** What tips would you give someone who wanted to lose weight?

Thinking Critically

5. **Explain** Why should a weight mainte-nance program include physical activity?
6. **Hypothesize** Why do you think weight lost on fad diets is usually regained?

Applying Health Skills

7. **Accessing Information** Use reliable on-line and print resources to research healthy weight-loss practices that have been scientifically proven. Share your findings with the class.

How Healthy Are Those FRIES?

The answer depends on what kind of oil the fries are cooked in.

When one major fast-food company announced that it was changing its cooking oil by reducing the amount of trans fats by 48 percent and increasing the amount of polyunsaturated fats by 167 percent, many consumers had no idea what the company was talking about.

It turns out it was a step in the right direction. Fast-food restaurants fry their foods in fats. Not all fats are created equal, however. Depending upon their chemical composition, some fats are healthier than others. Fats are made up of fatty acids, which may be saturated or unsaturated. Saturated fatty acids hold a full quota of hydrogen atoms in their chemical structure; unsaturated fatty acids do not. Consuming excess amounts of saturated fats raises blood levels of low-density lipoprotein (LDL) cholesterol—the "bad" cholesterol—which increases the risk of heart disease. Consuming unsaturated fats lowers LDL cholesterol and raises high-density lipoprotein (HDL) cholesterol (the "good" cholesterol), thereby reducing the risk of heart disease. Lard and butter are two examples of saturated fats. Soybean, olive, corn, and other vegetable oils are all unsaturated fats.

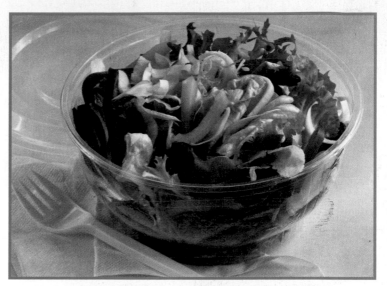

Many fast-food chains offer healthy options, such as salads.

A Partial Solution

In the past, fried fast-food products were cooked primarily in animal fats, which are generally saturated. Under pressure from consumers concerned about heart disease, many fast-food chains switched to unsaturated vegetable oils for frying. However, vegetable oils tend to be less stable and spoil more quickly than animal fats. So many chains switched again, turning to vegetable oils that have been partially hydrogenated—a process that fills unsaturated fat molecules with hydrogen atoms. Partial hydrogenation allows vegetable oils to stay fresh longer while still cooking up fries that are crisp and tasty.

For the fast-food industry, partially hydrogenated oils were doubly good. The companies got a cheap product with a long shelf life, and customers got vegetable oils, which they were demanding.

Unfortunately, the process of partial hydrogenation creates a new type of fatty acid known as a trans fatty acid. According to dietitian Liz Weiss, an expert on family nutrition, trans fats might be even worse for heart health than saturated fats. While saturated fats simply raise LDL cholesterol, Weiss explains, "trans fats appear to both raise bad (LDL) cholesterol and lower the good (HDL) cholesterol."

A fast-food restaurant's oil change will make its fried foods better for the hearts of the 46 million customers who eat there every day. What it won't do is turn any of those dishes into health foods. Fries cooked in the new oil will have the same amount of calories and will do nothing to trim America's growing waistline. So cut down on fries when eating out. Better still, try the salads! ■

TIME TO THINK...

About Fatty Acids

Look at the labels of at least 10 packaged food products that you normally eat, such as crackers, potato chips, desserts, and frozen meals. Note the amount of saturated fat in each product (it's usually listed in grams). List the five foods that have the greatest amount of saturated fat per serving, and five foods that have the least amount. Based on your findings, create an eating plan that significantly reduces your weekly intake of saturated fats. Share your plan with the rest of the class.

FAST FOOD: WHAT'S A HEALTHY CHOICE?

Model

Your decisions about what to eat can have a major impact on your health. Read about how Luke uses the decision-making process to choose healthful foods at a fast-food restaurant.

Luke considers several options, listed on the chart below. As he weighs these options, Luke thinks about the number of calories in each item. He also considers the amount of fat and sodium and the number of grams of protein. Then he considers his personal values and tastes. Luke cares about good nutrition and tries to eat fresh vegetables every day. He also likes chicken better than beef. After considering all these factors, Luke decides on a grilled chicken sandwich, a garden salad, and low-fat milk. He enjoys his meal and feels good about making an informed decision.

MENU ITEM	CALORIES	GRAMS OF FAT	NUMBER OF CALORIES FROM FAT	MILLIGRAMS OF SODIUM	GRAMS OF PROTEIN
Regular cheeseburger	320	13	120	820	15
Regular grilled chicken sandwich with mayonnaise, tomato, and lettuce	440	20	180	1040	27
Regular fish sandwich with tartar sauce and cheese	560	28	250	1060	23
Small french fries	210	10	90	135	3
Garden salad	35	0	0	20	2
Packet of fat-free vinaigrette dressing	50	0	0	330	0
Packet of ranch dressing	230	21	180	550	1
Medium cola	210	0	0	20	0
Small chocolate shake	360	9	80	250	11
Low-fat milk	100	2.5	20	115	8

Practice

Imagine that you have to choose a healthful fast-food meal. How well do you think you would choose? Look at the meals pictured below. Use the six steps of the decision-making process to make the most healthful choice. When you have made your decision, compare your choice with others in the class. Explain how you made your decision.

Apply/Assess

Research the nutrition facts from your favorite fast-food restaurant. Find the information on the Internet, or ask for nutrition information when you visit the restaurant. Compare the calories of the different foods. Consider the percentage of fat, protein, and carbohydrate that each food contains. Choose items from the menu that make a healthful meal you would enjoy. Write a paragraph about your decision. In your paragraph, explain: 1) the fast-food meals you considered; 2) the meal you chose; and 3) why you chose it.

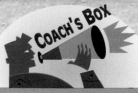

COACH'S BOX

Decision Making

1. State the situation.
2. List the options.
3. Weigh the possible outcomes.
4. Consider values.
5. Make a decision and act.
6. Evaluate the decision.

Self-✓Check

- Does my paragraph explain how I made my decision?
- Do I tell why my meal is a healthful choice?

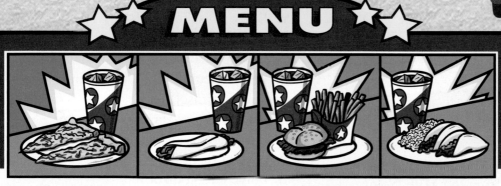

MENU

Two slices of thin-crust cheese pizza and a medium soft drink	Vegetable fajita and a medium soft drink	Bacon burger, french fries, and a medium diet cola	Two grilled chicken soft tacos, Mexican rice, and a medium cola
(620 calories, 18 g fat, 160 cal from fat, 1060 mg sodium, 24 g protein)	(620 calories, 19 g fat, 170 cal from fat, 967 mg sodium, 11 g protein)	(880 calories, 48 g fat, 430 cal from fat, 1670 mg sodium, 37 g protein)	(810 calories, 30 g fat, 200 cal from fat, 1607 mg sodium, 34 g protein)

After You Read

Use your completed Foldable to review the information on the six types of nutrients.

FOLDABLES™
Study Organizer

Reviewing Vocabulary and Concepts

On a sheet of paper, write the numbers 1–8. After each number, write the term from the list that best completes each statement.

- cholesterol
- fats
- fiber
- minerals
- vitamins
- nutrition
- Food Guide Pyramid
- calories

Lesson 1

1. Nutrients that strengthen muscles, bones, and teeth are called _____.
2. Eating foods high in _____ helps your body move wastes out of your system.
3. Sources of energy that also transport certain vitamins are _____.
4. Some _____ dissolve in water, while others dissolve in fat.
5. High _____ levels increase the risk of heart disease and stroke.

Lesson 2

6. The _____ recommends that teens eat three servings from the Milk, Yogurt, and Cheese Group every day.
7. _____ is the process of taking in food and using it for growth and good health.
8. Foods that are high in sugars and fats are generally high in _____ and low in nutrients.

On a sheet of paper, write the numbers 9–13. Write *True* or *False* for each statement below. If the statement is false, change the underlined word or phrase to make it true.

Lesson 3

9. You should eat <u>large</u> amounts of food from the Pyramid tip.
10. Your food choices should include many foods that are <u>nutrient dense</u>.

Lesson 4

11. The <u>liver</u> helps the small intestine by producing a blend of enzymes that breaks down proteins, carbohydrates, and fats.
12. <u>Kidneys</u> are a pair of organs that filter water and waste materials from the blood.
13. The <u>pancreas</u> is the place where most of the digestive process takes place.

Lesson 5

On a sheet of paper, write the numbers 14–16. After each number, write the letter of the answer that best completes each statement.

14. Which of the following is used to assess body size?
    a. Food Guide Pyramid
    b. Dietary Guidelines
    c. Body Mass Index (BMI)
    d. Nutritive Value Chart
15. An eating disorder in which a person has an intense fear of weight gain and starves herself or himself is
    a. anorexia nervosa.
    b. bulimia nervosa.
    c. bipolar disorder.
    d. binge eating disorder.
16. An eating disorder in which a person repeatedly eats large amounts of food and then purges is
    a. bulimia nervosa.
    b. anorexia nervosa.
    c. binge eating disorder.
    d. depression.

Thinking Critically

Using complete sentences, answer the following questions on a sheet of paper.

17. Assess If your body uses sugar for energy, why is eating large amounts of candy not good for your health?

18. Apply You need to eat breakfast on the go today. What will you choose to eat, and how will the nutrients in the food help your body?

19. Differentiate What are some factors that affect the food choices you make? Which factor do you think influences you most?

20. Hypothesize How might a person's body be affected by irregular eating patterns?

Career Corner

Dietitian Have you planned some of your family's meals? Are you concerned about people getting proper nutrition? Then you might enjoy a career as a dietitian. These professionals plan menus for people in hospitals, nursing homes, schools, or other facilities. To become a dietitian, you need a four-year college degree with a major in food and nutrition. You might volunteer for a community food-on-wheels program to prepare for this career. Visit Career Corner at health.glencoe.com to find out more about this and other health careers.

Standardized Test Practice

Reading & Writing

Read the paragraphs below and then answer the questions.

Why do you love some foods and dislike others? The answer to the first part of this question is easy—people generally like food that they have eaten and enjoyed in the past. The answer to the second part is not so simple, since people often dislike food that they have never tried. Why is this so?

People might find that the smell or texture of a certain food makes them dislike it. For example, they might enjoy eating a vegetable raw, but not like the feeling or taste of it when it is cooked. Others might refuse to eat a food that once made them sick. For instance, a person who felt ill after eating fish might not want to eat it again.

1. In the first paragraph of the passage the author uses a question to

   Ⓐ show that the passage is about people who hate food.

   Ⓑ explain why people like or dislike certain foods.

   Ⓒ tell why the author likes or dislikes certain foods.

   Ⓓ tell that the passage will be about food.

2. Which of the following best describes the organization of the second paragraph?

   Ⓐ comparing and contrasting different food favorites

   Ⓑ listing reasons for disliking a food

   Ⓒ stating a reason and giving an example of it

   Ⓓ stating a reason and telling why others disagree with it

3. Write a paragraph giving the reasons why you like and dislike certain foods.

 TH05_C2.glencoe.com/quiz

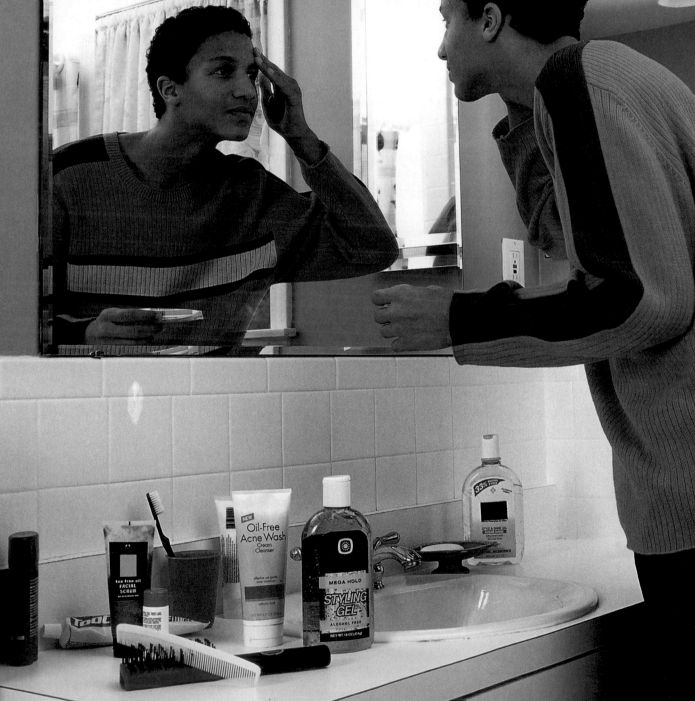

Personal Health and Consumer Choices

HEALTH Online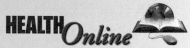

How well do you maintain your personal health and protect your senses? Are you a wise health consumer? To find out, take the Chapter 5 Health Inventory at health.glencoe.com.

FOLDABLES™ Study Organizer

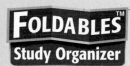

Before You Read

Make this Foldable to help you organize information on personal care, presented in Lesson 1. Begin with a plain sheet of 11″ × 17″ paper.

Step 1

Fold the short sides of the sheet of paper inward so that they meet in the middle.

Step 2

Fold the top to the bottom.

Step 3

Unfold and cut along the inside fold lines to form four tabs.

Step 4

Label the tabs as shown.

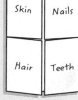

Skin | Nails

Hair | Teeth

As You Read

Record what you learn about the form, function, and care of teeth, skin, hair, and nails under the appropriate tab.

119

Caring for Your Teeth, Skin, Hair, and Nails

Quick Write

How do your personal grooming habits affect your appearance? Jot down a brief explanation.

LEARN ABOUT...

- keeping your teeth healthy.
- cleaning and protecting your skin.
- caring for your hair and nails.

VOCABULARY

- fluoride
- plaque
- tartar
- epidermis
- melanin
- pores
- dermis
- follicles
- ultraviolet (UV) rays
- dandruff
- head lice

Your Teeth

Healthy teeth and gums enable you to chew food thoroughly and speak clearly. Your teeth also give shape and structure to your mouth.

Tooth Care

To keep your teeth and gums healthy, brush and floss daily. Brush at least twice a day, but if possible, brush after every meal. Use a soft-bristled toothbrush, and replace it every two to three months or after an illness. Choose a toothpaste that contains **fluoride** (FLAWR·eyed), *a substance that helps prevent tooth decay.* If you can't brush after a meal, rinse your mouth with warm water. Flossing is also important. It removes food trapped between your teeth and along the gumline that rinsing and brushing miss. **Figure 5.1** on the next page shows how to brush and floss your teeth.

To fight tooth decay and keep your teeth and gums in good health, follow these guidelines.

- Eat at least five servings of fruits and vegetables each day. Also include foods that contain calcium, such as milk and yogurt.
- Limit your intake of sugar.
- Visit a dentist at least twice a year for regular cleanings and exams. Cooperate with the dentist by following the recommendations given to you during your health screening.

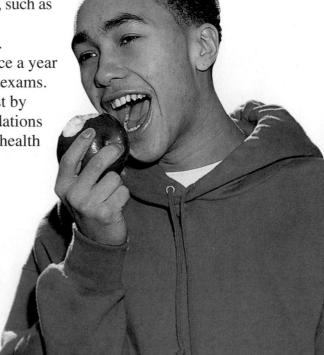

For a winning smile, be sure to make healthful snack choices. *Brainstorm a list of nutritious snacks.*

FIGURE 5.1

HOW TO BRUSH AND FLOSS

Proper brushing and flossing will keep your teeth healthy. *What else can you do to maintain the health of your teeth?*

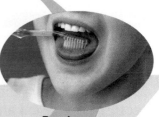

Brush your tongue and rinse your mouth.

How to Brush

Be sure to brush your teeth for at least two minutes—30 seconds for each area of your mouth.

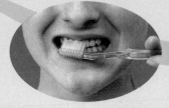

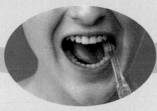

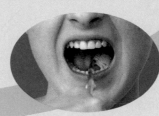

Brush the outer surfaces of your upper and lower teeth. Use a combination of up-and-down strokes and small circular or side-to-side strokes.

Thoroughly brush all chewing surfaces.

Brush the inside surfaces of your upper and lower teeth.

How to Floss

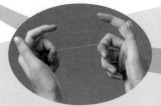

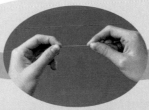

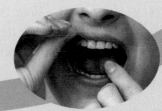

Forming a C with the floss around each tooth, keep sliding the floss back and forth gently as you move it up and down along the side of the tooth. Do the same for all of your teeth, using a clean section of floss for each tooth. When you've finished, rinse your mouth.

Wrap about 18 inches of floss around the middle finger of each hand.

Grip the floss firmly between thumb and forefinger.

Slide the floss back and forth between teeth toward the gumline until it touches the gumline.

HEALTH SKILLS ACTIVITY

ADVOCACY

Did You Brush Your Teeth?

As Timmy's baby-sitter, Leona is responsible for giving him an evening snack and getting him ready for bed. Timmy always wants soda and cookies and does not regularly brush his teeth before bed. Leona wants to encourage Timmy to take better care of his teeth so that he can avoid cavities.

WHAT WOULD YOU DO?

Write a dialogue between Leona and Timmy that shows her convincing him to eat more nutritious snacks and brush his teeth before going to bed.

CONNECT TO
Science

A WINNING SMILE
Some people have their teeth straightened and realigned by wearing braces. These devices, consisting of brackets and wires, can improve the look and function of teeth. Find out how teeth are treated with braces. In addition, research the latest advances in materials that are used to make braces.

Tooth Decay

Bacteria live in your mouth. When bacteria combine with saliva and the sugary substances that you eat, plaque forms. **Plaque** (PLAK) is *a thin, sticky film that builds up on teeth and contributes to tooth decay.* Once plaque is formed, the bacteria on the teeth produce an acid. This acid can eat a hole, or cavity, in the tooth's enamel—the hard material on the outer surface of the tooth. If a dentist does not treat the cavity, it gets bigger over time. The decay spreads, invading the tooth's dentin—bonelike material that surrounds the sensitive inner parts of the tooth. Decay can then spread to the pulp—tissue that contains nerve endings and blood vessels. If the cavity exposes a nerve, you'll know it. Eventually, you'll develop a toothache and will need to see the dentist right away.

Unremoved plaque may also harden and become tartar. **Tartar** (TAR·ter) is *hardened plaque that threatens gum health.* Only a dentist or dental hygienist can remove tartar completely.

Your Skin

Your skin is an organ, just like your lungs and heart. In fact, the skin is the body's largest organ. It is composed of three layers: the epidermis, the dermis, and a layer of fat cells. **Figure 5.2** shows the parts of the skin.

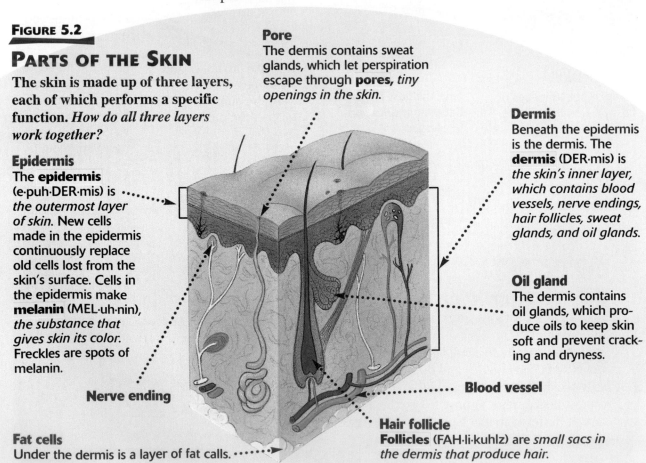

FIGURE 5.2

PARTS OF THE SKIN

The skin is made up of three layers, each of which performs a specific function. *How do all three layers work together?*

Epidermis
The **epidermis** (e·puh·DER·mis) is *the outermost layer of skin.* New cells made in the epidermis continuously replace old cells lost from the skin's surface. Cells in the epidermis make **melanin** (MEL·uh·nin), *the substance that gives skin its color.* Freckles are spots of melanin.

Nerve ending

Fat cells
Under the dermis is a layer of fat calls.

Pore
The dermis contains sweat glands, which let perspiration escape through **pores,** *tiny openings in the skin.*

Dermis
Beneath the epidermis is the dermis. The **dermis** (DER·mis) is *the skin's inner layer, which contains blood vessels, nerve endings, hair follicles, sweat glands, and oil glands.*

Oil gland
The dermis contains oil glands, which produce oils to keep skin soft and prevent cracking and dryness.

Blood vessel

Hair follicle
Follicles (FAH·li·kuhlz) are *small sacs in the dermis that produce hair.*

The skin has many important functions:

- **Waterproofing.** Your skin keeps water out of the body.
- **Vitamin D formation.** Your skin uses the sun's light to produce small amounts of vitamin D, which helps build bones and teeth.
- **Protection.** Skin protects you against germs and injuries.
- **Temperature control.** Blood vessels in the skin enable your body to retain or release heat, and perspiration helps keep your body cool.
- **Sensation.** The skin contains nerve endings that give you information about touch and temperature.

Acne

Acne is a skin condition that occurs when active oil glands cause hair follicles to become clogged. It often appears during puberty. The same hormones that cause your body to grow and mature during puberty also overstimulate some glands. Acne may affect the face, neck, back, chest, and shoulders. **Figure 5.3** shows how acne forms.

To deal with acne, gently wash the affected area at least twice daily with mild soap and warm water. Avoid touching the area, and avoid the use of heavy makeup or creams.

FIGURE 5.3

HOW ACNE FORMS

Whiteheads, blackheads, and pimples are three common kinds of acne.
What can you do to control acne?

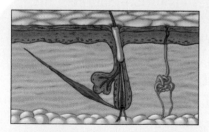 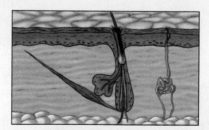 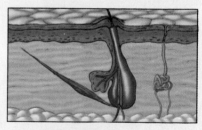

A Oil glands produce sebum, a substance that combines with dead skin cells to clog follicles. A whitehead results when a pore, or follicle opening, becomes plugged with sebum and dead skin cells.

B A blackhead forms when a whitehead is exposed to the air and darkens.

C If a clogged follicle ruptures and bacteria invade the skin, an infection occurs. The area becomes red, swollen, and filled with pus, producing a pimple.

Skin Care

Taking care of your skin can help you feel good about yourself. Here are some skin care tips.

- **Keep clean.** Bathe or shower daily. During your early teen years, oil and sweat glands are especially active. Washing with soap removes bacteria and excess oils from the surface of your skin. An underarm deodorant will also help to minimize body odors.

- **Eat properly and stay physically active.** Eat foods high in fiber, vitamins, and minerals. Green and yellow vegetables, milk, and eggs are high in vitamin A, which helps your skin stay healthy. Get regular physical activity, and get plenty of sleep.

- **Protect yourself from the sun. Ultraviolet (UV) rays** are *an invisible form of radiation from the sun that can penetrate and change the structure of skin cells.* UVB rays are the primary cause of sunburn. UVA rays make the skin age and wrinkle faster and also cause sunburn. Both types of UV rays increase the risk of skin cancer. To protect yourself from UV rays, try to stay out of the sun between 10:00 A.M. and 4:00 P.M. Remember that ultraviolet rays are just as strong on cloudy and hazy days.

- **If you're going to be in the sun, wear sunscreen and reapply it every hour.** Broad-spectrum sunscreens provide protection from both types of UV rays. Make sure that the sunscreen has an SPF (sun protection factor) of 15 or greater, depending on how easily you burn and how long you plan to be in the sun. Also be sure to wear a hat, T-shirt, and sunglasses, and drink plenty of fluids.

- **Avoid body decoration such as tattoos and piercing.** Less serious risks include scarring and minor infections. HIV, the virus that causes AIDS, and the virus that causes hepatitis, a dangerous inflammation of the liver, can also be spread through tattooing and piercing.

Your Hair

Hair can be styled, cut, colored, and changed in many ways. No matter how you wear it, keeping your hair clean and healthy is worth the effort. Hair care is part of personal grooming.

Many teens see their hair as a way to express themselves.

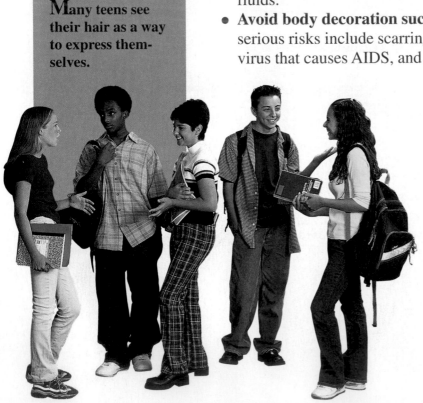

Hair Care

Daily brushing keeps your hair healthy by removing dirt and spreading oils from the roots to the ends. You should wash your hair regularly, using a gentle shampoo. How often you should wash depends on whether your hair tends to be dry or oily. People who have dry hair might not need to shampoo as often as people with oily hair do. After you have washed your hair, rinse it well to remove all the shampoo. If you blow-dry your hair, use a low-heat setting. Too much heat can cause the layered cells of your hair to split apart and even break off. Wind, chlorine, chemical treatments, and permanent hair dye can weaken hair in the same way. The result is dull, rough-feeling, sometimes even discolored hair.

Reading Check
Identify the main idea. Write a sentence describing the main idea of the first paragraph on this page.

Hair and Scalp Problems

Several problems can occur with the hair and the scalp, which is the skin beneath the hair. One is **dandruff**, *a flaking of the outer layer of dead skin cells on the scalp.* This condition is usually caused by dry skin. There is no cure for dandruff, but it can be controlled with special shampoos.

Another hair and scalp problem involves **head lice**, *parasitic insects that live on the hair shaft and cause itching.* Even though lice can't fly or jump from person to person, they are easy to catch from other people. To avoid getting lice, don't share combs, brushes, or hats with others. If you do get head lice, use a special shampoo (available at most drugstores) and wash your hair immediately. Any linens and clothes you have used should be washed in hot water or dry-cleaned.

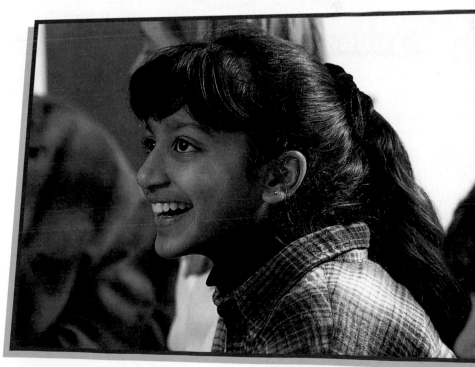

If you put your hair up in a ponytail, use a coated rubber band or soft cloth hair band. Noncushioned or uncovered elastic bands can cause severe breakage. *What are some other ways to prevent hair from breaking?*

Nail Care

Your finger- and toenails are made of the same cells that make up your hair. Your nails protect the sensitive tips of your fingers and toes. It's important to care for your nails—without proper attention, they can become weak, ingrown, or infected. Here are some nail-care tips.

- Clean and soften your hands in warm water. Notice the thin, skinlike layer at the base of each nail. This is the cuticle, a nonliving band of tissue. To keep your cuticles neat, push them back after soaking your hands, while they are soft. You may also use cuticle remover, a chemical that dissolves the cuticle.
- Trim your nails with nail scissors or clippers. Round your fingernails slightly, but cut your toenails straight across. Do not cut nails shorter than skin level.
- Smooth rough nail edges with a nail file or emery board.

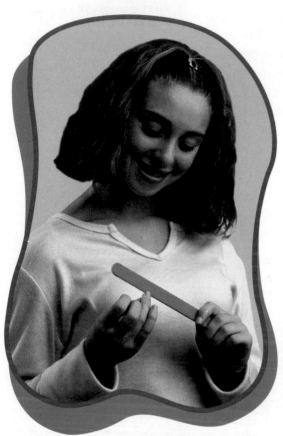

Keeping your nails clean, clipped, and smooth has health benefits. *How is this teen protecting her nails?*

Lesson 1 Review

Using complete sentences, answer the following questions on a sheet of paper.

Reviewing Terms and Facts
1. **Vocabulary** Define the terms *fluoride, plaque,* and *tartar.*
2. **Describe** What are the five functions of the skin?
3. **Explain** How does acne form?
4. **Recall** What can you do to care for your nails?

Thinking Critically
5. **Hypothesize** A friend says: "I don't have to go to the dentist because I've never had a cavity." Do you agree or disagree with your friend? Why?
6. **Hypothesize** How does taking care of your teeth, skin, hair, and nails affect all three sides of your health triangle?

Applying Health Skills
7. **Practicing Healthful Behaviors** Head lice spread easily among groups of younger children, especially in schools. With a partner, create a poster that suggests ways for younger children to avoid getting lice.

Caring for Your Eyes and Ears

Your Eyes

Your eyes tell you about the world—about light, shapes, colors, and movements. Your brain, which allows you to recognize a friend and understand the words on this page, interprets the data gathered by your eyes. **Figure 5.4** shows the parts of the eye.

FIGURE 5.4

STRUCTURE OF THE EYE

The eye works a lot like a camera. It takes in light and focuses it to create an image. The image is then sent to your brain, where the picture is "developed."

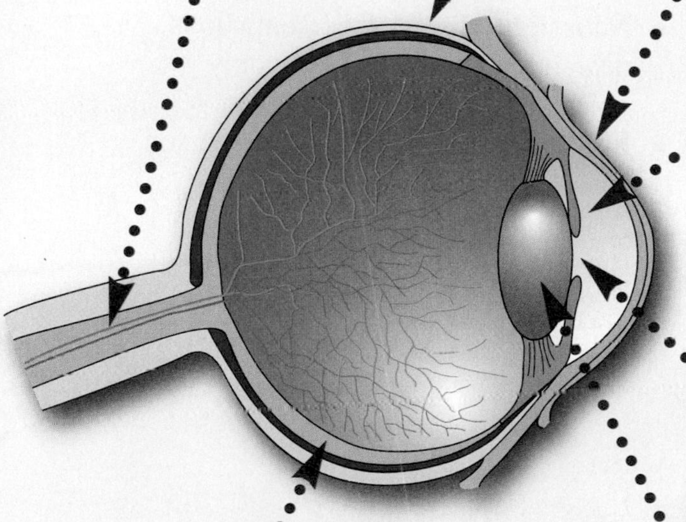

The sclera (SKLEHR·uh) is the white of the eye. It covers and protects the whole eye, except for the front.

The optic (AHP·tik) nerve is a bundle of nerve fibers that sends messages to the brain, which interprets them.

The cornea (KOR·nee·uh) is the clear section that lets in light at the front of the eye.

The iris (EYE·ris) is the colored part of the eye. It controls the size of the pupil.

The pupil (PYOO·puhl) is the dark opening in the center of the iris. It grows larger in dim light and smaller in bright light, so that the right amount of light enters the eye.

The retina (RE·tin·uh) is the light-sensing part of the inner eye.

The lens (LENZ) focuses the light on the retina.

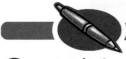

Quick Write

How do you think that taking care of your sight and hearing now will benefit you in the future?

LEARN ABOUT...

- keeping your eyes healthy.
- why people wear glasses or contact lenses.
- caring for your ears.

VOCABULARY

- optometrist
- ophthalmologist
- astigmatism
- decibel

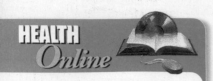

HEALTH *Online*

Topic: The eye

For a link to more information on the eye and vision, go to **health.glencoe.com**.

Activity: Using the information provided at this link, make a list of five facts about the eye.

Eye Care

Because your sense of sight is so important, you need to take care of your eyes. Below are some eye care tips.

- Make sure that you have enough light. Read and watch television in a well-lit room. If necessary, use a reading lamp.
- Avoid light that is too bright. Sit at least 6 feet away from the television set. Don't look directly at the sun or at any other bright light. When you are outside, wear sunglasses that protect against UVA and UVB rays.
- Avoid rubbing your eyes. If anything gets into your eyes, rubbing them may scratch the cornea. Instead, rinse your eyes with cool, clean water.
- Protect your eyes from injury. Wear protective gear when you play sports such as baseball and hockey. If you work with power tools or chemicals, wear protective glasses or goggles.

Eye Examinations

To make sure that your eyes are healthy, visit an eye care professional for regular examinations. An **optometrist** (ahp·TAH·muh·trist) is *a health care professional who is trained to examine the eyes for vision problems and to prescribe corrective lenses.* An **ophthalmologist** (ahf·thahl·MAH·luh·jist) is *a physician who specializes in the structure, functions, and diseases of the eye.* If you wear glasses or contact lenses, have your eyes checked once a year. Otherwise, have them checked every two years. Vision screening is also available at school. If this screening is not done routinely, students and their families can request a vision test by the school nurse. Some of the most common vision problems include the following:

Protective equipment is necessary for many activities. *Why do you think these teens need to protect their eyes?*

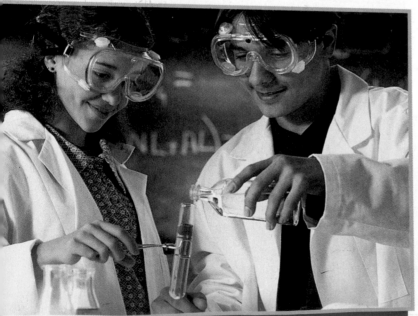

- **Nearsightedness**. A person who is nearsighted can see clearly only objects close to his or her eyes.
- **Farsightedness**. A farsighted person can see only distant objects clearly.
- **Astigmatism** (uh·STIG·muh·tiz·uhm), *an eye condition in which images are distorted, causing objects to appear wavy or blurry.*

Vision Correction

Many vision problems can be corrected with eyeglasses or contact lenses. Both glasses and contact lenses can correct nearsightedness, far-sightedness, and astigmatism.

Contact lenses rest on the corneas. They are available in several basic types. Hard lenses are made of slightly flexible plastic. They are easy to take care of, but some people find them uncomfortable. Soft lenses are made of soft, flexible plastic. These are easier to get used to but are more difficult to clean. Disposable contact lenses are worn for a set period of time, thrown out, and then replaced with a fresh pair of lenses.

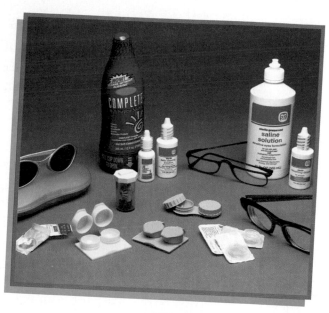

There are many ways to correct vision.

A type of corrective eye surgery called corneal modification alters the curve of the cornea so that light can focus directly on the retina. This procedure may eliminate the need for eyeglasses or contact lenses. This type of surgery is usually available to people 18 years and older. Remember always to get a second opinion—an opinion from another doctor—before having any optional surgery.

HEALTH SKILLS ACTIVITY

PRACTICING HEALTHFUL BEHAVIORS

Avoiding Eyestrain

Staring at a computer screen can strain and tire your eyes. The next time you surf the Internet or type a paper for school, take the following precautions to protect your eyes:

- Position the monitor 2 feet from your face and a few inches below eye level.
- Focus on a distant object for about 10 seconds every 10 minutes.
- Use an antiglare filter.
- Place the monitor well away from any windows to prevent glare.
- Never work on a computer in the dark.
- Adjust the monitor's brightness and contrast features so that you are comfortable.

- Wear computer glasses if necessary.
- Enlarge the font size on your computer.
- Remove dust from the screen regularly.

ON YOUR OWN

For a week, follow at least two or three of the suggestions listed here. Did you notice any difference in the way your eyes felt while you were working on the computer and afterward? Share your experience with the class.

Your Ears

Your ears allow you to hear, listen, and learn. They also help you keep your balance. **Figure 5.5** shows the structures of the ear and the way these parts work together.

Ear Care

Caring for your ears involves protecting them from loud sounds. *The unit for measuring the loudness of sound* is the **decibel**. Normal conversation is about 60 decibels. Sounds over 125 decibels are loud enough to be painful. Lower levels of sound can also harm the ears if the sounds continue over a long period of time. For example, prolonged sounds louder than 80 or 90 decibels, such as a rock concert or a jet plane taking off, can damage the tiny hair cells in your inner ear and lead to temporary or permanent hearing loss. Another way to care for your ears is to have periodic hearing tests administered. These can be obtained from the school nurse or from a speech therapist or audiologist.

To protect your ears from noise and to prevent other problems, keep the volume fairly low on your radio, CD player, cassette player, and television. This is an especially important precaution if you are using headphones. Wear earplugs or other hearing protection

FIGURE 5.5

HOW YOUR EARS WORK

Your ears not only allow you to hear, they also help you keep your balance.
What part of the ear is responsible for balance?

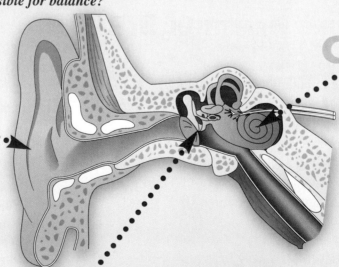

A The outer ear is shaped like a cup to pick up sound waves, which travel through the external auditory canal.

C In the inner ear, the fluid in the cochlea (KOK·lee·uh) moves. Tiny hair cells lining the cochlea vibrate in response, sending electrical messages to the auditory nerve. These messages travel to the brain, which identifies the sound.

B In the middle ear, sound waves make the eardrum vibrate. The vibrations move the hammer, the anvil, and the stirrup. These bones carry the vibrations to the inner ear.

Other structures in the ear are not directly involved in hearing. The eustachian (yoo·STAY·shuhn) tube keeps air pressure equal on both sides of the eardrum. The semicircular canals are filled with fluid and tiny hair cells. These hair cells send messages through nerves to the brain, helping your body keep its balance.

devices if you are going to be exposed to loud or pro-longed noise, such as the noise from a power lawn mower. Exposure to very loud noise can cause some people to lose part or all of their hearing or experience tinnitus (tin·EYE·tus), a constant ringing in the ears.

It's also important to clean and protect your ears. Some ways to keep your ears clean and to protect them are listed below.

- Clean the outside of your ears with a wet washcloth. Do not put a cotton swab or any other object into your ear canal. If earwax builds up inside your ears and becomes a problem, see a doctor to have it removed.
- On cold days, wear earmuffs or a hat that covers your ears. Cold air can irritate the middle ear and cause frostbite on the outer ear.
- If you think you have an ear infection, are experiencing pain in one or both ears, or have trouble hearing, tell your parents or guardians right away. They can help you seek care from a doctor or the school nurse.

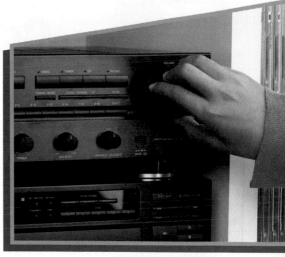

Protecting your ears from loud music helps prevent hearing problems. *What are some other ways to protect your ears?*

Lesson 2 Review

Using complete sentences, answer the following questions on a sheet of paper.

Reviewing Terms and Facts

1. **List** Name three ways in which you can protect your eyes.
2. **Vocabulary** What is the difference between an *optometrist* and an *ophthalmologist*?
3. **Explain** What happens to a person's sight as a result of *astigmatism*?
4. **Define** What is a *decibel*?
5. **Recall** Explain how the outer ear, middle ear, and inner ear work together to allow you to hear.

Thinking Critically

6. **Relate** What activities or situations in your life could be harmful to your hearing? What can you do to protect your hearing?

7. **Evaluate** How do you think your eyes and ears make you more aware of the world around you? Do you think that one of these sense organs is more beneficial than the other? Explain your answer.

Applying Health Skills

8. **Accessing Information** Advances in technology are constantly allowing doctors to find new ways to correct vision and hearing problems. Write letters to two national organizations that deal with vision and hearing disorders, and ask for pamphlets on the latest technologies. You might also look for this information on the Internet.

Consumer Choices and Your Health

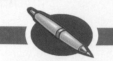

Choices That Affect Personal Health

When you go to a fast-food restaurant or into a store to buy a toothbrush, you are a consumer. A **consumer** (kuhn·SOO·mer) is *anyone who buys products and services.* A service is, for example, a haircut or a dental checkup. As a consumer, you need to be aware that many of the products and services you buy affect your health.

Being a responsible consumer involves thinking about your buying choices carefully. It means knowing what you are looking for in the products and services you purchase. Careful evaluation is especially important when you purchase health-related products and services. For example, when you choose a sunscreen, you should always select a broad-spectrum sunscreen because it will protect you from both UVA and UVB rays.

Understanding Your Consumer Choices

To select products and services wisely, you must have useful information about the items that you are thinking of buying. To get this information, you need to gather and evaluate the facts, make comparisons, and weigh your options. Some influences that affect your consumer choices are listed on the next page.

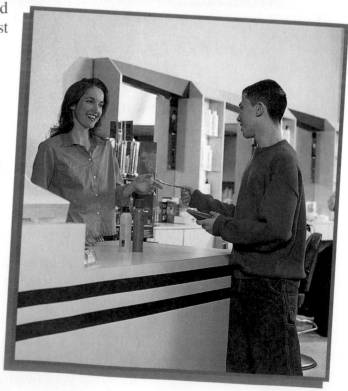

Buying decisions affect your physical, mental/emotional, and social health. *How do the personal products you buy affect your physical health?*

- **Personal factors.** Your personal beliefs, interests, and curiosity play a big part in your purchasing decisions.
- **Family background.** Your family and culture help to shape your buying decisions.
- **Peers.** Your friends' opinions might influence you when you consider buying a product or service.
- **Cost.** The price of a product or service can be a key determining factor. Shop for quality and value.
- **Advice of salespeople.** Store employees can assist you in making a purchasing decision, but the final choice should be based on your own needs and wants and on facts.
- **Advertising.** *Messages designed to cause consumers to buy a product or service* are called **advertising**. Ads can be a strong influence on your buying choices. Ads are powerful sales tools, and companies invest a lot of money in them to persuade you to buy products and services. Advertisers work closely with media programmers to make sure their ads reach target audiences. **Figure 5.6** shows the techniques advertisers use to sell their products to teens.

Types of Advertising

Advertisements usually fall into one of two groups: informational ads and image ads. Both types have the same basic purpose—to convince consumers to buy a product or service.

Informational ads rely mostly on facts. They may use statistics to back their claims, or they may include the advice of experts. A special kind of informational ad is an infomercial. An **infomercial**

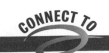

CONNECT TO

Language Arts

ARTICLE OR ADVERTISEMENT?
Some magazines include "special sections" that provide information and sell products. For example, a health section may give exercise tips while advertising certain equipment. Look for examples of special sections in magazines. *How are these sections more like advertising or more like articles?*

FIGURE 5.6

ADVERTISING TECHNIQUES AIMED AT TEENS

This table describes advertising techniques. *Why do you think such techniques can be successful?*

Advertising Technique	Image Used	Hidden Message
Bandwagon	Group of teens	Other teens use this product, so you should, too.
Beautiful People	A celebrity—a glamorous model or a famous athlete—giving a paid **endorsement** (in·DAWR·smuhnt), *a statement of approval.* Celebrities are usually paid a large amount of money for their endorsements.	You'll be like the people in the ad if you use this product.
Good Times	Teens having fun	You'll have a good time if you use this product.
Status	Brand name/designer clothing	You'll look "cool" if you wear these items.
Symbols	A well-known character	You'll be popular like this character if you use this product.

Reading Check

Understand shades of meaning. The word *infomercial* is a recent addition to the English language. List the two words that form the word *infomercial*.

(IN·foh·mer·shuhl) is *a long TV commercial whose main purpose seems to be to present information rather than to sell a product.* Many infomercials are misleading because they look like television programs.

Image ads pair a product or service with an attractive image. They may feature a famous athlete giving an endorsement. Their message is: "If you buy this product or service, this could be you!" They suggest that buying and using a certain product or service will improve your life.

Evaluating Advertisements

Although advertisements can provide consumers with important information on health-related products and services, they can also be misleading. They may exaggerate the good points of a product and omit or barely mention its negative aspects. They may blend fact with opinion, making it difficult to distinguish between the two. Part of being a wise consumer is recognizing your personal needs and wants. Ads will often try to convince you that what you need and what you want are the same thing, but sometimes they aren't.

When advertisers' claims sound too good to be true, they usually are. For example, product advertisements that promise "miracle" results in no time at all are usually misleading and often false.

Fraud is *deliberate deceit or trickery.* The makers of fraudulent products and the providers of such services may claim that they cure or prevent diseases and other health problems. While some of these products and services may not be completely worthless, their value is not as great as the company would like you to believe. Some may even be harmful to your health.

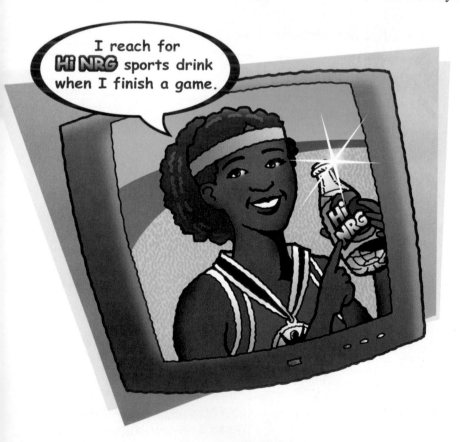

Advertisers often use celebrity endorsements to sell their products. *Why do you think celebrity endorsements might make people want to buy certain products or services?*

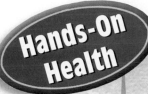

ADVERTISING TECHNIQUES

Some advertisements don't make their claims openly—they just suggest that something is true. Advertisers may use images or catchy phrases to imply that their product or service is the best, that everyone is using it, or that you will be happy or well liked or play a sport like a professional if you buy it.

WHAT YOU WILL NEED
- colored pencils, crayons, or markers
- magazines
- poster board
- scissors

WHAT YOU WILL DO
1. In small groups of three or four students, come up with an advertisement for a health or fitness product that advances one or more of the claims mentioned above.

2. Decide whether you want to create a newspaper or magazine ad, a script for a radio advertisement, or a series of sketches showing the action in a television ad. If you choose to create a visual advertisement, use either images clipped from magazines or your own drawings.
3. Make your advertisement and present it to the class.
4. Evaluate other groups' advertisements.

IN CONCLUSION
1. What did you learn by creating your own advertisement?
2. How do advertisements convince viewers to buy a product or make them change their minds about needing or wanting a product?

Lesson 3 Review

Using complete sentences, answer the following questions on a sheet of paper.

Reviewing Terms and Facts
1. **Vocabulary** Define the term *consumer.*
2. **Identify** List three influences on consumer choices.
3. **Recall** Describe two advertising techniques aimed at teens.
4. **Explain** How is an *infomercial* different from an advertisement?

Thinking Critically
5. **Evaluate** Rank these buying influences in order of their importance to you: personal factors, family background, peers, cost, advice of salespeople, advertising. Explain why you ranked these categories as you did.
6. **Explain** What can you do to avoid being a victim of fraud?

Applying Health Skills
7. **Analyzing Influences** Use critical thinking to analyze and use health information such as interpreting media messages: Find two ads for different brands of the same health care product. Review the information in the ads and write a brief paragraph explaining why you would choose one product over the other.

Lesson 4

Being an Informed Consumer

Quick Write

Imagine that you want to buy acne medication. The store has three different brands. How would you decide which one to buy? List several factors that would be important to you.

LEARN ABOUT...

- the questions to ask before you purchase a product.
- the factors you should consider when comparison shopping.
- why it is important to read product labels.
- what to do if you are dissatisfied with a product.

VOCABULARY

- comparison shopping
- generic products
- warranty

Teens as Consumers

Like most teens, you are a consumer. As you get older, you will have more money to spend. As your purchasing power increases, so does your responsibility. Your buying decisions reflect what is important to you.

Teens are a valuable consumer market for retailers. According to a study by Teenage Research Unlimited, U.S. teens spent $155 billion in the year 2000. **Figure 5.7** shows on what products and services teens spend their money.

FIGURE 5.7

TEEN PURCHASING POWER

This chart shows how teens ages 13 through 15 spent their money in 1999. *How close are these figures to your own spending patterns? How might the spending patterns of adults differ from the spending patterns of teens?*

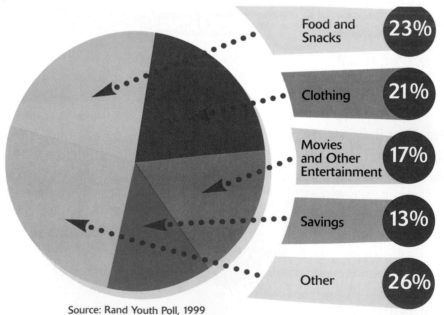

Food and Snacks **23%**

Clothing **21%**

Movies and Other Entertainment **17%**

Savings **13%**

Other **26%**

Source: Rand Youth Poll, 1999

Think Before You Buy

Every year consumers spend billions of dollars on health-related products such as toothpaste, shampoo, and skin cream. Companies invest money in advertising and promotions so that they can convince people to buy their products. As a consumer, how do you make wise buying choices? Below is a list of questions to consider before purchasing health products or any other item.

- Do I understand what the product does and how to use it?
- Is the product safe? Could the product or its packaging harm people or the environment?
- Is the product worth the price? Is there a similar product that costs less?
- What sets the product apart from similar products?
- Could the information on the package be misleading?
- Have I used other items made by the same company? Was I satisfied?
- What is the return policy of the company or store?

Comparison Shopping

Make a habit of **comparison shopping**, which means *accessing information, comparing products, evaluating their benefits, and choosing products that offer the best value.* For example, **generic** (juh·NEHR·ik) **products** are *products sold in plain packages at lower prices than brand name products.*

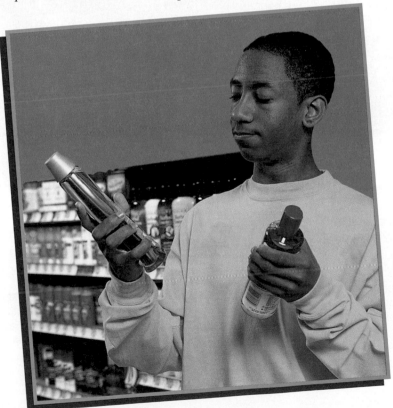

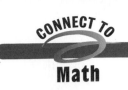
CONNECT TO

Math

COMPARING UNIT PRICES
Always check the unit price to determine which size product is the better buy. For example, a 6-ounce package selling for $3 has a unit price of $0.50 per ounce ($3.00 ÷ 6 = $0.50). An 8-ounce package selling for $3.60 has a unit price of $0.45 per ounce ($3.60 ÷ 8 = $0.45). *Calculate the unit price of two different sizes of a health product that you are thinking of buying. Which one is the better value?*

Suppose that you are at the store and have to choose between two bottles of shampoo. They're sold for about the same price. *What information on the two bottles could help you to make your decision?*

Generic products can save you money when they are equal in quality to brand name items. Look at labels to compare the ingredients in a generic product and a similar brand name product. **Figure 5.8** offers some other tips for comparison shopping.

Reading Product Labels

The labels on health products can help you make smart buying decisions. Labels also offer guidance for the safe and proper use of the product. **Figure 5.9** on the next page shows the information that labels typically provide. It also suggests how to use the information wisely. If a product label's information seems confusing or incomplete, speak with your doctor or pharmacist, or contact the manufacturer.

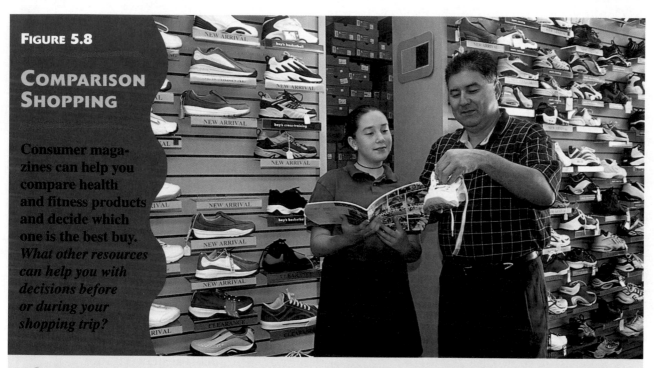

FIGURE 5.8

COMPARISON SHOPPING

Consumer magazines can help you compare health and fitness products and decide which one is the best buy. *What other resources can help you with decisions before or during your shopping trip?*

Cost
Compare prices of the same brand in different stores. Check newspapers for sales.

Features
Avoid paying for features that you don't need. However, do pay for features that you find especially useful or desirable.

Quality
Well-made products generally offer superior performance to those that are poorly made. A cheap product is no bargain if it falls apart or doesn't work.

Warranty
Before you buy a costly product, ask about the warranty. A **warranty** is *a company's or a store's written agreement to repair a product or refund your money should the product not function properly.* Always read the fine print on a warranty because it may cover only certain aspects of a product or its use.

Recommendations
Talk to people who have used the products that you are considering buying. These might be parents, guardians, or other trusted adults. You may also get information from the library or reliable media sources such as consumer reports. Ask questions and read articles to find out which products have earned recommendations.

Your Rights As a Consumer

The U.S. Constitution guarantees citizens basic rights such as freedom of speech and religion. Consumers also have certain rights, which are explained in **Figure 5.10** on the next page.

FIGURE 5.9

WHAT LABELS TELL YOU

Labels provide important product information.
Be sure to read the label before using a product.

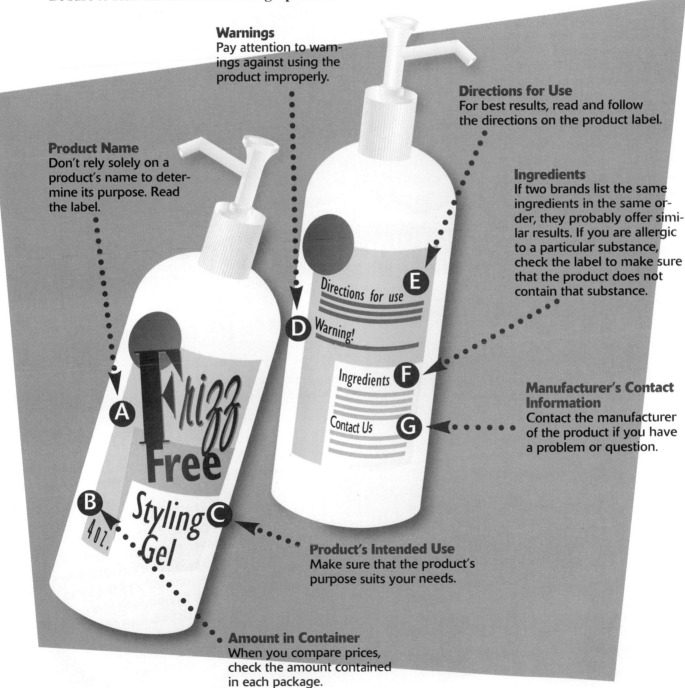

Warnings
Pay attention to warnings against using the product improperly.

Directions for Use
For best results, read and follow the directions on the product label.

Product Name
Don't rely solely on a product's name to determine its purpose. Read the label.

Ingredients
If two brands list the same ingredients in the same order, they probably offer similar results. If you are allergic to a particular substance, check the label to make sure that the product does not contain that substance.

Manufacturer's Contact Information
Contact the manufacturer of the product if you have a problem or question.

Product's Intended Use
Make sure that the product's purpose suits your needs.

Amount in Container
When you compare prices, check the amount contained in each package.

FIGURE 5.10

CONSUMER RIGHTS

See the list below to learn more about your rights as a consumer. *Why do you think these rights are important?*

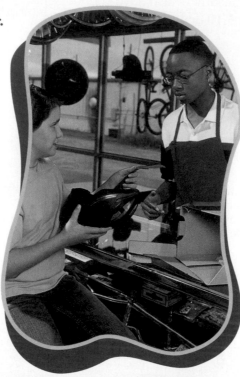

- **Consumers have the right to safety.** They should be able to purchase products and services that will not harm them.
- **Consumers have the right to choose.** They should have the opportunity to select from many products and services at competitive prices.
- **Consumers have the right to be informed.** They deserve truthful information about products and services.

- **Consumers have the right to be heard.** They should be able to join in the making of laws that affect them.
- **Consumers have the right to have problems corrected.** They have the right to complain when they have been treated unfairly.
- **Consumers have the right to consumer education.** They should have an opportunity to learn the skills necessary to help them make wise choices.

HEALTH SKILLS ACTIVITY

COMMUNICATION SKILLS

Exercising Your Consumer Rights

What would you do if you bought a defective product? If a product does not work, you have a right to complain. The following tips explain what you can do to make the process smoother.

- Keep all your sales receipts.
- Check any warranties on the product.
- Depending on the store's policy, you can ask for a refund or an exchange, or you can request that the product be repaired.
- If you would like a refund or an exchange, take the product to the store where you purchased it. Ask to speak to someone who can handle your complaint. State your problem calmly, and then offer your solution. If the person does not agree to your solution, ask to see a manager.

- If the store refuses to honor your request, you can take your complaint to a special consumer rights group.
- If you want the product repaired, take the product to an authorized service center, or mail it to the manufacturer.

ON YOUR OWN

Imagine that a health product you purchased was defective. Write a conversation between yourself and the store manager. Explain why you are dissatisfied with the product and request a repair, exchange, or refund.

Usually your rights as a consumer are recognized and respected wherever you purchase goods. Sometimes, however, more action is necessary. If you try to resolve a problem that you experience with a product and are dissatisfied with the result, you can seek help from any of the following groups.

- **Consumer advocates** are people or groups who devote themselves to helping consumers with problems. These include the Consumers Union and local consumer groups.
- **Business organizations** also assist consumers. The Better Business Bureau, for example, has a network of offices around the country that deal with complaints against local merchants.
- **Local, state, and federal government agencies** make sure that consumers' rights are protected. Among the federal agencies are the Food and Drug Administration and the Consumer Product Safety Commission.
- **Small-claims courts** are state courts that handle legal disputes involving amounts of money below a certain limit. The amount varies from state to state, ranging from $500 to $10,000. Both the consumer and the store present their cases to a judge, who hears both sides and makes a decision.

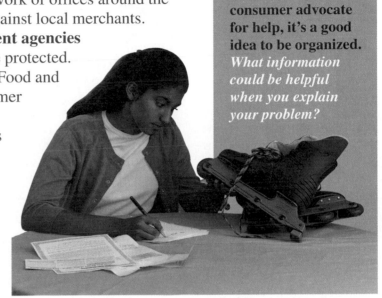

When you go to a consumer advocate for help, it's a good idea to be organized. *What information could be helpful when you explain your problem?*

Lesson 4 Review

Using complete sentences, answer the following questions on a sheet of paper.

Reviewing Terms and Facts
1. **Recall** What questions should you keep in mind when you're trying to decide whether or not to buy a product?
2. **Vocabulary** Define the term *comparison shopping.*
3. **Identify** What is a *warranty?*
4. **List** What are four types of groups that can assist consumers?

Thinking Critically
5. **Analyze** When would reading a product's label prevent injury?

6. **Apply** Choose two local stores and contact your local Better Business Bureau to find out about the experiences consumers have had with those stores.

Applying Health Skills
7. **Communication Skills** With a partner, write and act out a skit about returning a product, such as an appliance or toothpaste. Remember: The customer wants a good product. The store owner or manager wants to make money, run a responsible business, and keep the customer happy. Have your characters reach a fair solution.

5

Health Care Providers and Services

Quick Write

Why do you think there is a need for specialists in addition to family physicians?

LEARN ABOUT...

- the goals of health care.
- the types of health care providers and facilities.
- the types of insurance that help pay for health care.

VOCABULARY

- primary care provider
- specialist
- health insurance
- managed care
- health maintenance organization (HMO)
- preferred provider organization (PPO)
- point-of-service (POS) plan

The Goals of Health Care

When was the last time you visited a doctor's office or health clinic? Perhaps you had a sore throat and a fever, or maybe you sprained your wrist playing a sport. Health care professionals treat these and many other kinds of illnesses and injuries. In addition, health care professionals provide wellness exams to prevent diseases and injuries.

Health care professionals—including school nurses, counselors, health teachers, dental hygienists, and dietitians—also work to educate people and help them stay healthy. Numerous voluntary organizations, such as the American Heart Association and the American Cancer Society, offer health-related information and services. People donate time and money to these groups. The donated funds help to pay for medical research and treatment.

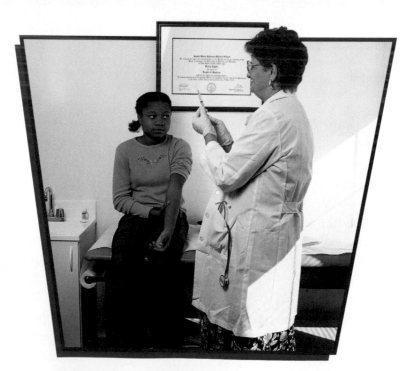

Immunization is a form of disease prevention, one of health care's two main functions. The other purpose of health care is the treatment of diseases and injuries. *Why do you think immunization is important?*

Some health care professionals provide general care, while others have special training to handle specific medical problems. **Primary care providers** are *the health care professionals who provide checkups and general care.* Family physicians and nurse practitioners are examples of primary care providers. For some problems, a doctor may recommend a specialist. A **specialist** (SPE·shuh·list) is *a health care professional trained to treat patients who have problems in specific areas.* Some examples of medical specialists are dermatologists, allergists, and ophthalmologists.

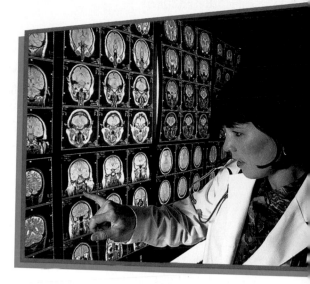

Health Care Facilities

Health care is available in many different places. Some of the most obvious sites that provide health care are school nurses' offices, doctors' offices, clinics, hospitals, and emergency rooms.

Health care facilities also include birthing centers, nursing homes, and drug treatment centers. Rehabilitation centers aid people in recovering from serious illness or injury. Hospices provide care and support for terminally ill (dying) patients.

Specialists' expertise is limited to specific areas of the body. *When might you consider going to a specialist instead of your family doctor?*

HEALTH SKILLS ACTIVITY

ACCESSING INFORMATION

Medical Specialists

Medical specialists deal with the functions, disorders, and care of specific areas of the body. Below is a list of medical specialists and their areas of expertise. Which of these specialists are familiar to you?

- **ALLERGISTS** treat people with asthma, hay fever, and other allergy-related disorders.
- **CARDIOLOGISTS** specialize in the heart and cardiovascular system.
- **DERMATOLOGISTS** specialize in the skin.
- **GYNECOLOGISTS** focus on the female reproductive system.
- **OPHTHALMOLOGISTS'** specialty is the eye.
- **ORTHOPEDISTS** specialize in bones, joints, and muscles.
- **PEDIATRICIANS** treat infants, children, and young teens.

- **PLASTIC SURGEONS** perform reconstructive and cosmetic surgery.
- **PSYCHIATRISTS** specialize in mental and emotional issues.
- **UROLOGISTS** specialize in the urinary system.
- **ORTHODONTISTS** are specialists in dentistry who focus on the alignment of the teeth and jaw.

ON YOUR OWN

Research one of the medical specialties listed here. Prepare a report about the reasons why a person might need to see such a specialist. Present your report to the class.

Health Insurance

Medical care is often very expensive. Surgery and hospital stays, for example, typically cost thousands of dollars. To pay for health care, many people buy health insurance. **Health insurance** is *a plan in which a person pays a set fee to an insurance company in return for the company's agreement to pay some or all medical expenses.* Although plans vary in what they cover, most of the cost of doctors' visits, hospital stays, and medication is usually included.

Private Health Care Plans

Many people receive health services through managed care plans. **Managed care** plans are *health plans that emphasize preventive medicine and work to control the cost and maintain the quality of health care.* Managed care is offered by health maintenance organizations (HMOs), preferred provider organizations (PPOs), and point-of-service (POS) plans.

A **health maintenance organization (HMO)** is a *health insurance plan that contracts with selected physicians and specialists to provide medical services.* Rather than pay for individual services, members pay a monthly fee. In addition, when a member visits a participating physician or specialist, he or she usually makes a copayment, a flat fee for a medical service that is covered under a health insurance plan.

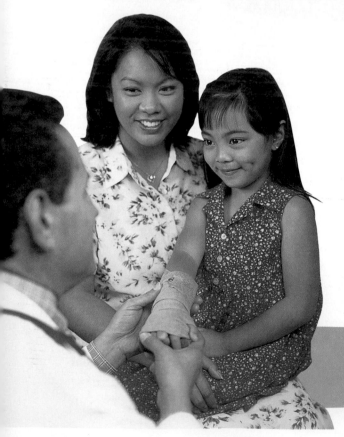

A **preferred provider organization (PPO)**, a variation on the HMO, is *a health insurance plan that allows its members to select a physician who participates in the plan or visit the physician of their choice.* Patients who decide to use their own doctors must pay a deductible, a portion of health care expenses that must be paid before the insurance coverage applies.

A **point-of-service (POS) plan** is *a health insurance plan that combines the features of HMOs and PPOs.* POS plans allow members to visit participating doctors or seek care outside the network at a higher cost.

Managed care plans emphasize preventive medicine and work to control the cost of health care.

Government Health Care Programs

Federal, state, and local governments each play a role in health care. All states, counties, and most large cities have health departments. These departments help develop health-related policies and laws, and work to maintain community health standards. For example, health department officials inspect restaurants to ensure that sanitary practices are being followed. Health departments also provide health-related information, services, and programs. These programs include immunizations and well-baby checkups.

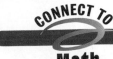

CONNECT TO **Math**

DOCTOR'S BILLS
Suppose that you are a member of a PPO. You are ill and visit your family physician. However, she is not a member of the PPO, so you will have to pay higher fees for medical services. The bill is $90. If the insurance company will pay only 70% of the cost, how much will you have to pay?

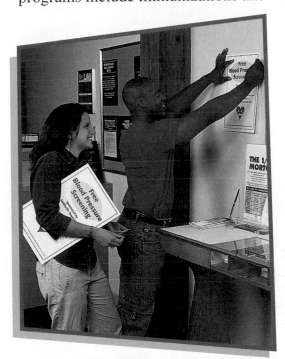

Local health department workers promote community health and prevent disease by talking with people and distributing information. *Look for at least one or two examples of community health services in your town or region.*

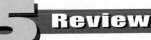

Lesson 5 Review

Using complete sentences, answer the following questions on a sheet of paper.

Reviewing Terms and Facts

1. **Vocabulary** Define the terms *primary care provider* and *specialist.*
2. **List** Identify three medical specialists, and explain their functions.
3. **Distinguish** What is the difference between an *HMO* and a *PPO*?
4. **Identify** What is a *POS plan*?
5. **Recall** What are two examples of programs provided by health departments?

Thinking Critically

6. **Apply** How can you cooperate with your health care provider during a health screening?
7. **Analyze** Explain the role of preventive health measures, immunizations, and treatment in disease prevention.

Applying Health Skills

8. **Accessing Information** Use Internet resources to find out about the American Heart Association or another voluntary health organization. What is the organization's purpose? How does it work? Share with your class what you've learned.

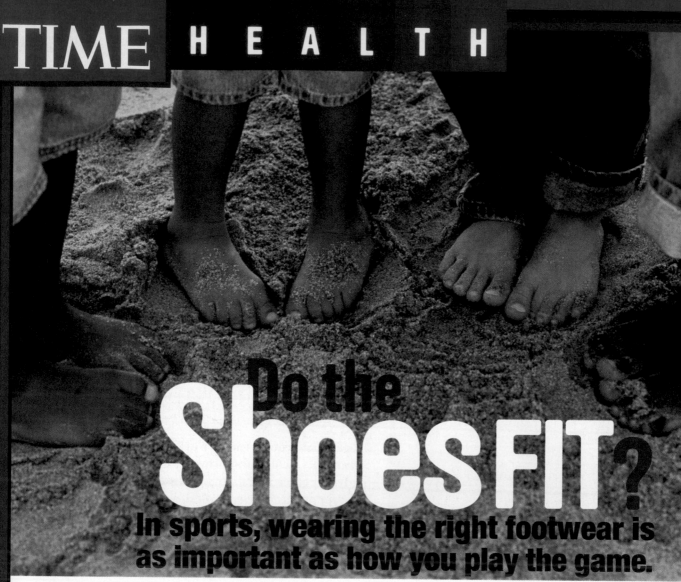

Do the Shoes FIT?

In sports, wearing the right footwear is as important as how you play the game.

You're playing basketball, when suddenly one of your big toes starts to ache. Like most athletes, you try to play through the pain—but by the end of the game, it's hard for you to even walk to the locker room.

"Jogger's toe" is a common sports injury. It happens when constant pounding of the toes against the toe box (front) of athletic shoes causes bleeding under the toenail. Wearing sneakers that are too big can cause jogger's toe, as this leaves room for the feet to slide forward.

According to the American Academy of Orthopedic Surgeons, 43 million Americans have foot problems. Yet, like jogger's toe, many foot injuries are preventable if you choose the right footwear for a particular activity.

Start by examining one of your sneakers on a flat surface. If the heel is worn more on the inside than the outside, you're a pronator. That means your feet roll inward each time your heel strikes the ground. Pronators need a shoe specially built to keep this from happening. If your heel is worn more on the outside, you're an underpronator, which means you need a shoe with more cushioning.

Not Just Any Shoe

As a general rule, if you do the same type of physical activity three or more times a week, you need a sport-specific shoe. The exceptions: basketball, running, and aerobics. These sports always require special shoes, regardless of how often you participate in them. Basketball and aerobics involve movements that demand good stability. Look for a sneaker with a high back, or "profile," that will keep your foot from rolling over. Otherwise you'll risk painful ankle sprains.

Many people assume that it's all right to walk in

Anatomy of a Sneaker

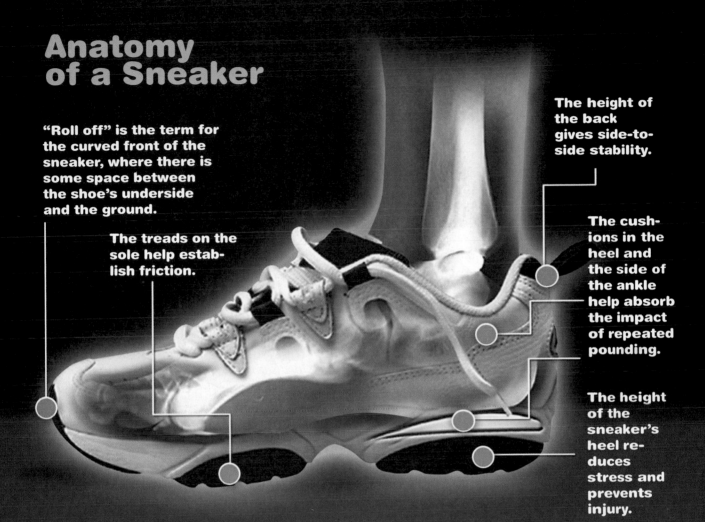

"Roll off" is the term for the curved front of the sneaker, where there is some space between the shoe's underside and the ground.

The treads on the sole help establish friction.

The height of the back gives side-to-side stability.

The cushions in the heel and the side of the ankle help absorb the impact of repeated pounding.

The height of the sneaker's heel reduces stress and prevents injury.

almost any shoe because walking is not as demanding as running. Not true, according to Dr. Carol Frye of the orthopedic academy: "Walking shoes should be at least two and a half inches thick in the heel area, giving you comfortable cushioning," she says. "They should also have a rocker-sole design that encourages the foot's natural roll as you move."

Runners need even more cushioning because they're constantly pounding their feet. The front of running shoes should be flexible, because runners tend to push out with each stride. It also helps if the outer soles have deep, wide treads.

Shoe-Shopping Tips

When you're shopping for sneakers, try them on 30 minutes to one hour after you've exercised. That way, the foot is still fully expanded. Always wear the type of socks you'll be wearing during the sport or activity. Check that you have a thumb's width—about one-half inch—of space between the front of the sneaker and the tip of your toes, or enough room for your toes to wiggle.

Follow these tips to help keep the tips of your toes—and the rest of your feet—injury free! ◪

TIME TO THINK...

About Athletic Shoe Fit

Imagine that you are working in a store that sells athletic shoes. You want to create a list of helpful guidelines for customers who are trying on shoes. Using this article as a resource, create a checklist for consumers that features important points to remember when searching for a properly fitting athletic shoe.

FINDING HYGIENE FACTS

Model

Part of practicing personal hygiene (cleanliness) is getting accurate, reliable information. Read about how Samantha uses the skill of accessing information before making a health decision.

Samantha wants to get the top of one ear pierced. She has saved up enough money from her allowance to pay for the procedure, but her parents want to know more about it before they give her permission. Samantha makes a list of questions and gets information from several sources. She talks to her doctor, friends who have had that part of their ears pierced, and the employees of a jewelry store. She goes to the local library and photocopies magazine articles by health experts, and she also reviews several health-related Web sites.

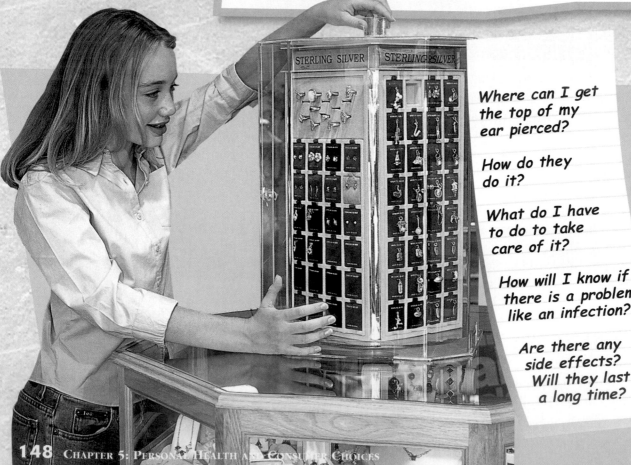

Where can I get the top of my ear pierced?

How do they do it?

What do I have to do to take care of it?

How will I know if there is a problem, like an infection?

Are there any side effects? Will they last a long time?

Practice

Read about Ian, a teen who is considering making a change that could affect his health, and answer the questions below.

Although Ian likes wearing his glasses, he feels that they are in the way now that he has joined the basketball league. He worries about someone knocking into him and breaking them. Ian would like to get contact lenses, but he's not sure of the pros and cons of glasses and contact lenses. Moreover, Ian doesn't know much about the types of lenses that might be best for him or how sensitive his eyes are.

1. Where can Ian go to find reliable information about contact lenses?
2. How can he be sure that the information he finds is accurate and objective?

Apply/Assess

Imagine that you are in a situation similar to Ian's. First, develop guidelines for evaluating health information. Then find sources of information regarding one of the following hygiene-related products: tooth whitener, acrylic nails, hair dye, self-tanning cream.

Remember to identify all of your sources and explain why they are reliable and accurate. Consult trusted adults, such as your parents or guardians, and use resources such as the Internet, magazines, newspapers, books, and printed materials from recognized organizations. You can also talk to someone who has had experience with the product that you're interested in. Present your findings to the class in a one-page report.

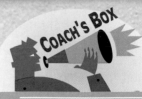

COACH'S BOX

Accessing Information

Ask yourself these questions about any source of information.
- Is it scientific?
- Does it give only one point of view?
- Is it trying to sell something?
- Does it agree with other sources?

Self-√Check
- Did I find sources of information on a hygiene-related product?
- Did I check the accuracy of the sources that provided information on the product that I chose?
- How did I determine that the information was accurate?

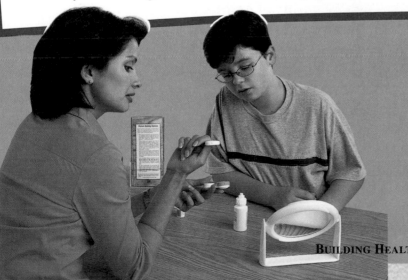

After You Read

Use your completed Foldable to review the information on caring for teeth, skin, hair, and nails.

FOLDABLES™
Study Organizer

Reviewing Vocabulary and Concepts

On a sheet of paper, write the numbers 1–9. After each number, write the term from the list that best completes each statement.

- ophthalmologist
- melanin
- decibels
- follicles
- dandruff
- head lice
- pores
- epidermis
- dermis
- ultraviolet rays

Lesson 1

1. _____ is the substance that gives skin its color.
2. The layer of skin that contains blood vessels is called the _____. It is covered by the _____.
3. Hair grows from structures called _____.
4. Tiny openings in the skin are _____.
5. _____ can increase the risk of skin cancer.
6. _____ is a flaking of the outer layer of dead skin cells on the scalp.
7. _____ are tiny insects that live on the hair shaft.

Lesson 2

8. A(n) _____ is a physician who specializes in diseases of the eye.
9. The loudness of sound is measured in _____.

On a sheet of paper, write the numbers 10–18. Write *True* or *False* for each statement below. If the statement is false, change the underlined word or phrase to make it true.

Lesson 3

10. Deliberate deceit or trickery in advertising is known as <u>fraud</u>.
11. An <u>infomercial</u> is a statement of approval.
12. <u>Advertising</u> consists of messages that try to convince you to buy a product or service.

Lesson 4

13. <u>Brand name</u> products come in plain packages.
14. Important factors in <u>comparison shopping</u> include the cost, features, quality, and warranty of the product or service.

Lesson 5

15. A nurse practitioner is an example of a <u>specialist</u>.
16. <u>Orthopedists</u> are specialists in dentistry who focus on the alignment of the teeth and jaw.
17. <u>Health insurance</u> is a plan in which a person pays a set fee to an insurance company in return for the company's agreement to pay some or all medical expenses.
18. <u>Managed care</u> is a health plan that emphasizes preventive medicine and that strives to manage the cost and maintain the quality of health care.

Thinking Critically

Using complete sentences, answer the following questions on a sheet of paper.

19. **Explain** How are healthy teeth the result of both good hygiene and a well-balanced diet?
20. **Predict** How might allowing eye or ear problems to go untreated affect other areas of your health?

21. Synthesize How can analyzing advertising claims for health care products help you make wise purchasing decisions?

22. Assess Do you think that companies should be required to provide health insurance for employees and their families? Why or why not?

Career Corner

Audiologist A teen who hears a ringing in his or her ears after attending a loud concert may need to seek help from an audiologist. Audiologists treat people who have suffered a hearing injury or who have a hearing disorder. These professionals also test noise levels in workplaces to determine whether these levels are safe for workers.

Audiologists have four years of college and a two-year advanced degree. Find out more about this and other health careers by clicking on Career Corner at health.glencoe.com.

Standardized Test Practice

Reading & Writing

Read the paragraphs below and then answer the questions.

What causes goose bumps? Wind and cold weather stimulate receptors in your skin, and these receptors send a signal to your brain. Your brain sends a signal back to your skin, causing the blood vessels there to expand and the tiny muscles on each hair follicle to contract. These almost invisible hair follicles stand up straight, resulting in goose bumps.

Something similar happens when you shiver. Cold air hits your skin, receptors in the skin send a message to your brain, and your brain signals muscles all over your body to contract and relax repeatedly. All this muscle work helps generate heat to keep you warm.

1. Because cold air stimulates receptors in your skin, the
   A receptors expand.
   B receptors contract.
   C receptors send a message to your heart.
   D receptors send a message to your brain.

2. The author develops the second paragraph by
   A describing shivering.
   B comparing goose bumps and shivering.
   C explaining what makes you shiver.
   D describing how you keep warm.

3. Write a paragraph describing how the skin regulates body temperature.

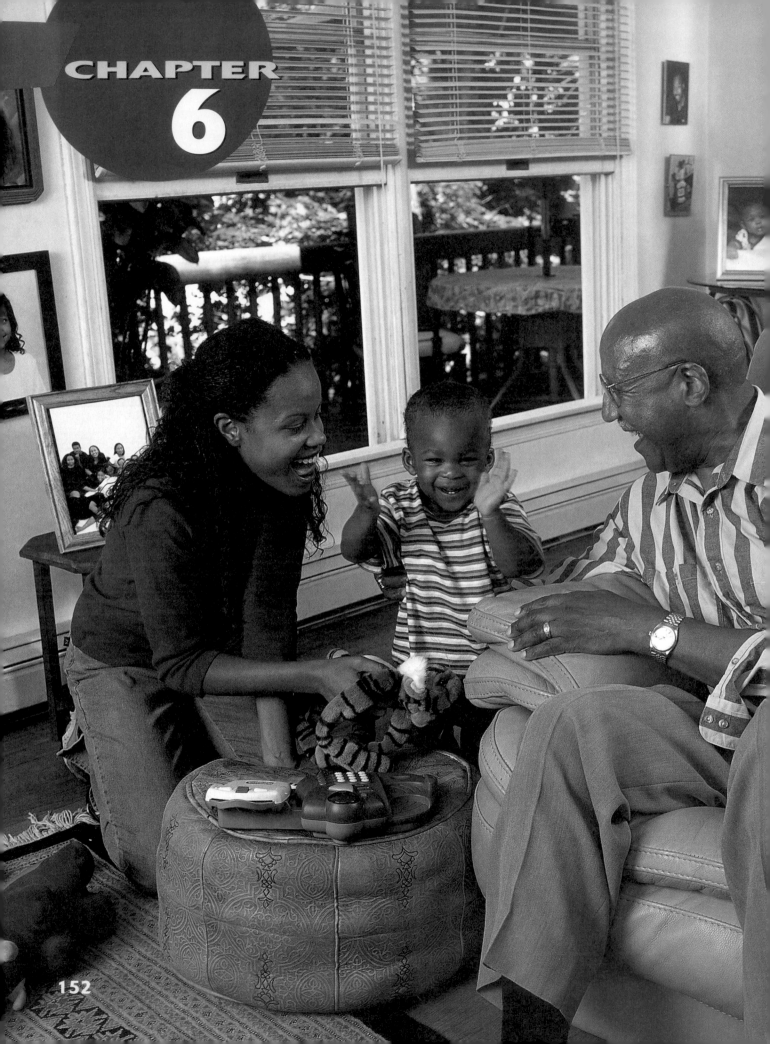

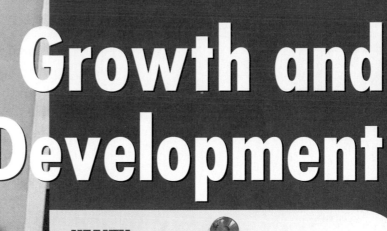

Growth and Development

HEALTH *Online*

Do your choices, attitudes, and behaviors show that you are preparing for adulthood? Find out by taking the Chapter 6 Health Inventory at health.glencoe.com.

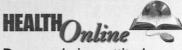

FOLDABLES™
Study Organizer

Before You Read

Make this Foldable to help you organize what you learn in Lesson 1 about the changes of adolescence. Begin with a plain sheet of 8½″ × 11″ paper.

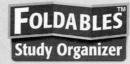

Step 1

Fold the sheet of paper along the long axis, leaving a 2″ tab along the side.

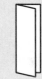

Step 2

Turn the paper and fold it into thirds.

Step 3

Unfold and cut the top layer along both fold lines. This makes three tabs.

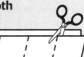

Step 4

Label the tabs as shown.

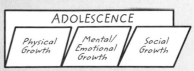

ADOLESCENCE

Physical Growth | Mental/Emotional Growth | Social Growth

As You Read

Define key terms and record what you learn about the changes that take place during adolescence.

Adolescence

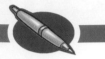

Quick Write

Briefly describe what new interests you have found in the past year. How do your new interests show that you've changed?

LEARN ABOUT...

- the influence of the endocrine system on growth and development.
- the physical, mental/ emotional, and social changes that occur during adolescence.

VOCABULARY

- adolescence
- hormones
- endocrine system
- metabolism
- puberty

Growing and Changing

During your teen years your body will change in many ways. The physical changes, such as outgrowing your clothes, will be obvious. You will experience mental and emotional changes, too. You may begin to have new thoughts and feelings.

Changes are a normal part of adolescence. **Adolescence** (a·duhl·EH·suhns) is *the stage of life between childhood and adulthood, usually beginning somewhere between the ages of 11 and 15.* Many of the changes you will experience during adolescence are brought about by hormones. **Hormones** (HOR·mohnz) are *chemical substances produced in certain glands that help to regulate the way your body functions.* A gland is a group of cells or an organ that secretes hormones and/or other powerful chemical substances that the body needs. The release of hormones helps to prepare your body for adulthood.

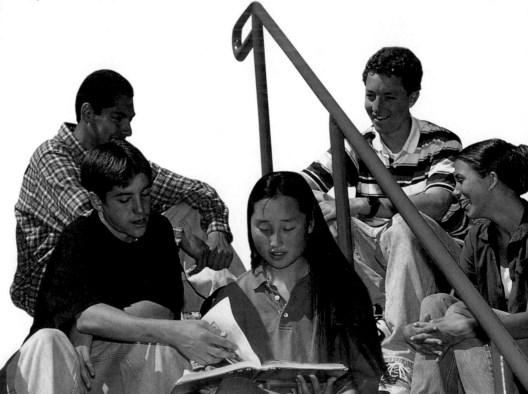

A person's circle of friends changes throughout life.

The Endocrine System

The hormones that cause the physical and emotional changes of adolescence are produced by your endocrine system. The **endocrine** (EN·duh·kruhn) **system** consists of *glands throughout the body that regulate body functions.*

Your endocrine system produces hormones that go directly into your bloodstream. The hormones are then carried to different parts of the body to control various functions. For example, some hormones regulate growth. Others help the body to digest food and adjust its balance of salt and water. **Figure 6.1** describes the major glands of the endocrine system and the body functions they regulate.

Reading Check
Make predictions. What problems might develop if your endocrine system wasn't working properly?

FIGURE 6.1

THE ENDOCRINE SYSTEM

The glands of the endocrine system help to regulate many of the body's functions, including growth and development. *What operations do the adrenal glands regulate?*

Pituitary gland
The pituitary gland at the base of the brain produces several hormones that control the work of other glands and organs, such as the thyroid gland, adrenal glands, and kidneys. Pituitary gland hormones also regulate the body's growth and development.

Parathyroid glands
The parathyroid (par·uh·THY·royd) glands are located within the thyroid gland. They regulate the levels of calcium and phosphorous in the blood.

Thyroid gland
The hormone produced by the thyroid gland regulates body growth and the rate of **metabolism**, *the process by which the body gets energy from food.* The thyroid is located alongside the trachea, or windpipe.

Adrenal glands
The adrenal (uh·DREE·nuhl) glands produce hormones that help regulate the balance of salt and water in the body. The adrenal glands also aid in digestion and control the body's response to emergencies and excitement. They are located on top of the kidneys.

Pancreas
The pancreas, located behind the stomach, controls the level of sugar in the blood and provides the small intestine with digestive chemicals called enzymes.

Ovaries (in female)
Ovaries (OH·vuh·reez) are the female reproductive glands. Hormones produced in the ovaries control sexual development and the maturing of eggs.

Testes (in male)
The testes (TES·teez) are the male reproductive glands. The hormone produced in the testes controls sexual development and the production of sperm.

Respect

Show that you
respect your health
by making responsi-
ble decisions. When
you eat nutritious
foods, stay alcohol-
and drug-free, and
avoid risk behaviors,
you show that you
value your health.
*What other behaviors
show self-respect?*

Physical Development

You may already have noticed some of the changes that adolescence brings. Teen boys will find their voices becoming deeper.
Their muscles develop and their shoulders may broaden. Teen girls
will notice changes in their body shape. These are just some of the
physical signs of puberty.

Puberty (PYOO·buhr·tee) is *the time when you develop physical characteristics of adults of your own gender.* **Figure 6.2** lists
the types of physical changes that occur during puberty.

Once the growth spurt of puberty starts, physical growth generally occurs at a rapid pace. However, it is important to remember
that growth patterns differ among adolescents. Girls usually grow
2 to 8 inches taller between the ages of 11 and 14. Boys usually
begin their growth spurt later than girls do. They may grow 4 to 12
inches between the ages of 13 and 16. After their initial growth
spurts, adolescents of both genders often keep growing for several
more years.

FIGURE 6.2

Your Changing Body

Many types of physical
changes occur during
puberty.

- Male hormone produc-
  tion increases.
- Sudden, rapid growth
  occurs.
- All permanent teeth
  come into place.
- Acne may appear.
- Underarm hair appears.
- Pubic hair appears.
- Perspiration increases.

- External genitals enlarge.
- Breasts may enlarge
  somewhat.
- Shoulders broaden.
- Muscles develop.
- Sperm production starts.
- Facial hair appears.
- Larynx gets larger, and
  voice deepens.

- Female hormone pro-
  duction increases.
- Sudden, rapid growth
  occurs.
- All permanent teeth
  come into place.
- Acne may appear.
- Underarm hair
  appears.
- Pubic hair appears.

- Perspiration increases.
- External genitals
  enlarge.
- Breasts develop.
- Hips become wider.
- Body fat increases.
- Ovulation occurs.
- Menstruation starts.
- Uterus and ovaries
  enlarge.

Mental Development

The changes you experience during adolescence aren't only physical ones. You also develop more complex thinking skills. You learn to analyze and solve complicated problems. You also come to understand that many questions do not have simple right or wrong answers. Because of this insight, you learn that you will have to rely on values to make responsible decisions.

Adolescence is when you begin to recognize that other people have points of view that may be different from your own. You also realize that you have the power to make choices that can affect your life. You recognize that your actions have consequences and that it's important to take responsibility for these consequences.

Emotional Development

The teen years are a time of emotional changes as well. As a child, you probably tried hard to win your parents' approval. While this is still important to you, during adolescence the approval and acceptance of your peers also begin to matter. You may also begin to feel attracted to members of the opposite gender. These feelings are part of growing up, too.

Teens grow and mature at different rates. This may affect personal health. For example, teens who experience early growth may feel different or more mature than their peers. Those who experience later growth may be worried about looking younger than their peers. It is important to recognize and accept that body types and levels of maturity differ during adolescence. Respect and appreciate these differences.

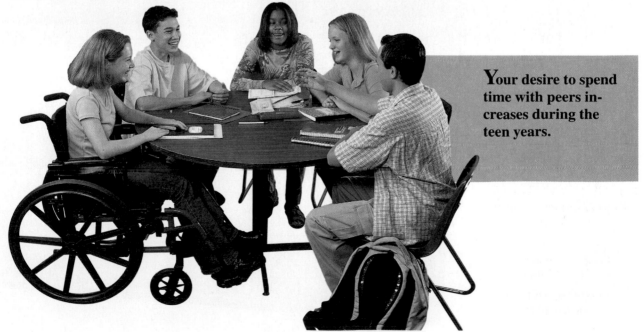

Your desire to spend time with peers increases during the teen years.

Emotional Changes

Many teens find that adolescence brings on powerful emotions. Sometimes you feel happy, excited, and full of life. At other times you may be sad, scared, and ready to cry. You may even notice that you experience a confusing mix of all of these emotions in a single day. Mood swings are a natural part of being a teen. They are caused by the release of hormones as well as the changes—physical and otherwise—that you are going through.

These fluctuations in your emotions are signs that you're maturing emotionally. During adolescence you may find that you're growing closer to your friends. You're probably also beginning to understand others' emotional needs better.

Expressing Your Emotions

Learning how to manage and express strong feelings healthfully is another way in which you grow during adolescence. No matter what you are feeling, it is important to express your emotions in constructive and appropriate ways. Try to face feelings of anger, sadness, or frustration instead of hiding them. Tell someone if a problem is bothering you or if you often feel sad; talk to your parents, another trusted adult, or a friend. If you are angry or upset with someone, take time to consider the other person's point of view.

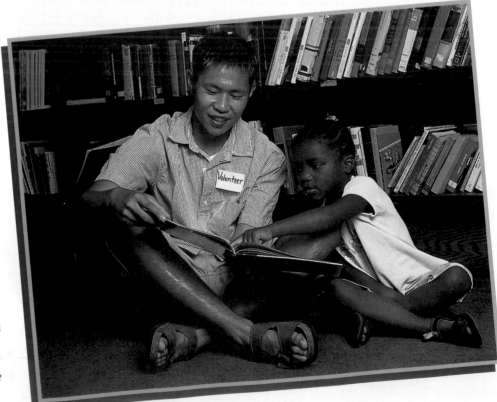

Volunteering is not only a great way to make use of your skills and talents, it can also help you meet your own emotional needs. *What abilities could you put to use through volunteering?*

Social Development

As you progress through the teen years, you are constantly learning about yourself and others. You are figuring out how you fit into society and discovering what makes you unique. For years the attitudes and values of your family and friends shaped the way you saw yourself. They will continue to have a strong influence on you, but your sense of identity is likely to undergo major changes. As a result, you will probably become part of new social groups. This is an important part of growing up.

Your growth and development during adolescence will take many paths. Identify your interests, and think about the activities that you enjoy. This will help you discover who you are and what is important to you. The interests and activities that you pursue in adolescence, your attitudes, and your values will help shape the type of person you will become as an adult.

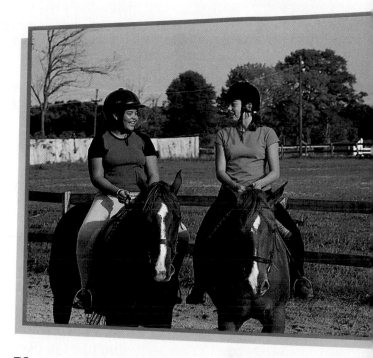

Your interests and activities tell others a great deal about who you are and what is important to you. *Name some entertainment choices that promote mental and physical health.*

Lesson 1 Review

Using complete sentences, answer the following questions on a sheet of paper.

Reviewing Terms and Facts

1. **Vocabulary** What are *hormones?*
2. **Recall** Describe the influences of the endocrine system on growth and development.
3. **Distinguish** What is the difference between *adolescence* and *puberty?*
4. **List** Compare and contrast changes in males and females during puberty. List three physical changes that are similar for males and females, three changes that occur only in males, and three changes that occur only in females.
5. **Explain** What emotional changes do teens experience during puberty?

Thinking Critically

6. **Consider** Appraise the importance of social groups.
7. **Analyze** Which of the many changes of adolescence do you think are most challenging for teens to cope with? Explain your choices.

Applying Health Skills

8. **Analyzing Influences** Think of five aspects of your life that influence you most right now. You might include specific people you know; groups and activities you are involved in; or music, TV shows, or movies that you like. Next, try to remember the five factors that influenced you most two years ago. Have the lists changed? Why do you think this is so?

The Male Reproductive System

The Human Reproductive System

Reproduction (ree·pruh·DUHK·shuhn) is *the process by which living organisms produce others of their own kind.* Reproduction is essential to all living things. Without it, groups of organisms would disappear over time.

Human life results from the union of two cells: one from the male and one from the female. These cells are produced by structures in the male and female reproductive systems. The human **reproductive** (ree·pruh·DUHK·tiv) **system** consists of *body organs and structures that make it possible to produce young.* Most human body systems are alike in both males and females. However, this is not the case for the male and female reproductive systems. Each of the two systems is specially suited to perform its role in reproduction.

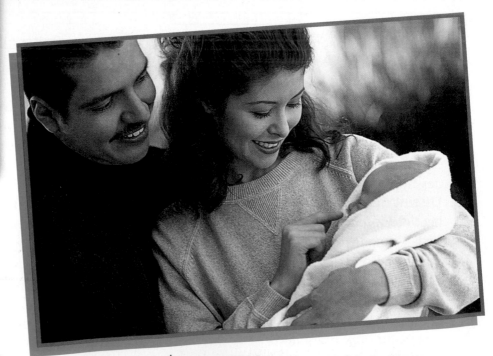

A baby is produced by the union of a male cell and a female cell. *Why is reproduction essential to all living things?*

The Male Reproductive System

Figure 6.3 shows the internal and external parts of the male reproductive system. This system's function is to produce sperm and transmit them to the female reproductive system. **Sperm**, *the male reproductive cells,* are first produced during puberty—usually between ages 12 and 15.

In males, the process of reproduction begins in the testes. The **testes** are *the pair of glands that produce sperm.* When a male is sexually stimulated, sperm leave the testes through tubes that lead to the urethra. Along the way, the sperm mix with fluids that protect them and help them to travel. This *mixture of sperm and fluids* is called **semen** (SEE·muhn). Semen is released from the urethra through the penis (PEE·nuhs). The muscular action that forces semen through the urethra and out of the penis is called ejaculation (i·ja·kyuh·LAY·shuhn).

FIGURE 6.3

PARTS OF THE MALE REPRODUCTIVE SYSTEM

These illustrations show the internal and external parts of the male reproductive system. *What is the function of the epididymis?*

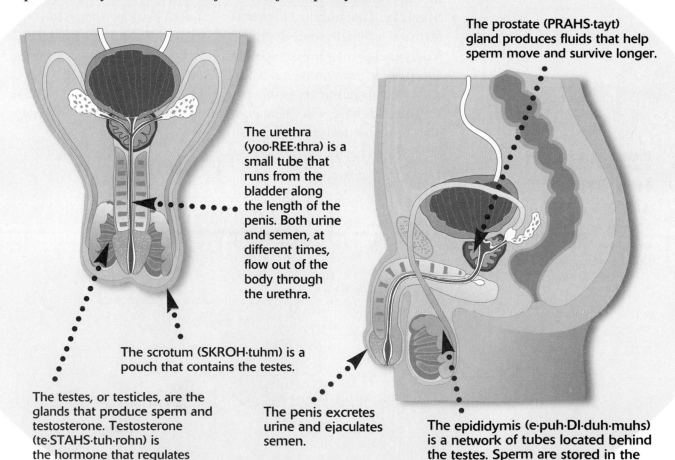

The prostate (PRAHS·tayt) gland produces fluids that help sperm move and survive longer.

The urethra (yoo·REE·thra) is a small tube that runs from the bladder along the length of the penis. Both urine and semen, at different times, flow out of the body through the urethra.

The scrotum (SKROH·tuhm) is a pouch that contains the testes.

The testes, or testicles, are the glands that produce sperm and testosterone. Testosterone (te·STAHS·tuh·rohn) is the hormone that regulates male sexual development.

The penis excretes urine and ejaculates semen.

The epididymis (e·puh·DI·duh·muhs) is a network of tubes located behind the testes. Sperm are stored in the epididymis.

Male Health Concerns

Several disorders can affect the male reproductive system. The following are some of the most common:

- **Inguinal hernia.** If a boy or man strains his abdominal muscles, he can weaken the muscles that hold his intestine in place. This can allow the intestine to push through, as shown in **Figure 6.4**, creating an inguinal hernia (ING·gwuh·nuhl HUHR·nee·uh). A boy or man who has a hernia may notice a bulge in his groin or scrotum. Only surgery can repair a hernia.

- **Testicular cancer.** Cancer of the testes is rare, but it is the most common cancer in American males between the ages of 15 and 35. Symptoms may include a lump or swelling in the scrotum, pain or tenderness in one of the testicles, or a dull ache in the lower abdomen and groin. If it is detected in its early stages, testicular cancer can usually be cured. Regular self-examinations as well as health screenings can help boys and men to discover this disease.

- **Prostate cancer.** This type of cancer usually affects men over the age of 55. Cancer of the prostate gland is the second most common form of cancer in men. Current treatments include surgery to remove all or part of the prostate gland, radiation therapy, and hormone therapy.

- **Sterility.** The inability to produce enough healthy sperm to fertilize a female reproductive cell is a condition called sterility. Many factors can impair sperm production. These factors include exposure to environmental hazards, such as radiation, lead, X rays, and certain chemicals (some pesticides, for example). Males who smoke and those who have contracted mumps after puberty may also become sterile.

FIGURE 6.4

INGUINAL HERNIA

Although hernias are common and are not serious right away, they can eventually cause serious injuries to the intestines and testicles.

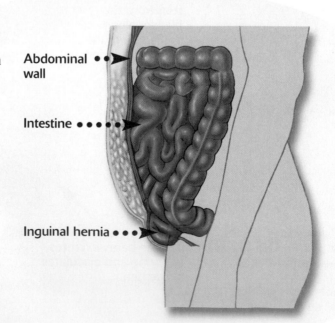

Abdominal wall

Intestine

Inguinal hernia

Caring for the Male Reproductive System

Males can keep their reproductive systems healthy by

- performing a testicular self-examination each month. This exam involves checking the testes for lumps or swelling. Soreness or a dull ache in the groin can also be a sign of problems with the reproductive system. A doctor and the American Cancer Society can provide information on how to perform the procedure.
- taking a shower or bath daily to keep the external reproductive organs clean. Males should bathe or shower more often when they get sweaty.
- always wearing protective gear when they participate in contact sports, such as football.
- having regular health screenings and cooperating with health care providers regarding any treatment.

Males should discuss with parents or guardians any questions they have about their reproductive systems or sexuality in general. Talking openly and honestly about these issues is a way to communicate effectively.

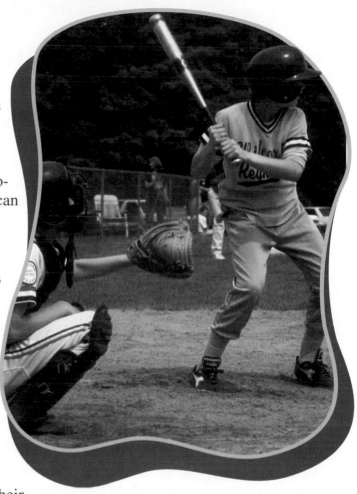

Wearing protective gear can help boys and men prevent injuries to their reproductive organs. *What else can males do to take good care of their reproductive organs?*

Lesson 2 Review

Using complete sentences, answer the following questions on a sheet of paper.

Reviewing Terms and Facts

1. **Vocabulary** Describe the function of the human *reproductive system.*
2. **Distinguish** What is the difference between *sperm* and *semen?*
3. **Identify** Name the parts of the male reproductive system.
4. **Recall** Identify three disorders of the male reproductive system.

Thinking Critically

5. **Consider** Why are regular self-examinations of the testes important?
6. **Explain** What glands do the male reproductive system and the endocrine system share?

Applying Health Skills

7. **Accessing Information** Call or write to the American Cancer Society to find out the proper way to perform a self-examination for testicular cancer. Create a pamphlet that explains the procedure.

The Female Reproductive System

Quick Write

Write down one fact you know about menstruation.

LEARN ABOUT...

○ the functions of the female reproductive system.
○ the organs and structures of the female reproductive system.
○ the process of menstruation.
○ the care of the female reproductive system.

VOCABULARY

○ fertilization
○ ovulation
○ menstruation
○ ovaries
○ uterus
○ gynecologist

The Female Reproductive System

The female reproductive system has four main functions. First, it produces the hormones estrogen (ES·truh·juhn) and progesterone (pro·JES·tuh·rohn), which are necessary for female sexual development and for reproduction. Second, it stores and releases female reproductive cells, called egg cells or eggs. Third, this system allows fertilization to take place. **Fertilization** (fuhr·tuhl·uh·ZAY·shuhn) is *the joining of a male sperm cell and a female egg cell to form a new human life.* Fourth, the female reproductive system nourishes and protects the developing child until it is able to survive outside the female's body. **Figure 6.5** shows the female reproductive system.

The Menstrual Cycle

Ovulation (ahv·yuh·LAY·shuhn) may start as soon as a girl reaches puberty. **Ovulation** is *the process by which the ovaries release a single mature egg.* Just prior to ovulation, the lining of the uterus thickens. If fertilization occurs, this lining will develop further and nourish the fertilized egg. If fertilization does not occur, the lining breaks down into blood, tissue, and fluids. The body sheds the lining through the vagina. **Menstruation** (men·stroo·WAY·shuhn) is *the flow of the uterine lining material from the body.* For most girls, menstruation starts between ages 9 and 16. When a woman is pregnant, the lining is not shed, so she does not menstruate.

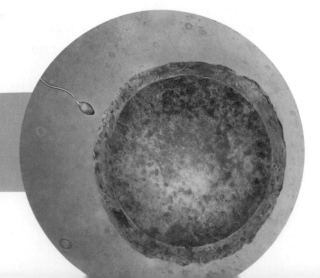

Fertilization occurs when a male sperm cell penetrates a female egg cell. Only one sperm cell can enter one egg cell. *Where are the sperm cells produced?*

FIGURE 6.5

PARTS OF THE FEMALE REPRODUCTIVE SYSTEM

Fertilization and pregnancy occur in the female reproductive system.
What role do the fallopian tubes play in reproduction?

At puberty the **ovaries**, the *two female reproductive glands,* start to release eggs, or ova. The ovaries also increase production of estrogen and progesterone, hormones that are necessary for female sexual development.

The cervix (SUHR•viks) is the opening at the bottom of the uterus.

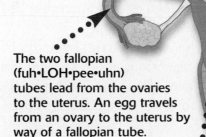

The two fallopian (fuh•LOH•pee•uhn) tubes lead from the ovaries to the uterus. An egg travels from an ovary to the uterus by way of a fallopian tube. Fertilization takes place in a fallopian tube.

Labia (LAY•bee•uh) are folds of skin that cover the opening of the vagina.

A fertilized egg becomes implanted in the **uterus** (YOO•tuh•ruhs), *a pear-shaped organ in which a developing child is nourished.* The uterus is also called a womb (WOOM).

The vagina (vuh•JY•nuh) is a muscular passageway that leads from the uterus to the outside of the body. Menstrual flow leaves the body through the vagina. In addition, a baby is pushed out of its mother's body through the vagina.

Menstruation usually occurs approximately every 28 days. A menstrual (MEN·stroo·uhl) period lasts for about 5 days. However, the length of both the menstrual cycle and the period can vary from female to female. A teen girl's menstrual cycle may change from month to month. This should not be a cause for concern unless menstruation stops for months at a time. **Figure 6.6** on page 166 describes the timing of events in a typical menstrual cycle.

Reading Check

Think about the topic. Why do you think it is important for you to study the reproductive system at your age?

Fertilization

Sperm entering the vagina travel through the uterus to the fallopian tubes. Fertilization takes place in a fallopian tube when a male sperm cell and a female egg cell unite. The fertilized egg then moves through the fallopian tube to the uterus, where it becomes implanted. In the uterus, the fertilized egg gradually grows and develops.

Using tampons incorrectly increases the risk of TSS. *What are some of the symptoms of TSS?*

Female Health Concerns

Several disorders can affect the female reproductive system. These include the following:

- **Vaginitis.** Pain, itching, and discharge are symptoms of vaginitis (va·juh·NY·tuhs), an infection of the vagina. This problem is treated with medication.
- **Premenstrual syndrome (PMS).** Some women may experience physical and emotional discomfort before menstruation begins each month. Symptoms of premenstrual (pree·MEN·struh·wuhl) syndrome include headaches, breast tenderness, fatigue, irritability, acne, and abdominal cramps. These symptoms may be mild or severe. Regular exercise and dietary changes can often ease PMS, but serious cases may require medical attention.
- **Toxic shock syndrome (TSS).** This rare bacterial infection has been linked to tampon use. It can be serious and even fatal if not treated. Symptoms include high fever, a rash, and vomiting. Females can protect themselves by following the directions for tampon use carefully.
- **Cancer.** The breasts, ovaries, uterus, and cervix can all be affected by cancer, although this is rare in teens. Regular health screenings and self-examinations can detect cancer early, greatly increasing the possibility of recovery.
- **Infertility.** The inability to produce children is called infertility (in·fuhr·TI·luh·tee). Surgery or hormone treatment can treat some types of infertility.

FIGURE 6.6

THE MENSTRUAL CYCLE

A girl's menstrual cycle is often irregular for the first year or two. After that, a menstrual cycle is generally about 28 days long.

Ovulation: A mature egg is released from the ovary into a fallopian tube.

Menstrual flow stops after about 5 days.

Menstrual flow begins.

If fertilization has not occurred, the uterine lining begins to break down.

Fertilization is most likely to occur during these days.

Caring for the Female Reproductive System

Females can keep their reproductive systems healthy by

- showering or bathing daily to keep external reproductive organs clean.
- scheduling regular health screenings by a gynecologist, beginning at the age recommended by a doctor. A **gynecologist** (gy·nuh·KAH·luh·jist) is *a doctor who specializes in the female reproductive system.*
- examining their breasts monthly for any unusual lumps or discharge. A doctor and the American Cancer Society can provide information on the breast self-exam.
- keeping a record of their menstrual cycles. Cycles may be irregular at first. Females should see a doctor if they experience severe or unusual pain or excessive bleeding during menstruation. Females should cooperate by following the doctor's recommendations for treatment.

Females may have questions or concerns about their reproductive systems or other aspects of sexuality. If so, they should discuss these issues openly and honestly with parents or guardians.

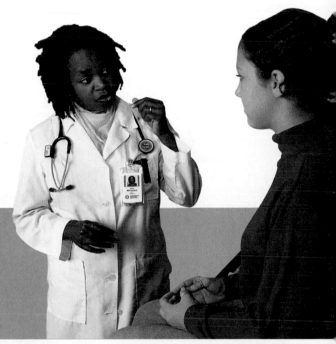

Regular health screenings can help detect problems of the female reproductive system. *Why is early detection important?*

Lesson 3 Review

Using complete sentences, answer the following questions on a sheet of paper.

Reviewing Terms and Facts

1. **Vocabulary** Define the terms *fertilization* and *ovulation.*
2. **Identify** What is *menstruation?*
3. **Recall** List three problems that can affect the female reproductive system.
4. **List** Name four ways to keep the female reproductive system healthy.

Thinking Critically

5. **Analyze** How are ovulation, fertilization, and menstruation related?
6. **Consider** Why is it important for a female to see a doctor if she stops menstruating for several months?

Applying Health Skills

7. **Accessing Information** Use Internet or library resources to find information on problems of the female reproductive system. Write a paragraph explaining your findings, and share it with the class.

Human Development

Quick Write

Think of a family that you know whose members have similar physical features. In what ways do they resemble each other?

LEARN ABOUT...

- the basic unit of life.
- development before birth.
- the factors that affect development before birth.

VOCABULARY

- cell
- tissue
- organ
- body system
- embryo
- fetus
- chromosomes
- genes

Building Blocks

Your body is made up of tiny "building blocks" called cells. A **cell** is *the basic unit of life.* Microscopic cells form your tissues, organs, and body systems. **Figure 6.7** shows how these cells make up the parts of your body.

FIGURE 6.7

BUILDING BODY SYSTEMS

Tiny cells are grouped together to build your body's complex systems.

A **body system** is *a group of organs that work together to carry out related tasks.* Examples include the digestive system and the endocrine system.

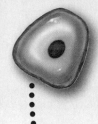

Cells come in many different forms and shapes. Each type of cell has a particular function. This is a cell from the lining of the stomach.

Tissues are *groups of similar cells that do a particular job.* Each type of tissue is designed to perform one function. The tissue that forms the stomach lining, for example, protects the stomach from the acid in gastric juice.

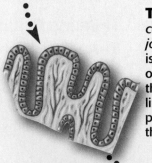

Organs are *body parts made up of different tissues joined together to perform a function.* For example, the stomach is an organ made up of muscle, mucous membranes, and other types of tissue. These tissues work together to help digest food.

Development After Fertilization

The human body begins as a single fertilized cell, the result of the union of a sperm and an egg. The fertilized cell then starts to divide; over a period of hours, one cell becomes two, two become four, four become eight, and so on. These cells are referred to as an **embryo** (EM·bree·oh), the name for *the developing organism from fertilization to about the eighth week of development*. After about a week the embryo attaches itself to the lining of the uterus. After the eighth week the embryo is called a **fetus** (FEE·tuhs), the name for *the developing organism from the end of the eighth week until birth*. From the moment of fertilization until birth, the cells develop into tissues, organs, and body systems. **Figure 6.8** shows how the fetus develops during pregnancy.

Pregnancy generally lasts a little over nine months. From the start, the developing fetus receives nutrients and oxygen from its mother through a tube called the umbilical (uhm·BI·li·kuhl) cord, which is attached to its abdomen.

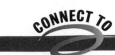

CONNECT TO

Math

THEY GROW SO FAST! The months a fetus spends developing in the uterus are a time of rapid changes. Using the information from Figure 6.8, calculate the number of inches the developing fetus grows at each three-month stage. Then calculate the weight the average fetus gains during the same stages of development.

FIGURE 6.8

THE DEVELOPING FETUS

Pregnancy lasts approximately nine months. *What must happen to an egg cell in order for pregnancy to begin?*

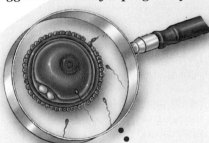

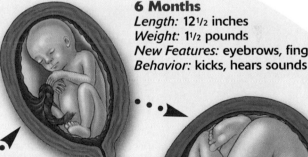

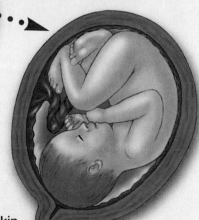

6 Months
Length: 12½ inches
Weight: 1½ pounds
New Features: eyebrows, fingernails
Behavior: kicks, hears sounds

Fertilization
A sperm cell unites with an egg cell. This union forms an embryo that is microscopic in size.

3 Months
Length: 3 inches
Weight: 1 ounce
New Features: arms, legs, fingers, toes, brain, nerves; heartbeat can be heard using a special instrument
Behavior: begins to move

9 Months
Length: 18–20 inches
Weight: 7–9 pounds
New Features: smooth skin
Behavior: eyes open, fingers can grasp, body organs and systems can work on their own

Care During Pregnancy

An expectant mother needs to create a healthy environment for her fetus. **Figure 6.9** lists ways she can do this. The mother must also take care of her own health needs. Many physiological and emotional changes occur during pregnancy, including weight gain, fatigue, and mood swings. These changes are normal.

Heredity

Traits such as eye color are inherited. Structures within cells influence heredity. **Chromosomes** (KROH·muh·sohmz) are *threadlike structures that carry the codes for inherited traits*. Almost all human cells contain 46 chromosomes in 23 pairs. Each chromosome is divided into small parts called genes. **Genes** are *the basic units of heredity*. Children inherit genes for each trait from each parent. This results in a particular set of inherited characteristics.

FIGURE 6.9

HEALTHY MOTHER, HEALTHY BABY

During pregnancy a mother can help ensure her fetus's good health.

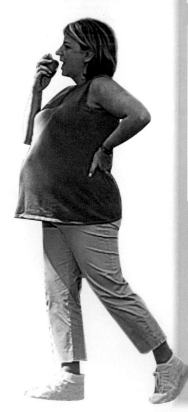

DO ✓

Eat Healthful Foods
The fetus's nourishment comes directly from its mother. A nutritious eating plan is essential to the health of both the mother and the fetus. ✓

Have Regular Checkups
A female should see a doctor as soon as she suspects that she is pregnant. If she is, the doctor will set up a schedule of appointments throughout the pregnancy to monitor both the mother's health and the fetus's development. ✓

Beware of Infections
Certain diseases such as rubella (German measles) and some sexually transmitted diseases pose severe danger to a fetus. A vaccine is available to protect against rubella. A doctor can explain how best to avoid other dangerous infections. ✓

DON'T ✓

Smoke or Use Tobacco
Chewing tobacco or inhaling tobacco smoke (even breathing in smoke from other people's cigarettes or cigars) can harm a developing fetus. ✓

Drink Alcohol
Any alcohol a pregnant female drinks enters the fetus's system. This can cause the fetus to develop many physical and mental problems; this is known as fetal alcohol syndrome or fetal alcohol effects. ✓

Take Any Unnecessary Drugs
All medicines, even those available without a prescription, can affect a developing fetus. A pregnant female should take medication only if absolutely necessary, and only with a doctor's approval. She should avoid all illegal drugs. ✓

Unlike other body cells, sperm and egg cells do not have 46 chromosomes. Each has 23 chromosomes. When the sperm and egg cells unite during fertilization, they produce an embryo that contains 46 chromosomes, as shown in **Figure 6.10** on page 172. The chromosomes in the sperm determine whether the child will be a boy or a girl. Each egg cell contains one X (female) chromosome. Each sperm cell contains either an X (female) or a Y (male) chromosome. An XX chromosome combination will produce a female child; an XY combination will produce a male child.

Hands-On Health

ANALYZING INHERITED TRAITS

Has anyone ever told you that you have "your mom's dimples" or "your dad's chin"? You share such traits with your family members because physical characteristics are inherited. Heredity can explain why you have a smooth or dimpled chin, attached or detached earlobes, and even the ability to roll your tongue!

WHAT YOU WILL NEED
- paper
- pen or pencil

WHAT YOU WILL DO
1. Survey ten people who are not related to you to see if they have any of the following five traits: attached earlobes, dimples, hitchhiker's thumb, widow's peak, or dimpled chin.
2. Ask the people in your survey whether one or both of their parents have any of these traits.
3. Make a table that includes a column for each trait and a row for each person you survey.
4. Fill in the table, making a check mark for each trait that is present next to the name of the person who has that trait. Write an *M* for mother, an *F* for father, or both an *M* and an *F* (if appropriate).

5. Share your findings with the class.

IN CONCLUSION
1. Which trait was most common among members of your study group? Which was the least common?
2. How often did you find that one or both parents also had a trait that your subject had? What can you conclude about heredity from this information?

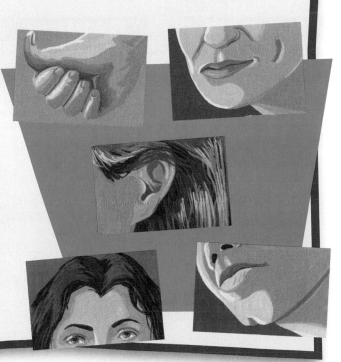

Genetic problems can cause serious disorders. Down syndrome, for example, is a genetic disorder in which a person's cells have 47 chromosomes instead of 46. Such disorders can affect physical or mental development, or both. Genetic disorders may be mild or severe; a few are fatal.

FIGURE 6.10

COMBINING CHROMOSOMES

During fertilization the sperm adds its 23 chromosomes to the 23 chromosomes in the egg to form an embryo that contains all 46 chromosomes.

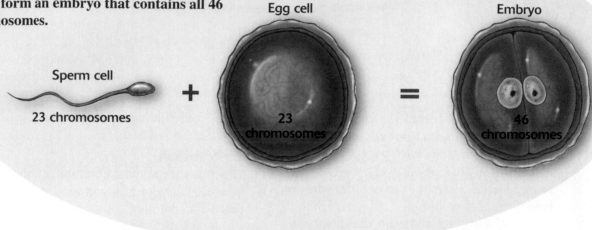

Sperm cell

23 chromosomes

+

Egg cell

23 chromosomes

=

Embryo

46 chromosomes

Lesson 4 Review

Using complete sentences, answer the following questions on a sheet of paper.

Reviewing Terms and Facts

1. **Vocabulary** Define the terms *cell* and *body system*.
2. **Distinguish** Explain the difference between an *embryo* and a *fetus*.
3. **Identify** List three ways in which a pregnant woman can help ensure her fetus's good health.
4. **Restate** Describe one physiological and one emotional change that occurs during pregnancy.

5. **Recall** Explain how chromosomes determine whether a child is male or female.

Thinking Critically

6. **Speculate** Why does a woman need to consume more calories while she is pregnant?
7. **Explain** Why should a woman be under a doctor's care while she is pregnant?

Applying Health Skills

8. **Advocacy** Research the effects of secondhand smoke—tobacco smoke in the air—on a developing fetus. What advice would you give to a pregnant woman who lives with someone who smokes?

Making the Most of Your Teen Years

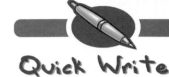

Changes Throughout Life

The teen years are a time of rapid changes. You'll see the effects of these changes in the way you look, the way you think and feel, and the way you interact with others. Adolescence is not the only time physical, mental/emotional, and social changes occur, however. Changes take place at all stages of the life cycle, beginning at birth.

Birth and Infancy

About nine full months after fertilization, a fetus is completely developed and ready to be born. During the birth process, the mother has strong contractions that push the baby out of her body.

Infancy (IN·fuhn·see), *the first year of life,* is a time of amazing growth. During infancy a baby's weight triples, and his or her size increases by half. Even before infants learn to sit, crawl, and stand, they participate actively in their world. They reach for objects. They smile and laugh. They imitate sounds and may say a few words.

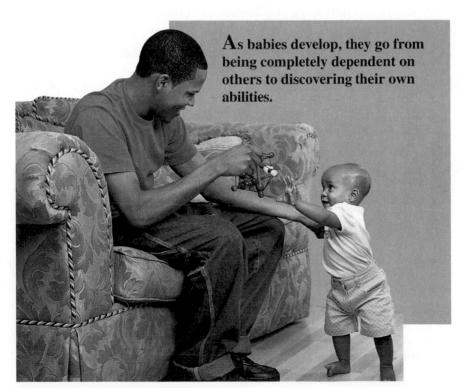

As babies develop, they go from being completely dependent on others to discovering their own abilities.

Quick Write

What are some common stereotypes people have about teens? Do you think that these ideas are fair or justified? Explain.

LEARN ABOUT...

- the stages of the life cycle.
- what it means to be an adult.
- the ways in which adolescence will prepare you for adulthood.

VOCABULARY

- infancy
- toddler
- preschooler

Childhood

After his or her first year, an infant enters a new stage of life as a toddler. A **toddler** is *a child between the ages of one and three.* Early childhood is an exciting time. Toddlers learn to walk, talk, and use the toilet. They learn that they can do many things for themselves. As they become independent, they begin to actively explore their surroundings. Toddlers are eager to master new tasks, and they take pride in their accomplishments.

A child between ages three and five is called a **preschooler.** Children at this stage rapidly develop physical and mental skills. Preschoolers like to sing and make up elaborate stories. They enjoy imitating their siblings and parents by playing "dress-up" and using toy versions of kitchen equipment, tools, and telephones.

Children continue to develop during a stage called late childhood, the period between ages 6 and 11. This is a time when children go to school, expand their knowledge, and strengthen their social skills. Interaction with friends becomes more and more important. **Figure 6.11** shows the stages of life from birth through adulthood.

Adolescence and Adulthood

Except for infancy, at no time during your life do you grow and change as much as you do during adolescence. The physical, mental/emotional, and social changes you experience during your teen years serve as a bridge from childhood to adulthood. The decisions you make now, such as eating healthful foods; engaging in sports or other physical activity; and avoiding tobacco, alcohol, and other drugs, will affect the person you become as an adult.

FIGURE 6.11

FROM BIRTH THROUGH ADULTHOOD

At all stages of the life cycle, people learn, change, and develop. The ages shown here are approximate; people move through these stages at their own pace.

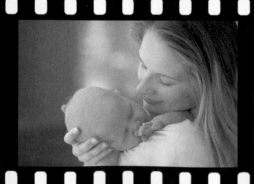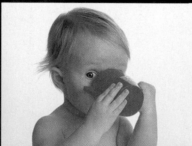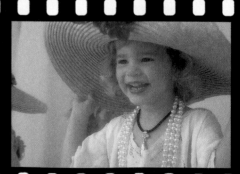

Infancy (birth to age 1) During this period infants develop trust and are dependent on others.

Early Childhood (ages 1-3) In the toddler years children learn that they can do simple tasks without help.

Middle Childhood (ages 3-5) Increased mental skills during the preschool period give children the ability to play make-believe and imitate real-life situations.

The early adulthood stage begins at age 19. Adulthood is a time of increased independence, but it is also a time to develop deeper relationships with others. You will meet many kinds of people, some of whom may not share your values and views of life. Maintaining your sense of identity and personal beliefs will help you interact with others and solve problems. Most people begin a career in their twenties, and some choose to marry and start a family.

People in their thirties, forties, and fifties are in their middle adult years. During these years most adults concentrate on their jobs and children. They may take classes to gain new skills.

In late adulthood some people look forward to retirement. Others may be continuing their careers or starting new ones. Many people in their mid-sixties and beyond also take this time to volunteer in their communities, develop new hobbies, or travel.

The life cycle of a human being includes the aging process, dying, and death. It is important for families to talk about dying and death, as they are a natural part of the life cycle.

Preparing for Adulthood

The changes you go through as an adolescent prepare you for adulthood. Changes in your thinking abilities will lead you to consider more factors when you face complex situations. You begin to ask yourself "what if" questions: What if I skip breakfast? What if I fix up my old bike instead of buying a new one? Asking yourself questions about the consequences of your actions will help you make safe and healthful choices.

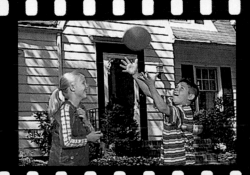

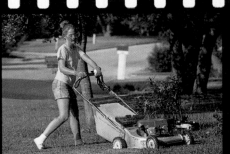

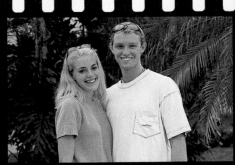

Late Childhood (ages 6-11) In this stage children begin to interact more with their peers. They gain mastery over objects and activities.

Adolescence (ages 12-18) During this period teens take on greater responsibility and begin to develop their adult personalities.

Adulthood (age 19 and onward) During adulthood people work to develop relationships, to achieve goals, and to understand the meaning of their lives.

Reducing Risk

Making the most of your teen years requires you to think ahead and consider the consequences of possible decisions. Follow the strategies below to reduce the risk of injury and illness.

- **Keep yourself safe from injuries.** Always wear a safety belt when riding in a car. Practice safety at home. The most common causes of accidental death in the home are falls, fires, and poisoning. Wear appropriate protective gear to participate in a sport.
- **Protect your body and mind from illegal drugs.** Using marijuana, Ecstasy, cocaine, and other illegal drugs can cause serious damage to your developing body and mind.
- **Protect your mouth, throat, and lungs from tobacco.** Smoking or chewing tobacco products of any kind can cause many health problems, especially cancer.
- **Protect yourself from alcohol.** Drinking alcohol can seriously harm your digestive system and your liver. Alcohol also affects your judgment and slows down your reflexes.
- **Practice abstinence to protect yourself from sexually transmitted diseases, pregnancy, and emotional trauma.** Becoming sexually active creates the risk of contracting HIV or other sexually transmitted diseases. Moreover, as a teen, you're not ready to become a parent.

HEALTH SKILLS ACTIVITY

DECISION MAKING

Developing New Interests

Brianna is excited by the idea of learning to play the guitar this year. However, she is wondering how taking lessons will affect her life. She thinks: "My music teacher says I have some musical talent. Learning to play the guitar will put that talent to good use and could be fun. Will I, however, have enough time to take lessons and handle my responsibilities at home and at school? What if the guitar lessons get to be too hard? Will I want to continue if I don't feel like I'm doing a good job?" She asks her parents for advice. They feel that she should decide for herself. Should she take guitar lessons this year?

WHAT WOULD YOU DO?

Apply the six steps of the decision-making process to Brianna's situation. Explain to the class how you arrived at your decision.

1. **STATE THE SITUATION.**
2. **LIST THE OPTIONS.**
3. **WEIGH THE POSSIBLE OUTCOMES.**
4. **CONSIDER VALUES.**
5. **MAKE A DECISION AND ACT.**
6. **EVALUATE THE DECISION.**

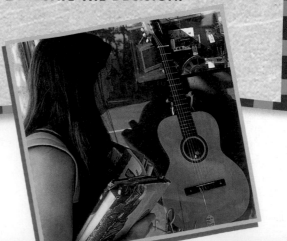

Moving Toward the Future

You will grow and develop in many new ways during your teen years. The experiences you have and the knowledge you gain as a teen will help you deal with the challenges of adulthood. An interest you have now may later blossom into a satisfying career. Your teen years open the door to your future. In the coming years you will

- learn to accept your body and its characteristics.
- develop self-confidence and discover what makes you unique.
- become more independent in your thoughts and feelings.
- learn to solve problems and make decisions in a mature way.
- learn to accept responsibility for your actions.
- establish more mature relationships.
- develop a greater interest in, and awareness of, your community and the world.
- plan for your future beyond high school.

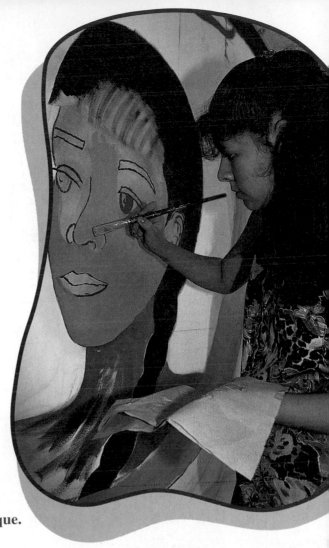

In adolescence you will make exciting discoveries about who you are and what makes you unique.

Lesson 5 Review

Using complete sentences, answer the following questions on a sheet of paper.

Reviewing Terms and Facts

1. **Vocabulary** Define the term *infancy*. Then name two ways in which a baby changes during that time.
2. **Distinguish** Explain the difference between a *toddler* and a *preschooler*.
3. **Recall** Identify three actions you can take to reduce your risk of injury and illness.

Thinking Critically

4. **Analyze** What are some specific ways in which parents can help their children move successfully through the stages of childhood?
5. **Evaluate** Trust is learned in infancy. How important do you think trust is in adolescence? Explain your answer.

Applying Health Skills

6. **Refusal Skills** With one of your classmates, role-play a situation in which you use refusal skills to say no to someone who is trying to convince you to do something that would harm your health, such as smoking cigarettes or becoming sexually active.

Food for the Heart

How can you keep your heart pumping strong far into the future? Feed it right!

You've heard the saying: You are what you eat. Take time to consider a new twist on that old saying: You *will be* what you eat. Healthy growth and development depend on a solid nutritional foundation. In other words, eating nutritious foods now will keep you healthy in the years to come.

According to the American Heart Association (AHA), all we have to do is look inside our hearts (literally) for a solid example of how food can make us stronger.

Know What You Eat by Heart

The AHA has released recommendations on what we should be eating to keep our hearts healthy. This time the AHA played down confusing numbers and complicated percentages. They focused instead on plain old foods—fruits, vegetables, beans, whole grains, and fish—that will help most Americans prevent heart disease, high blood pressure, and stroke.

Some AHA Guidelines

The AHA now recommends that people eat at least two 3-ounce servings of fatty fish (tuna, salmon, mackerel) a week. The type of fatty acids found in these fish, known as omega-3 fatty acids, appears to protect against heart disease. Canned tuna, salmon, and sardines all count—so this kind of fish is easy to include in your eating plan.

Limit the amount of trans fatty acids in your diet. Trans fatty acids are found in anything that contains partially hydrogenated oil, such as many prepared baked goods, fast foods, and some margarines. Consuming excess amounts of trans fatty acids has been linked to an increased risk of heart disease.

High-protein diets may work in the short run, but there's no evidence that they lead to lasting weight loss or improve your health. In fact, many high-protein foods are also high in saturated fat, which can increase the risk of heart disease.

Weight Loss = Heart Wins

Of course, even with such basic guidelines from the AHA, portion control is still critical. To get maximum benefit from any eating plan, you need to limit what you consume and make sure you don't take in more calories than your body can burn.

If you do need to lose weight, don't try to drop too much weight too fast. Aim for no more than 1 pound a week. It takes patience, but such slow progress is safer than crash dieting and more likely to produce lasting results. ■

EAT MORE

Like any other healthy eating recommendations, the AHA guidelines emphasize certain foods. However, any food, if eaten to excess, can harm your health. Here's a checklist to live by:

FRUITS AND VEGETABLES Apples, pears, oranges, peas, and broccoli are just a few examples of these nutritional powerhouses. Fruits and vegetables are chock-full of nutrients and fiber. Try to eat at least five servings a day.

GRAINS These include breads, cereals, rolled oats, rice, and pasta. Choose mostly whole grains, and aim for about six servings a day. An eating plan rich in grains (particularly whole grains) can decrease the risk of heart disease.

DAIRY PRODUCTS Milk, yogurt, cottage cheese, and other dairy products contain bone-building calcium. Stick to low-fat or fat-free dairy products—the whole-fat versions contain too much saturated fat, which is linked to the development of heart disease.

PROTEIN Beans, fish, skinless poultry, and lean meats are all good sources of protein. Six ounces a day is usually enough to keep muscles and tissues healthy.

FATS AND OILS Olives, walnuts, canola oil, and sunflower oil are some examples. Eaten in moderation, they can, among other things, reduce the risk of heart disease by boosting levels of high-density lipoprotein (HDL), the "good" cholesterol.

TIME TO THINK...

About Eating for Your Future

In small groups, choose a body organ, such as the brain or the stomach. Using reliable online and print resources, research what foods might promote the health of that organ. Create a menu that features those foods. Present your menu to the class and explain how the foods benefit the health of your chosen organ.

SAYING NO TO SEXUAL ACTIVITY

Model

During the teen years, positive and rewarding friendships are essential. Teens need time to grow and develop without the health risks of early sexual activity.

Dylan and Ashley really like one another. On Friday night Ashley plans to have dinner with Dylan and his dad. Then Dylan's dad is supposed to drop them off at the movies with some friends. Just before Ashley is supposed to arrive, however, Dylan's dad calls to say that he's stuck at work. As Dylan hangs up the phone, Ashley arrives. Dylan explains the situation. Ashley suggests that they hang out until his dad gets home. Dylan thinks for a minute and then replies, "No. Let's see if Oscar and Dana want to meet us at the pizza place. That way, we won't put ourselves in a bad situation." Ashley agrees. They call Oscar and Dana and agree to meet. Dylan calls his dad to let him know. Later, Dylan's dad drives the group to the movies.

Practice

In a small group, read the following situations. Then discuss how you could say no using S.T.O.P. Share your solutions with the class.

Situation 1: *You have permission from your parents to spend time with someone you care about. After a few months, this person begins pressuring you to engage in sexual activity.*

Situation 2: *You are at the local library studying with your boyfriend or girlfriend. You have been seeing each other for several weeks and really like spending time together. Your girlfriend or boyfriend says, "Let's go over to my house and listen to some CDs. No one is home, and we could be alone for a change."*

Apply/Assess

Divide into groups of three or four students. Analyze and list reasons why it is important for teens to abstain from sexual activity. Choose from the following categories: personal reasons and values, relationship reasons, financial reasons, and social reasons. Then work with your group to write scenarios that show teens refusing to become sexually active. Use the reasons you've listed as well as S.T.O.P. to show why and how the teens are refusing to become sexually active.

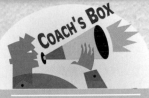

COACH'S BOX

Refusal Skills

S.T.O.P. is an easy way to remember how to use refusal skills.
S Say no in a firm voice.
T Tell why not.
O Offer another idea.
P Promptly leave.

Self-✓ Check

- Did our group list several reasons why teens should abstain from sexual activity?
- Did our scenarios show teens refusing to become sexually active by using S.T.O.P.?
- Did our scenarios include the reasons we came up with?

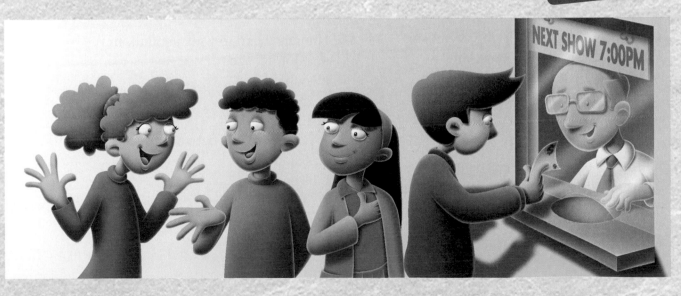

CHAPTER 6 ASSESSMENT

After You Read

Use your completed Foldable to review the information on the changes of adolescence.

FOLDABLES™
Study Organizer

Reviewing Vocabulary and Concepts

On a sheet of paper, write the numbers 1–6. After each number, write the term from the list that best completes each statement.

- metabolism
- pituitary
- hormones
- reproduction
- sperm
- endocrine

Lesson 1

1. _____ are chemicals that help to regulate the way your body functions.

2. The _____ system consists of glands that regulate body functions.

3. The _____ gland is located at the base of the brain.

4. The process by which your body gets energy from food is called _____.

Lesson 2

5. The process by which living organisms produce others of their own kind is _____.

6. _____ are the male reproductive cells.

Lesson 3

On a sheet of paper, write the numbers 7–10. Write *True* or *False* for each statement below. If the statement is false, change the underlined word or phrase to make it true.

7. The flow of the uterine lining material from the body is <u>reproduction</u>.

8. At puberty, the <u>testes</u> start to release eggs.

9. A fertilized egg grows in the <u>uterus</u>.

10. A <u>gynecologist</u> is a doctor who specializes in the female reproductive system.

On a sheet of paper, write the numbers 11–15. After each number, write the letter of the answer that best completes each statement.

Lesson 4

11. A tissue is
- **a.** a developing child.
- **b.** a group of similar cells that do a particular job.
- **c.** a group of organs working together to carry out related tasks.
- **d.** the basic unit of heredity.

12. The basic units of heredity are
- **a.** genes.
- **b.** cells.
- **c.** chromosomes.
- **d.** embryos.

13. A body part made up of different tissues joined together to perform a function is called a(n)
- **a.** chromosome.
- **b.** fetus.
- **c.** body system.
- **d.** organ.

Lesson 5

14. Humans learn to walk and talk in
- **a.** adolescence.
- **b.** puberty.
- **c.** childhood.
- **d.** infancy.

15. A preschooler is between the ages of
- **a.** 6 and 11.
- **b.** 1 and 3.
- **c.** 3 and 5.
- **d.** 12 and 18.

Thinking Critically

Using complete sentences, answer the following questions on a sheet of paper.

16. **Explain** How do the changes of adolescence prepare you for adulthood?
17. **Apply** How can a teen use effective communication skills to discuss with parents or other trusted adults the changes that occur during adolescence?
18. **Summarize** Describe the life cycle of human beings, including birth, dying, and death.

Career Corner

Pediatrician Babies and children grow so fast. Pediatricians help keep track of this rapid growth and development. These professionals are medical doctors who specialize in the care of children from birth to 14 years of age. To become a pediatrician, you'll need a four-year college degree, four years of medical school, and one to seven years of residency training. Visit Career Corner at health.glencoe.com to learn more about this and other health careers.

Standardized Test Practice

Math

Read the data table below and then answer the questions.

The table below lists the average size of a fetus at the end of each month of development.

Growth of a Fetus	
Months After Fertilization	Size (cm)
1	0.6
2	4
3	7.5
4	15
5	25
6	30
7	35
8	40
9	51

1. Which type of graph would *least* likely be used to represent these data on the growth of the fetus?
   - **A** bar graph
   - **B** circle graph
   - **C** line graph
   - **D** histogram

2. How many more centimeters did the fetus grow from 8 to 9 months than from 3 to 4 months?
   - **A** 3.5 cm
   - **B** 5.5 cm
   - **C** 7.5 cm
   - **D** 9.5 cm

3. Explain in words the patterns in growth rate seen in the data table.

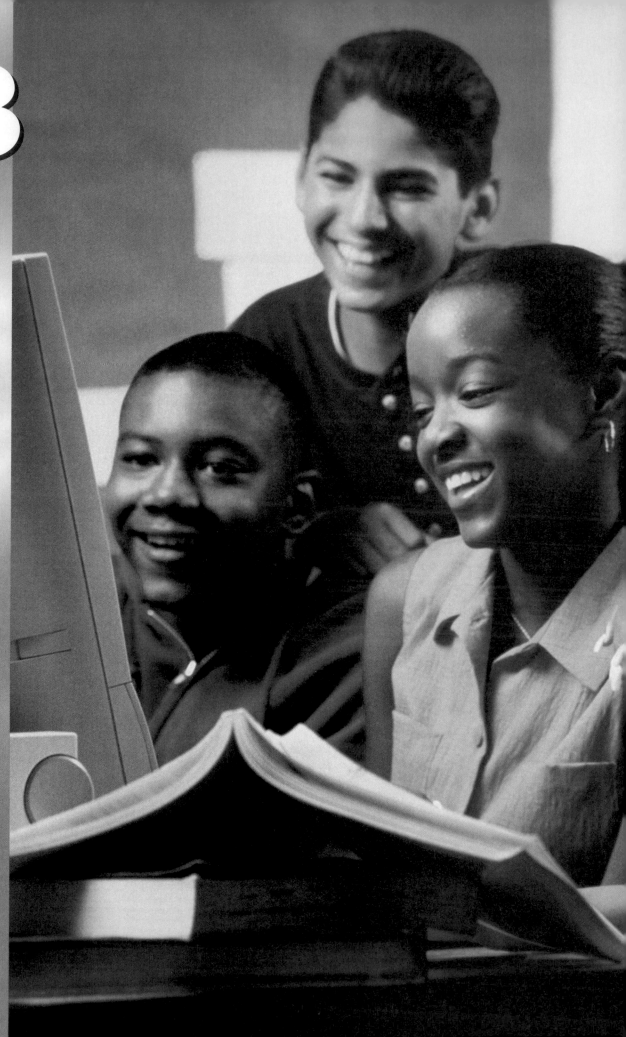

3

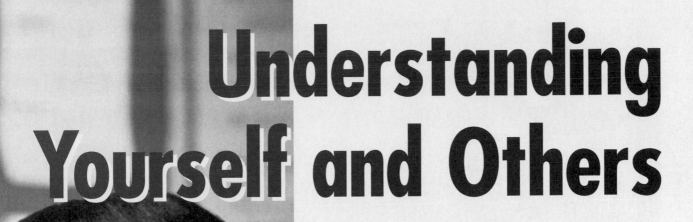

Understanding Yourself and Others

HEALTH in Action

How is your community like a computer network?

Working together is the key to success, for people as well as computers in a network. Your parents or guardians, family members, friends, teachers, and other trusted members of your community are there to offer help when you need it—just as you can be there to offer help when it's needed. Communicating clearly, resolving conflicts, and respecting yourself and the needs of others keep all systems running smoothly!

CHAPTER 7

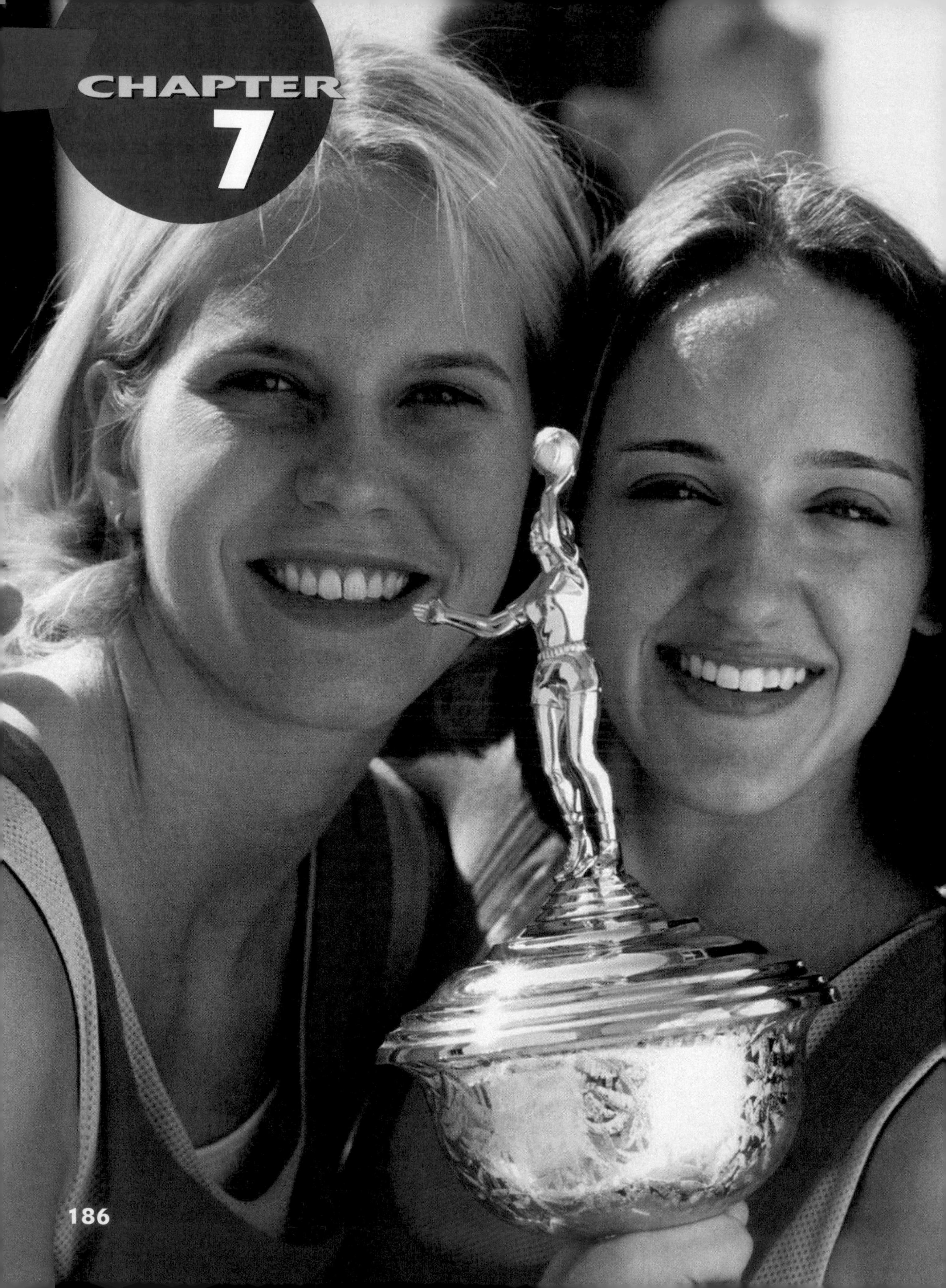

Mental and Emotional Health

HEALTH *Online*

Go to health.glencoe.com and take the Health Inventory for Chapter 7 to evaluate your mental and emotional health.

FOLDABLES™ Study Organizer

Before You Read

Make this Foldable to help you record what you learn about mental/emotional health in Lesson 1. Begin with a plain sheet of 8½″ × 11″ paper.

Step 1

Line up one of the short edges of the sheet of paper with one of the long edges to form a triangle. Fold and cut off the leftover rectangle.

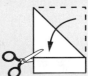

Step 2

Fold the triangle in half, and unfold. The folds will form an X dividing four equal sections.

Step 3

Cut up one fold line and stop in the middle. This forms two triangular flaps. Draw an X on one tab, and label the other three as shown.

Step 4

Fold the X flap under the other flap, and glue together to make a three-sided pyramid.

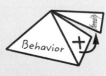

As You Read

Take notes on the three factors that shape personality.

What Is Mental and Emotional Health?

Quick Write

Do you view disappointments as a part of life or do you tend to dwell on them? Write a short paragraph explaining how you deal with disappointments.

LEARN ABOUT...

- the characteristics of good mental and emotional health.
- the factors that shape your personality.
- the advantages of a positive self-concept and high self-esteem.
- developing good mental and emotional health.

VOCABULARY

- mental and emotional health
- resilient
- personality
- self-concept
- self-esteem
- empathy

Understanding Mental and Emotional Health

This chapter focuses on your mental and emotional health. **Mental and emotional health** is *your ability to deal in a reasonable way with the stresses and changes of daily life.* People who are in good mental and emotional health usually

- have a positive attitude and outlook on life.
- accept their limitations and set realistic goals.
- have a positive view of themselves and others.
- are **resilient**, or *able to bounce back from a disappointment, difficulty, or crisis.*
- act responsibly at school, at home, and in social situations.
- are aware of their feelings and are able to express those feelings in healthy ways.
- accept constructive feedback—messages that evaluate a person and his or her actions—without becoming angry.

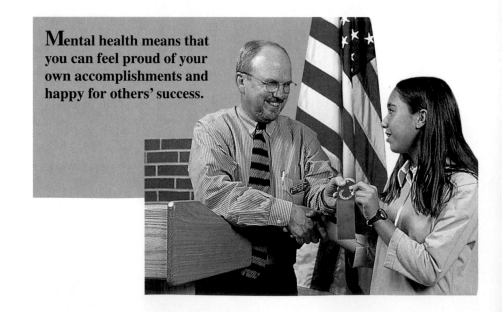

Mental health means that you can feel proud of your own accomplishments and happy for others' success.

Understanding Who You Are

Part of good mental and emotional health is understanding and accepting yourself. This means that you recognize your strengths and work to improve your weaknesses. Good mental and emotional health also means that you recognize that you are a unique individual.

Have you ever thought about the characteristics you have that make you different from everyone else? These characteristics form your personality. **Personality** is *a special mix of traits, feelings, attitudes, and habits.* It plays a key role in your mental and emotional health. Your personality is unique; it makes you who you are.

Factors That Shape Your Personality

Many factors influence your personality, but the three most important are heredity, environment, and behavior. To some extent these factors will continue to shape you throughout your life. Although you have no control over your heredity and probably have little control over your environment, you *can* control your behavior. You can decide which of your qualities to focus on and whether to try to improve situations when possible. You can make decisions that will positively affect your health and demonstrate good character. In short, you can decide how to *act.*

HEALTH SKILLS ACTIVITY

ANALYZING INFLUENCES

What Shapes Your Personality?

Your personality includes your attitudes, thoughts, feelings, and other traits. Many aspects of your personality can be traced to particular factors, such as heredity, environment, and behavior.

- Heredity is the passing on of traits from your parents. You inherit features such as your height; body type; and the color of your skin, hair, and eyes.
- Environment is your surroundings. Your community, family, friends, role models, and experiences, as well as the media and technology, are all part of your environment.

- Behavior is the way you act in the many different situations in your life. How you take care of yourself, how you show you care for others, and whether your actions reflect core ethical values all shape your personality.

ON YOUR OWN

List ten of your personality traits. Then make a chart with three columns, headed heredity, environment, and behavior. In each column, write which of your personality traits reflect that influence. You may list a trait in more than one column.

Understanding Self-Concept

Think about how you would describe yourself. Are you confident, fun to be with, intelligent, honest? Your description paints a picture of how you view yourself and how you believe that others view you. *The view that you have of yourself* is called your **self-concept**. You may have a realistic self-concept—a fairly accurate awareness of your strengths and weaknesses. Some teens, however, have unrealistic self-concepts. Unfortunately, they may focus only on what they see as their faults, usually exaggerating them.

The ways in which people act toward you can reinforce the view you have of yourself. A person who receives support and love tends to develop a positive self-concept. A person who is neglected or criticized often tends to develop a negative self-concept.

FIGURE 7.1

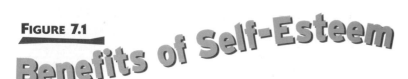
Benefits of Self-Esteem

A high level of self-esteem benefits your total health.

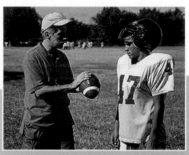

Accepting constructive feedback You can accept and learn from constructive feedback.

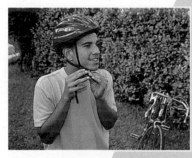

Respecting your health and the health of others
When you respect yourself, you pay attention to your health, safety, and appearance.

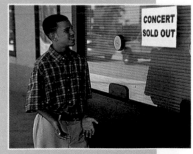

Seeing the positive side
When negative events occur, you have a positive attitude and outlook.

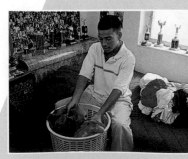

Showing responsibility
You accept responsibility for yourself and act responsibly toward others.

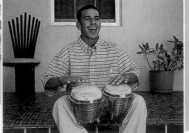

Having self-confidence You believe in your abilities and are willing to try new activities, even if you do not always succeed.

Your Self-Esteem and Self-Confidence

One factor that is closely related to your self-concept is self-esteem. **Self-esteem** is *the confidence and pride you have in yourself.* The way you feel about your body, your mind, your emotions, and your interactions with others are all part of your self-esteem. Some of the benefits of high self-esteem are shown in **Figure 7.1** on page 190. High self-esteem enhances *self-confidence*—your belief in your strengths and abilities.

Your self-esteem, like your self-concept, comes from positive and negative messages that you receive from others. It is also affected by messages you send to yourself. Negative messages you send to yourself can block out positive messages from others.

Developing Mental and Emotional Health

People with high self-esteem are more likely to practice good health habits and avoid harmful behaviors. You can work to improve self-esteem.

Improving Self-Esteem and Self-Confidence

Sometimes you'll have low self-esteem. These times usually don't last long. However, if you find that you feel unworthy most of the time, talk with a trusted adult, such as a parent, a religious leader, or a school counselor. To build your self-esteem and self-confidence, try these lifetime strategies:

- **Set realistic goals for yourself.** Meeting a goal takes planning and effort. Break down long-term goals into short-term goals. This will help you see that you are making progress.
- **Recognize your strengths.** Make a list of what you're good at, and work to develop new skills. Recognize and accept your limitations, too—no one is perfect.
- **Ask for help when you need it.** When you are trying to learn something new, accept your limitations and find someone who can help you reach your goal.
- **Learn to accept constructive feedback.** Try to focus on the problem and not to take the criticism personally. Listen carefully, and ask questions if you need to.
- **Learn from your mistakes and failures, but don't dwell on them.** Take responsibility for your actions, and don't be afraid to admit when you are wrong. Look at mistakes as opportunities to grow and improve.
- **Develop positive character traits.** Personal characteristics that contribute to self-esteem and self-confidence include being honest, having *integrity* (standing by your values), being responsible, and respecting the dignity of others.

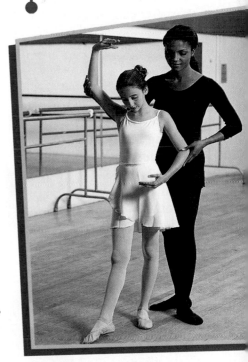

Learning to accept constructive feedback can help you improve your skills and your self-esteem. *Describe a technique for responding appropriately to constructive feedback.*

Respecting Individual Differences

You can boost your own mental health by showing respect for people's individual differences. Here are some strategies: Try to avoid judging people according to your own culture, environment, age, and background. Recognize that, in addition to core ethical values, people have values that have been formed by their families, personal experiences, and other sources. Appreciate the qualities that make individuals unique. Following these strategies will enhance your relationships and your health.

An important part of respecting others is showing empathy. **Empathy** is *the ability to identify and share another person's feelings.* When you are making a decision that might affect someone else or are thinking about what to say to someone, try to consider the other person's views and feelings.

Another strategy for showing respect for others is to focus on their strengths, not their weaknesses. This positive view will benefit your mental and emotional health as well as theirs.

FIGURE 7.2

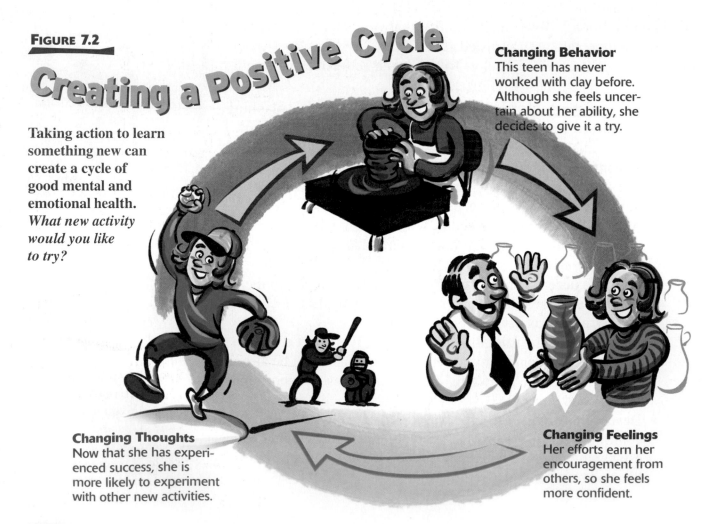

Creating a Positive Cycle

Taking action to learn something new can create a cycle of good mental and emotional health. *What new activity would you like to try?*

Changing Behavior
This teen has never worked with clay before. Although she feels uncertain about her ability, she decides to give it a try.

Changing Feelings
Her efforts earn her encouragement from others, so she feels more confident.

Changing Thoughts
Now that she has experienced success, she is more likely to experiment with other new activities.

Attitudes and Behavior

Your attitudes and behavior affect your mental and emotional health. The effects can be beneficial when positive attitudes lead you to practice behaviors that promote your health. For instance, if you see obstacles in your life as challenges that you can conquer, you are probably successful at getting past bumps in the road to reach the goals you set for yourself. On the other hand, negative thoughts and feelings may lead you to behave in ways that harm your mental and emotional health. For example, if you think you can't do anything well, you may avoid trying new activities. This may deepen your belief that you're no good at anything. **Figure 7.2** on page 192 shows how you can learn to approach challenges in a positive way. This attitude will help you the next time you encounter a problem. Others may notice your positive attitude and work to improve their own.

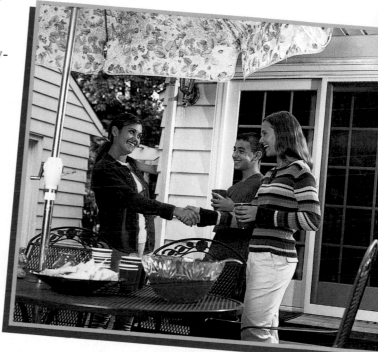

Try approaching new situations with a positive attitude. *How can a positive attitude help you when you meet new people?*

Lesson 1 Review

Using complete sentences, answer the following questions on a sheet of paper.

Reviewing Terms and Facts

1. **Vocabulary** Define *mental and emotional health.* What are three characteristics of a person who is in good mental and emotional health?
2. **List** What are the three most important factors that shape personality?
3. **Explain** What is a *self-concept?*
4. **Identify** Name four ways to build self-esteem and self-confidence.
5. **Recall** Describe strategies for showing respect for individual differences, including age differences.

Thinking Critically

6. **Analyze** Why do you think your attitude toward other people affects your mental and emotional health?
7. **Describe** How can practicing health-promoting behaviors be a positive way to gain attention from others?

Applying Health Skills

8. **Communication Skills** Think of a caring adult who has been important in your life and has given you encouragement. Write a letter to thank this person for caring. Explain in the letter how this encouragement has affected your self-concept and self-esteem.

Your Emotions

Quick Write

Do people usually know when you are happy, angry, or sad? What do you do that lets people know how you feel?

LEARN ABOUT...

- the different types of emotions.
- how to express emotions in a healthy way.
- ways to cope with loss.

VOCABULARY

- emotions

Understanding Your Emotions

Think about what you're feeling right now. Are you happy, sad, nervous, or excited? Perhaps you are experiencing several different emotions. **Emotions** are *feelings such as love, joy, or fear.* Your emotions affect every aspect of your health and well-being.

Emotions themselves are not positive or negative, although you may find them scary or unpleasant sometimes. All the emotions you have are normal. Although you can't stop yourself from feeling emotions, you can figure out healthy ways to deal with them.

Recognizing Your Emotions

Before you can manage and express your emotions in positive ways, you need to recognize what you feel. That sense of accomplishment you feel after making the honor roll could be pride. That queasy feeling as you think about an upcoming test may be anxiety. Although you can often identify emotions such as happiness, sadness, anger, fear, and love, you may sometimes find that many different emotions are tangled up together. When that happens, stop and think about what you are feeling and why. Then you can begin to deal with your emotions.

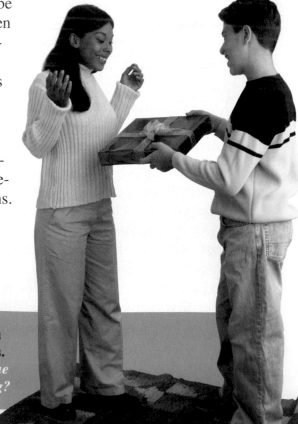

Your emotions change as you encounter different situations. *What emotions do you think the teens in this picture are feeling?*

Expressing Your Emotions

Everyone reacts differently to certain situations. Where you may react to disappointment by becoming quiet, your friend might cry. Often you express emotions in the same ways that family members do. Some people have no difficulty talking about their feelings. Others may reveal their emotions in subtle ways through their body language. For example, you may know that your teammate is nervous because of his hunched shoulders and clenched teeth. No matter how you have been taught to manage your emotions, you can learn to express them in healthy ways. You can even learn to manage strong emotions such as fear or anger.

Dealing with Fear and Anger

Fear and anger can be unpleasant emotions to experience. Both feelings can lead to harmful behaviors if you do not manage them effectively. To manage fear, try talking about it. Try to laugh, relax, or plan ahead of time how you will deal with a situation that frightens you. To handle anger in a healthful way, take a deep breath and calm down. Focus on what made you angry, and think of how to express your true feelings. If you are angry with someone, calmly tell that person how you feel. If you are angry about a situation, talk it over with a parent or other trusted adult, or with a friend.

Reading Check
Identify main ideas. Find the sentence that best tells the idea in each paragraph on these two pages.

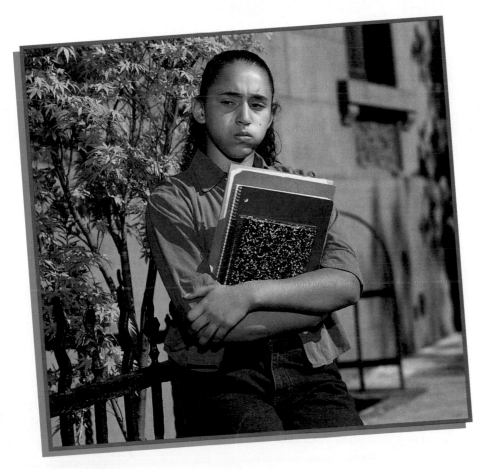

Taking a moment to take a deep breath or count to ten can help you deal with anger. *How do you manage feelings of anger?*

COMMUNICATION SKILLS

Standing Up to Bullies

Mei's classmates always make fun of a new student who speaks with an accent. She feels that it isn't right to pick on someone for being different. She has also seen the new student crying after being teased. Mei is afraid that if she says anything to her classmates, the teasing will become even worse, or the bullies may start picking on her.

What Would You Do?

Suppose that you are Mei and that you have decided to speak to one of your classmates about your concern. List the points you want to communicate. With a partner, role-play the situation, using speaking and listening skills. Then switch roles.

SPEAKING SKILLS
- Think before you speak.
- Use "I" messages.
- Be direct, but avoid being rude or insulting.
- Make eye contact and use appropriate body language.

LISTENING SKILLS
- Use conversation encouragers.
- Pay attention.
- Show empathy.
- Avoid interrupting, but ask questions when appropriate.

Coping with Change

Everyone experiences change—it is a part of life. Changes often have positive results, but each one also involves some type of loss. Sometimes the loss you experience causes you to feel grief or sorrow.

Although the emotions associated with grief may be unpleasant, they all have value and can help you come to terms with your loss. In order to do this, you need to experience and work through emotions such as hurt, anger, and fear. Ignoring them will not help you overcome them. Below are emotional and physical reactions involved in the grieving process:

- **Shock and denial.** You refuse to accept the reality of the loss.
- **Anger and resentment.** You are angry about the loss, and you may direct your anger at other people.
- **Hurt.** You feel mental and emotional pain over the loss.
- **Inadequacy.** You feel that you cannot deal with the loss.
- **Fear and anxiety.** You feel afraid.
- **Guilt.** You blame yourself for the loss or feel that you could have done something to prevent it.
- **Depression.** You feel intense sadness.
- **Physical symptoms.** You feel ill.
- **Acceptance.** You accept the reality of the loss, adjust to it, and make peace with yourself and others.

Avoiding Unhealthful Behaviors

When teens become confused by their emotions, they may deal with their feelings in unhealthful ways. Their fear, sense of rejection, sadness, or boredom may lead them to use drugs or alcohol, strike out at others, overeat or refuse to eat, or engage in other risk behaviors. Teens with low self-esteem may be especially in danger of making unhealthful choices when faced with confusing emotions. In turn, their self-esteem plunges even lower. These unhealthful behaviors can also damage other areas of their physical, mental/emotional, and social health.

If you have engaged in risk behaviors, remember that it is never too late to change. When you need to blow off steam or combat boredom, try exercising or talking to a friend. Writing in a journal can sometimes help you figure out what you feel and why. Doing volunteer work or taking up a new hobby can help you redirect your emotion into positive activities. These coping strategies can also help you maintain a positive attitude, which will help you the next time your feelings upset you.

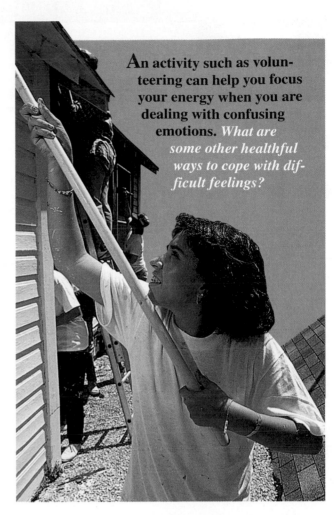

An activity such as volunteering can help you focus your energy when you are dealing with confusing emotions. *What are some other healthful ways to cope with difficult feelings?*

Lesson 2 Review

Using complete sentences, answer the following questions on a sheet of paper.

Reviewing Terms and Facts

1. **Vocabulary** Define the term *emotions*.
2. **Recall** Describe a strategy for managing anger effectively.
3. **Identify** What are the emotional and physical reactions of people who are experiencing grief?

Thinking Critically

4. **Apply** What coping strategies would you suggest to a person who uses alcohol or other drugs to deal with anger or fear?

5. **Analyze** Describe two methods of communicating emotions constructively.

Applying Health Skills

6. **Accessing Information** Find out about support groups in your community for people who have gone through significant changes in their lives, such as moving to a new area. What kinds of groups are available? How do they help people deal with change? Write a short report on your findings.

Managing Stress

Quick Write

List three sources of stress in your life. Next to each source, name the physical and emotional signs that tell you that this is a source of stress.

LEARN ABOUT...

- sources of stress.
- how people respond to stress.
- healthy ways of managing stress.

VOCABULARY

- distress
- eustress
- stressor
- adrenaline
- fatigue
- physical fatigue
- psychological fatigue
- coping skills

What Is Stress?

Stress is a part of life. Major events can cause stress, and so can everyday irritations such as missing a bus. Stress is your body's response to changes around you. Stress can have a negative effect on individual and family health. For example, you may get a stomachache because you are worried about an upcoming event. Negative stress, or **distress**, is *stress that prevents you from doing what you need to do or that causes you discomfort.*

Some stress is considered positive. Positive stress, or **eustress** (YOO·stres), is *stress that can help you to accomplish goals.* Think about how you feel before a big game or when you are about to perform in the school band. You're excited, challenged, and motivated—this is eustress.

Everyone experiences different sources of distress and eustress. For example, one person may be distressed by the idea of having to speak in public, whereas another might enjoy it. Moreover, people react to different **stressors**, or *triggers of stress.* **Figure 7.3** lists some common sources of stress.

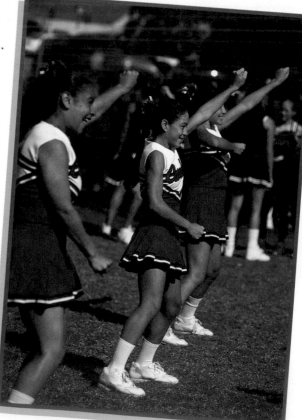

Any change or major event, even one that is generally considered positive, can cause your body to experience stress. *What positive events in your life have been sources of stress?*

FIGURE 7.3

SOURCES OF STRESS

Some events are definitely more stressful than others. You may react
to a specific stressor differently from the way your friend would.
*How are emotions and stress related? How might stress affect personal
and family health?*

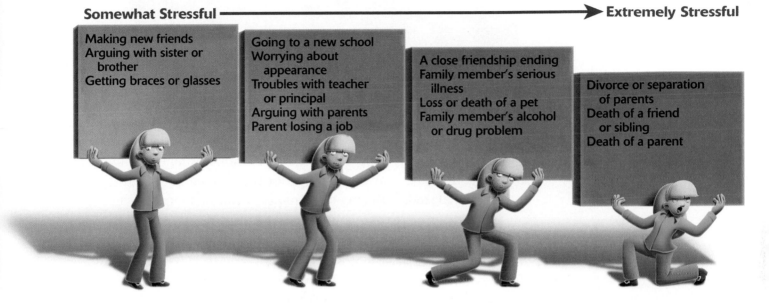

Somewhat Stressful ———————————————————→ **Extremely Stressful**

Making new friends
Arguing with sister or
  brother
Getting braces or glasses

Going to a new school
Worrying about
  appearance
Troubles with teacher
  or principal
Arguing with parents
Parent losing a job

A close friendship ending
Family member's serious
  illness
Loss or death of a pet
Family member's alcohol
  or drug problem

Divorce or separation
  of parents
Death of a friend
  or sibling
Death of a parent

The Stress Response

Your body cannot tell the difference between distress and eustress. Because your body responds to every change, any change—
negative or positive—causes stress. Anticipating your first
performance in the school play can be a stressor. Figuring out how
to manage your time so that you can study for a test and attend
softball tryouts can be another.

Your body responds to stressors by getting ready to act. This response is called the "fight-or-flight" response because your body
prepares to fight the stressor or flee from it. One part of this reaction is the release of adrenaline into your bloodstream. **Adrenaline**
(uh·DRE·nuhl·in) is *a hormone that increases the level of sugar in
your blood, thereby giving your body extra energy.* The following
list explains some other physical responses to a stressor.

- More blood is directed to your muscles and brain.
- Your heart beats faster.
- Your muscles tighten up and are ready for action.
- Your senses sharpen. You become more alert.
- Your air passages widen so that you can take in more air.

Reading Check

Understand *adrenaline*.
List the effects of adrenaline on the body. How
can these effects be both
positive and negative?

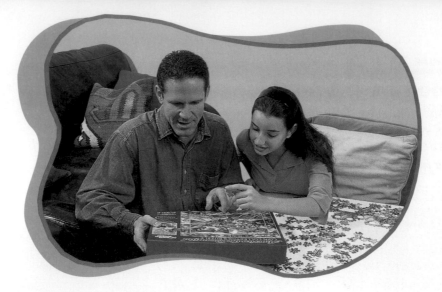

Working on a project can help to relieve psychological fatigue. *What activities do you do to refresh yourself?*

Stress and Fatigue

After a stressor is gone, your body's response to it usually stops. However, if you are experiencing extreme or long-lasting stress, the response may continue. After a time your body can become exhausted. **Fatigue**, or *extreme tiredness,* then sets in.

Two types of fatigue exist. **Physical fatigue** is *extreme tiredness of the whole body.* It usually occurs after vigorous activity or at the end of a long day. Your muscles may feel overworked and sore, and your body feels tired all over. When you experience physical fatigue, you need rest. The other type of fatigue is **psychological** (sy·kuh·LAH·ji·kuhl) **fatigue**, or *extreme tiredness caused by your mental state.* Stress, worry, boredom, or depression can cause psychological fatigue. To relieve this kind of fatigue, you might try an activity such as exercising or working on a hobby. Activities like these can take your mind off the stress and energize you.

Avoiding Stress

Sometimes you can avoid situations that cause stress. Think about what makes you feel uncomfortable or anxious. Can you eliminate these sources of stress? Obviously, you can't avoid some sources, such as having to take a test. However, in those situations you can decrease the stress by being well prepared.

Some stressors are exciting events that you don't want to avoid, such as running for your school's student council. During such times, cut down on other sources of stress to make sure that you don't become overwhelmed. For example, to prevent the stress of being rushed or feeling as if you have too much to do, plan ahead so that you can get everything done. If you feel stressed because you are starting a new school, try to meet some of your classmates before school starts. Use common sense to avoid other types of stress. For example, if you know that there might be pressure to try alcohol or drugs at a party, make other plans for that evening.

Ways to Manage Stress

Stress can affect your physical, mental/emotional, and social health. That is why it is important to develop effective **coping skills**, or *ways of dealing with and overcoming problems*. Here are some coping strategies that can help you manage stress.

- **Eat nutritious foods.** During periods of stress, it's especially important to eat nutritious foods. Doing so will give you energy and help you stay healthy.
- **Get enough sleep.** Research has shown that teens need at least nine hours of sleep each night to function at their best. Getting an adequate amount of sleep will keep up your energy level, allowing you to deal with stressful situations.
- **Relax.** Take a few moments to breathe deeply and slowly. Working your way up from your feet to your head, tighten and then relax one group of muscles at a time. Try imagining that you are in a peaceful place. As you relax, empty your mind of troubling thoughts.
- **Maintain a positive outlook.** Thinking positively can help to reduce stress. Try to keep stressful situations in perspective. Is not getting a perfect score *really* the worst thing that could ever happen to you? Also, make sure that you have some fun. After a stressful day, spend some time joking around with friends or see a funny movie. Laughter is a great stress reliever.
- **Be physically active.** As you've learned, stress can increase your body's energy level. A good way to channel this energy is to be physically active. Engaging in physical activity helps reduce tension and makes you feel more relaxed.
- **Manage your time.** List all the tasks you need to do. Think about what each one involves and how much time you will need to accomplish it. Plan your schedule so that you have enough time to complete each task. Knowing that you have time to do whatever you need and want to do reduces stress.
- **Talk.** Just talking your concerns out with another person can relieve stress. Other people can often see solutions to your problems that you can't.

Talking with someone can relieve stress. *How else can you manage stress effectively?*

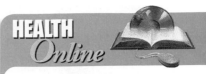

HEALTH *Online*

Topic: Stress

For links to more information on managing stress, go to health.glencoe.com.

Activity: Using the information provided at these links, create a comic strip showing how one teen uses healthful strategies to cope with a stressful situation.

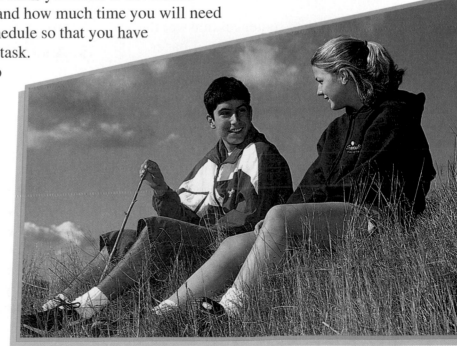

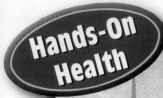

MANAGING YOUR TIME

When you learn to manage your time, you are better able to eliminate the stress and worry that comes from feeling that you can't accomplish everything you need to.

WHAT YOU WILL NEED
- paper
- pencil or pen
- ruler

WHAT YOU WILL DO
1. Using a ruler, make a chart showing each day of the week.
2. On a separate sheet of paper, list all of the activities you would like to fit in during the week. Be realistic.
3. Identify the activities on your list as either obligations or choices. Then decide which of the choices are most important to you, and put a check mark next to them.
4. On your chart, block out the time you will need for your obligations.
5. Estimate the time you will need for each of your remaining activities.
6. Schedule in your choices, starting with the ones you marked as important.

IN CONCLUSION
1. What did your schedule for the week reveal to you about your use of time?
2. How can planning in advance help you decide what new commitments to accept?

Lesson 3 Review

Using complete sentences, answer the following questions on a sheet of paper.

Reviewing Terms and Facts
1. **Vocabulary** Define the terms *distress* and *eustress*. Use each term in an original sentence.
2. **Explain** What is a *stressor?* How does your body respond to a stressor?
3. **Distinguish** What is the difference between physical fatigue and psychological fatigue?
4. **List** Name five ways to manage stress.

Thinking Critically
5. **Analyze** How does the release of adrenaline help you deal with stress?
6. **Describe** Name a situation that is stressful for most teens. Describe how coping skills can be applied to manage this situation.

Applying Health Skills
7. **Stress Management** For one week, record every instance of stress that you feel. List the stressor, how your body and mind reacted to it, and how you handled it. What coping strategies did you demonstrate?

Mental and Emotional Problems

Types of Mental and Emotional Problems

It's normal to feel sad, anxious, or fearful from time to time. However, if such feelings continue for days or weeks, they may signal a mental or emotional problem. The cause of a mental or emotional problem cannot always be identified. Sometimes there is a physical cause, such as inherited genetic traits. Emotional causes are harder to pinpoint. A person may develop a mental or emotional problem because of stress, a lack of coping skills, or a negative experience. It's important to identify lifetime strategies for prevention and early identification of mental and emotional disorders that may lead to long-term disability.

Anxiety Disorders

In some people, nervousness or fear takes the form of an anxiety disorder. An **anxiety disorder** is *a disorder in which intense anxiety or fear keeps a person from functioning normally.* The following are examples of specific anxiety disorders.

- **Phobias** are inappropriate or exaggerated fears of something specific. Some phobias can interfere with normal activities.
- **Obsessive-compulsive disorder** is a condition in which a person cannot keep certain thoughts or images out of his or her mind. The person may then develop repetitive behaviors, such as constant handwashing, to relieve the anxiety.
- **Various stress disorders** may affect people who have been through overwhelming experiences, such as a violent attack. Symptoms may include flashbacks to the event, nightmares, and intense fear.

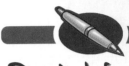

Quick Write
Is it easy for you to ask for help with problems? Why or why not?

LEARN ABOUT...

- types of mental and emotional problems.
- the warning signs of serious mental and emotional problems.
- how to help yourself or a friend with mental or emotional problems.

VOCABULARY

- anxiety disorder
- mood disorder
- depression
- support system
- suicide

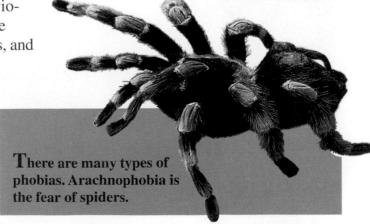

There are many types of phobias. Arachnophobia is the fear of spiders.

Mood Disorders

Another category of mental and emotional problems is mood disorders. A **mood disorder** is *a disorder in which a person undergoes mood changes that seem inappropriate or extreme.* As a teen, you experience normal mood swings in response to the stress in your life. However, the mood changes of a person with a mood disorder are not necessarily reactions to events in their lives.

Depression is *a mood disorder involving feelings of hopelessness, helplessness, worthlessness, guilt, and extreme sadness that continue for periods of weeks.* Depression is a very serious condition that may leave a person completely unwilling or unable to function. Severely depressed people may even think about ending their own lives.

Another mood disorder is bipolar disorder, in which a person has extreme mood swings for no apparent reason. A person who has bipolar disorder usually alternates between periods of hyperactivity (mania) and depression. Such a person will often take dangerous risks during the hyperactive periods.

FIGURE 7.4

WARNING SIGNS OF MENTAL OR EMOTIONAL PROBLEMS

Certain signs may indicate the presence of a mental or emotional problem. If you believe that you or someone you know may have a mental or emotional problem, seek help from a trusted adult. Deciding to get help is an important lifetime strategy for early identification of disorders such as anxiety or depression.

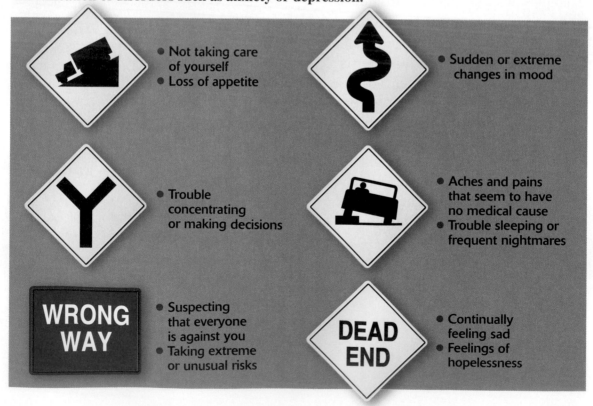

- Not taking care of yourself
- Loss of appetite

- Sudden or extreme changes in mood

- Trouble concentrating or making decisions

- Aches and pains that seem to have no medical cause
- Trouble sleeping or frequent nightmares

WRONG WAY
- Suspecting that everyone is against you
- Taking extreme or unusual risks

DEAD END
- Continually feeling sad
- Feelings of hopelessness

Treating Mental and Emotional Problems

Mental and emotional problems are linked to a complex network of causes and effects that occur throughout a person's life. These problems can be successfully treated with counseling and/or medication.

When to Seek Help

Being able to ask for help is a sign that you are taking responsibility for your health. **Figure 7.4** on the previous page shows some warning signs that often signal serious mental or emotional problems.

Where to Find Help

If you feel that you or a peer may have a mental or emotional problem, talk to someone about it. This is often the first step in reaching a solution and is an important strategy to use throughout your life. Although talking about your problem will not make it go away instantly, it will reassure you that you are not alone. **Figure 7.5** lists people you can turn to for help with a mental or emotional problem.

HEALTH Online

Topic: Depression

For links to more information on how to get help for depression, go to **health.glencoe.com**.

Activity: Using the information provided at these links, create a brochure featuring ways to get help for depression.

FIGURE 7.5

SOURCES OF HELP

Many resources are available for those with mental or emotional problems. Getting help early may prevent long-term disability.

Parent, Guardian, or Other Family Member
Families are built-in support systems. A **support system** is *a network of people available to help when needed.* A parent, older brother or sister, or grandparent can be a great source of help.

Mental Health Professional
These people are specially trained to deal with mental and emotional problems. Your family doctor or school counselor can recommend a professional or program for you.

Teacher
A teacher whom you like and trust could help you when you are in need.

School Nurse or Counselor
School nurses and guidance counselors are specially trained to understand and deal with the problems of teens. They can help you and will respect your privacy.

Religious Leader
The leader of a church, synagogue, or mosque may be a good person to talk to. Many religious leaders are experienced in counseling people.

Reading Check

Create your own main idea statements. Use the following words to create your own sentences about teen suicide: *listen, secret, indications, intervention, comfort.*

Teens and Suicide

Suicide is *the act of intentionally killing oneself.* Suicide is the third leading cause of death in the United States among young people ages 10 to 24. Every day, 14 teens or young adults take their own lives. Most of the time, these young people don't want to die; they just want their problems to go away. Quick intervention can prevent suicidal teens from choosing this permanent escape from their problems. If someone threatens suicide, get help immediately. Encourage the person to talk to a concerned adult or professional counselor. Tell an adult about the situation yourself.

Sometimes a person who doesn't actually use the word *suicide* gives serious indications that he or she is thinking about it. If you notice any of the following signs in yourself or others, seek help:

- Talking about death or mentioning methods of suicide
- Avoiding activities that involve family or friends
- Showing a low level of energy
- Taking greater risks than usual, such as using illegal drugs
- Losing interest in hobbies, sports, or school
- Giving away prized personal possessions
- Having a history of suicide attempts

HEALTH SKILLS ACTIVITY

DECISION MAKING

Helping a Troubled Friend

Paul notices that his friend Ken has become moody and withdrawn. When he asks Ken what is wrong, Ken just says, "It doesn't matter. No one can help me." Paul thinks that Ken may have a serious emotional problem, but he isn't sure how to help. He thinks that maybe he should try harder to get Ken to talk to him, or tell an adult about Ken's behavior. However, he doesn't want to invade his friend's privacy. What should Paul do?

What Would You Do?

Imagine that you are Paul, and use the six steps of the decision-making process to decide what you would do in his situation.

1. STATE THE SITUATION.
2. LIST THE OPTIONS.
3. WEIGH THE POSSIBLE OUTCOMES.
4. CONSIDER VALUES.
5. MAKE A DECISION AND ACT.
6. EVALUATE THE DECISION.

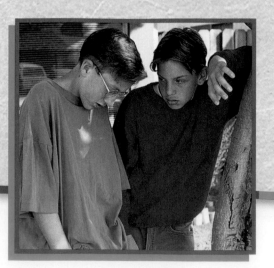

Helping a Friend

If someone you know talks about suicide, you must take it very seriously. One of the first things to do is listen. Let the person talk, which shows that you care. Remain calm—this will be a source of comfort to your friend. Do not, however, promise to keep the discussion secret. After you've listened, talk to your friend. Never make remarks such as "You can't be serious," or "You don't have the nerve." Rather, tell your friend that his or her life is very important to you. Point out that this bad time will pass, and urge your friend to go with you now to get some help. Let your friend know that you will stand by her or him.

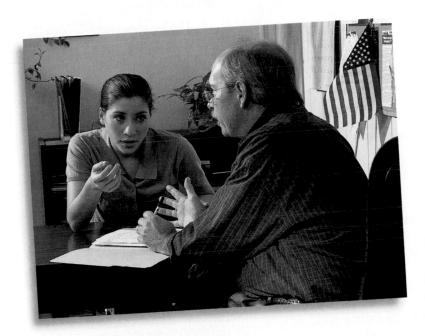

If a friend mentions suicide, it is important to get help immediately. A school nurse or guidance counselor is a good source of assistance in this situation.

Lesson 4 Review

Using complete sentences, answer the following questions on a sheet of paper.

Reviewing Terms and Facts

1. **Vocabulary** Define *anxiety disorder.*
2. **List** Describe two mood disorders and the characteristics associated with them.
3. **Recall** Name four types of people to whom you can go for help with mental or emotional problems.
4. **Identify** What signs might indicate that someone is thinking about committing suicide?

Thinking Critically

5. **Explain** Why might someone with a mental or emotional problem need to see a psychologist?
6. **Analyze** What would you do if a friend talked about committing suicide?

Applying Health Skills

7. **Advocacy** Write an article for the school paper about mental and emotional problems. Discuss whether these disorders are preventable, why early identification is important, and where people can get help.

Gray Matters

Are you using your mind to maximum advantage? Take our quiz and find out!

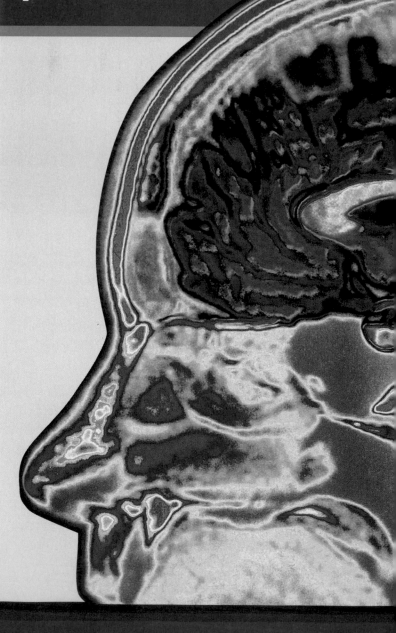

Quiz

1. Your brain is fully developed by the time you reach your teens.
   a. **True**   b. **False**

2. Which activity could cause new brain cells to grow?
   a. **Exercise**
   b. **Watching television**

3. People use only 10 percent of their brains.
   a. **True**   b. **False**

4. Alcohol kills brain cells.
   a. **True**   b. **False**

5. If you spend the summer in front of the television, you might feel as though you've lost some brainpower when you go back to school.
   a. **True**   b. **False**

6. Which of the following foods is good for your brain?
   a. **Fish**
   b. **Cereal**
   c. **Almonds**
   d. **All of the above**

7. As long as you study during the day, staying up all night won't affect your academic performance.
   a. **True**   b. **False**

Answers: 1. b.; 2. a.; 3. b.; 4. a.; 5. a.; 6. d.; 7. b.

Check out the explanations on the next page!

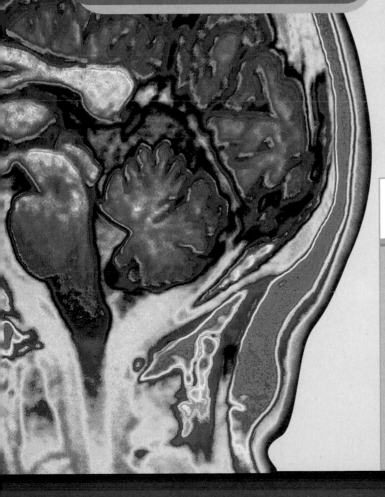

Explanations

1. Researchers were shocked to discover that **the brain goes through a second period of growth during puberty.** Learning new skills during this time can give brainpower a big boost. The positive activities that you devote your mental energy to now—sports, music, studies—will strengthen nerve-cell connections and become "wired" into your brain!

2. **Exercise may not only build biceps, but also brain cells,** or neurons. Researchers at the Salk Institute in La Jolla, California, discovered that the brains of mice that ran on an exercise wheel produced more neurons than the brains of mice that didn't exercise. The active mice also performed complex tasks better than the inactive mice. The lesson? Keep moving, and you might ace those midterms.

3. **It's a myth that people use only a certain percentage of their brain.** As long as you keep using your noggin, whether it's by doing a crossword puzzle or painting a picture, you'll maximize your brain power.

4. **Drinking alcohol can shrink or destroy nerve cells.** This can have serious consequences. A University of California at San Diego study found that alcohol decreases teens' ability to remember and solve problems. While neurons that have shrunk return to normal once someone stops drinking, dead ones can't be brought back to life.

5. **You don't actually lose brain cells** by taking the summer off, but you do get out of some good mental habits. To stay in top form, challenge yourself. You don't have to do something as dry as reading the dictionary, but try to keep up with news events or visit a museum.

6. **Running a brain requires a balanced diet.** Small portions of high-protein foods like fish can give your brain a boost, due to the amino acid tyrosine. Carbohydrates are crucial, especially those in whole grains, fruits, and vegetables. Carbs supply you with glucose, the basic energy source needed for all body processes, including thinking.

7. A study conducted by Carlyle Smith of Trent University in Peterborough, Ontario, Canada, found that **sleep deprivation may disrupt your brain's ability to retain certain kinds of information.** In the study, students were taught a complex logic game, then deprived of sleep. When retested a week later, the students had forgotten up to half of what they had learned.

TIME TO THINK...

About Your Brain

Create an exercise program—for your brain. Write down specific activities, such as reading and solving puzzles, that can help increase brainpower, as well as the amount of time you will devote to these activities. Also include the physical activities you will participate in and the foods you will eat to nourish your brain. Present your ideas to the class, and add ideas from your classmates' programs to improve your brain workout.

LEARNING TO HANDLE STRESS

Model

Mason felt as if his whole world had turned upside down when his parents got divorced. He knew his younger sister was upset too. His problems seemed to be getting worse.

Mason decided to deal with his stress. First, he told his parents about his feelings, and they suggested seeing a family counselor together. Mason also began taking walks with his sister so that they could share their thoughts and feelings. He made sure he ate well and got enough physical activity. Although Mason was still sad about the divorce, he now had an easier time adjusting to the changes and feelings it caused.

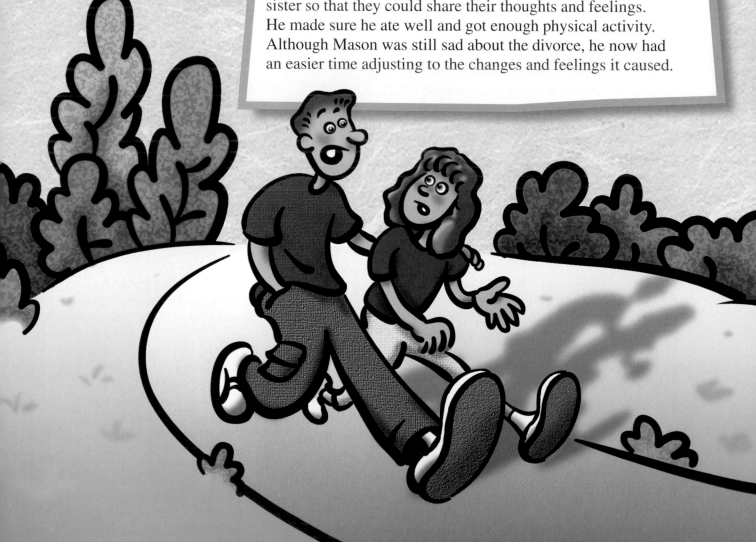

Practice

Read the following scenario about a teen who needs to manage the stress in her life.

People tell Chelsea all the time that she worries too much. Chelsea doesn't see how she can help it. She wants to do well in school, on the soccer team, and in her dance class. It seems to Chelsea that when she isn't worrying about one area of her life, she is distressed about another. Recently she has noticed that she has days when she doesn't feel much like eating because she is feeling stressed. She knows that this isn't good for her health, but she doesn't know what to do.

On a sheet of paper, identify the cause of Chelsea's stress. Develop a plan to help Chelsea by listing four specific actions she could take to manage the stressful feelings she experiences.

Apply/Assess

How do you deal with stress in your life? Sharing helpful tips with others in your class can give you more ideas about healthful ways to manage stress.

Working in groups of four, take turns describing what causes stress in your life. Then explain what helps each of you relax or feel better when you are stressed. As a group, create a poster showing four causes of stress and four healthful ways in which a person can cope with stress.

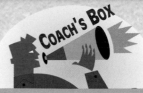

COACH'S BOX

Stress Management

When you experience stress, do one or more of the following.
- Stay healthy.
- Relax.
- Think positively.
- Be physically active.
- Manage your time.
- Talk.

Self-✓Check
- Did we show four causes of stress?
- Did we identify healthful ways to deal with stress?

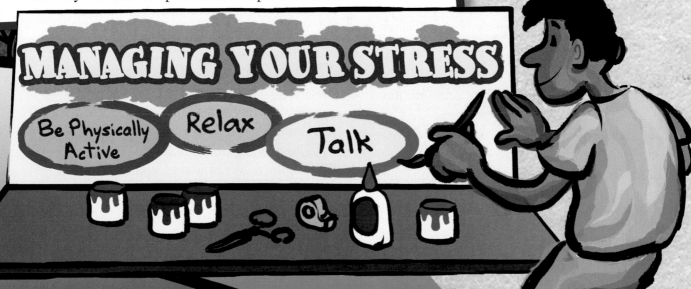

CHAPTER 7 ASSESSMENT

After You Read

Use your completed Foldable to review the information on the factors that shape personality.

FOLDABLES™
Study Organizer

Reviewing Vocabulary and Concepts

On a sheet of paper, write the numbers 1–7. After each number, write the term from the list that best completes each statement.

- behavior
- emotions
- loss
- guilt
- personality
- resilient
- self-esteem

Lesson 1

1. If you are _____, you are able to bounce back from a disappointment, difficulty, or crisis.
2. _____ is the mix of traits, feelings, attitudes, and habits that makes you the person you are.
3. _____ is the factor contributing to personality that you can control.
4. The confidence and pride that you have in yourself is called _____.

Lesson 2

5. Happiness, sadness, anger, and fear are all _____.
6. The changes that happen in your life cause you to experience _____.
7. During the grieving process, some people experience _____, blaming themselves for the loss.

On a sheet of paper, write the numbers 8–15. Write *True* or *False* for each statement below. If the statement is false, change the underlined word or phrase to make it true.

Lesson 3

8. Your body <u>can</u> distinguish between positive and negative stress.
9. When your body releases adrenaline, the level of sugar in your blood <u>decreases</u>.
10. If you are under extreme or long-lasting stress, you may experience <u>fatigue</u>.
11. Ways of dealing with and overcoming problems are known as <u>handling</u> skills.

Lesson 4

12. A phobia is an example of <u>a mood disorder</u>.
13. <u>Depression</u> involves feelings of hopelessness, helplessness, worthlessness, guilt, and extreme sadness that continue for periods of weeks.
14. <u>Giving away prized personal possessions</u> may be a warning sign that a person is thinking of committing suicide.
15. A <u>support system</u> is a network of people who are available to help when needed.

Thinking Critically

Using complete sentences, answer the following questions on a sheet of paper.

16. **Synthesize** How is good mental health related to self-esteem?
17. **Apply** How would understanding the feelings associated with grief enable you to help someone who has experienced a loss?
18. **Analyze** How can stress be a positive influence in your life?
19. **Explain** What would you do to get help if you thought that you were developing a phobia?

20. Evaluate How might traits such as honesty, integrity, responsibility, and respecting the dignity of others contribute to self-esteem and self-confidence? What actions could a teen take to demonstrate each of these positive characteristics?

21. Suggest Identify and describe lifetime strategies for prevention and early identification of disorders such as depression and anxiety that may lead to long-term disability.

Career Corner

Psychiatrist Psychiatrists are medical doctors who diagnose and treat people with mental health problems. They may specialize in child and adolescent psychiatry, geriatrics, or addictions.

Psychiatrists complete a four-year college degree, four years of medical school, and one to seven years of residency training. Learn more about this and other health careers by clicking on Career Corner at health.glencoe.com.

Standardized Test Practice

Reading & Writing

Read the paragraphs below and then answer the questions.

It is time for some new thinking on the subject of suspending students from school. Suspension is not an appropriate or effective punishment. Why not require students to perform community service instead?

Community service would give students a chance to learn something new. It would also allow them to contribute to society. Students assigned to a local soup kitchen or community center would return to the classroom with a better sense of what the outside world is like. Time away from the classroom would benefit students and teachers. While disruptive students are performing community service, classroom teachers and other students would have a break from the stress of interrupted class work.

1. Which statement best summarizes this passage?
- **A** Students who misbehave should be required to perform community service.
- **B** Community service is better than suspension for disciplining students.
- **C** Students who are suspended should also perform community service.
- **D** Only by performing community service can students learn to behave.

2. What is the purpose of this passage?
- **A** to inform readers about suspension problems
- **B** to persuade readers to think about an alternative idea
- **C** to express an opinion about current suspension rules
- **D** to explain why community service is worthwhile

3. Write a paragraph suggesting an alternative solution for classroom discipline problems.

HAPPY
BIRTHDAY!

Social Health: Family and Friends

HEALTH *Online*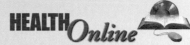

Rate your social health habits by taking the Health Inventory for Chapter 8 at health.glencoe.com.

FOLDABLES™
Study Organizer

Before You Read

Make this Foldable to help you organize what you learn about verbal and nonverbal communication in Lesson 1. Begin with a plain sheet of 8½″ × 11″ paper.

Step 1

Fold the sheet of paper in half along the long axis.

Step 2

Turn the paper and fold it into thirds.

Step 3

Unfold and cut the top layer along both fold lines. This makes three tabs.

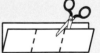

Step 4

Draw two overlapping ovals, and label as shown.

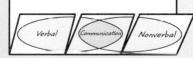

Verbal *Communication* *Nonverbal*

As You Read

Write down the definitions and examples of verbal and nonverbal communication under the appropriate tab. Under the middle tab, describe how both types of communication help to convey feelings, thoughts, and information.

Developing Communication Skills

Quick Write

Compose a short dialogue between two good friends. One friend is worried about taking next week's science test. The other is a sympathetic listener.

LEARN ABOUT...

- ways in which people communicate.
- how verbal communication differs from nonverbal communication.
- how to be an effective speaker and listener.

VOCABULARY

- communication
- verbal communication
- nonverbal communication
- body language
- tact

Communicating with Others

You hang up the telephone and smile with relief. Your friend Tyler has just explained a math homework problem that really had you stumped. What happened? You and Tyler communicated. **Communication** is *an exchange of thoughts, feelings, and beliefs among people.*

Communication requires a sender, a receiver, and a message. To exchange ideas, both the sender and the receiver must try to keep the message clear. Senders must express themselves clearly. Receivers must listen carefully. Unfortunately, people don't always say what they really mean, and listeners may hear only what they want to hear. The result can be a failure to communicate.

Effective communication means that you can express yourself clearly and understand others. This builds positive relationships and creates a healthy social environment. People can enjoy being

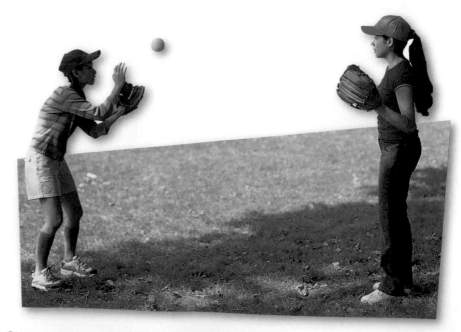

Communication is a little like playing catch. It involves a sender transmitting something to a receiver.

themselves while they understand and value one another. Good communication skills will help you succeed in all areas of your life.

Verbal Communication

You and Tyler used words to discuss your math homework. This paragraph uses words to give you information. When you write a book report, you use words to express your ideas. These are all examples of verbal communication. **Verbal communication** means *using words to express yourself, either in speaking or in writing.* When people think of communication, they think of verbal communication first. Verbal communication makes it possible to

- read a book, newspaper, magazine, Internet site, or sign.
- keep in touch with others through letters and e-mail.
- talk with someone in person, on the telephone, or over the Internet.
- appreciate speakers and performers on TV and on the radio.

Nonverbal Communication

People also communicate without words. **Nonverbal communication** includes *all the ways you can get a message across without using words.* Nonverbal communication can give your words more meaning. It can also replace words. Think of the messages you send with a wave of your hand, a smile, or a shrug. **Body language** is *a type of nonverbal communication that includes posture, gestures, and facial expressions.*

Developing Good Character

Caring

Show that you care about others. Make and effort to interact with many different people, including members of other ethnic and cultural groups. Try to adapt group activities so that a variety of people can be included. *Give two examples of how group activities might be adapted to include a variety of people.*

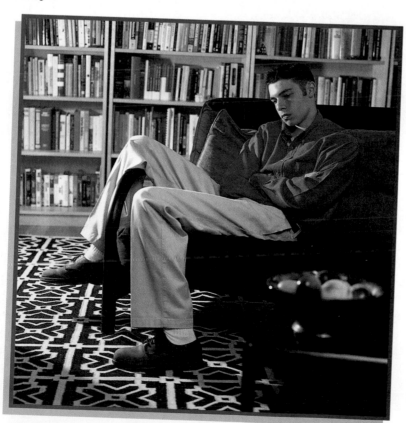

What do you think this teen's body language says about what he's feeling?

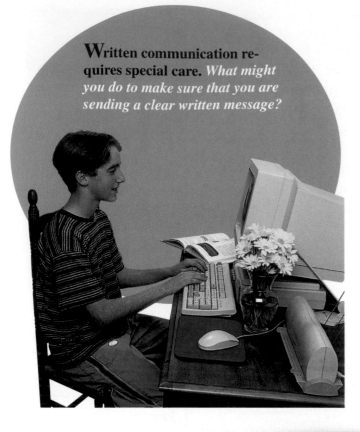

Written communication requires special care. *What might you do to make sure that you are sending a clear written message?*

Skills for Effective Communication

Good communication skills make good relationships possible. When you express yourself clearly, you help others understand you. When you listen carefully, you show people that you value their thoughts and feelings. See **Figure 8.1** for some tips on how to communicate effectively.

Although honesty is important, bluntly expressing your opinions or feelings can sometimes hurt other people's feelings. Ask yourself: Would I be hurt if someone said this to me? If the answer is yes, find another way to make your point. Use **tact**—*the quality of knowing what to say to avoid offending others.*

HEALTH SKILLS ACTIVITY

COMMUNICATION SKILLS

Handling Constructive Feedback

Constructive feedback can be helpful by pointing out weaknesses, but it can also cause the person who is receiving it to feel defensive. Here are some techniques for using constructive feedback effectively.

WHEN GIVING CONSTRUCTIVE FEEDBACK

- Avoid giving constructive feedback to anyone in front of other people. Criticism is not to be used to make fun of others.
- Avoid criticizing a person's past actions or remarks that can't be changed. Focus on what can be done in the future.
- Praise the good points of an idea or behavior before pointing out weaknesses.
- Focus on the specific problem, not the person. Offer help if you can.

WHEN RECEIVING CONSTRUCTIVE FEEDBACK

- Consider the reason for the feedback. The person probably cares a great deal about you.
- Focus on the message. Before responding to the criticism, determine whether the person is criticizing you for no reason or is being helpful.
- Ask for clarification if you don't understand what someone is trying to tell you. Even helpful messages can be confusing or poorly delivered.

WITH A GROUP

Perform a skit to show how to offer feedback in a positive way. Invent a situation in which one person has done something poorly and two friends give constructive feedback. Show the positive response to the feedback.

FIGURE 8.1

SPEAKING AND LISTENING STRATEGIES

Here are some strategies for effective communication.

Speaking Skills

- Think before you speak.
- Use "I" messages to express thoughts, feelings, needs, and wants.
- Make clear, simple statements. Be specific when giving suggestions or expressing ideas.
- Be honest and direct, but use tact. Avoid being rude or insulting.
- Use appropriate body language. Make eye contact with the other person and use suitable gestures as needed to clarify your meaning.
- Let your listener respond to see what you need to make clearer.

Listening Skills

- Use appropriate body language. Lean forward slightly, and make eye contact with the speaker. Use suitable facial expressions or gestures, or nod your head to show that you are listening.
- Use conversation encouragers—words that prompt a speaker to continue—to show that you are paying attention. Try saying, "Really?" or "Go on."
- Mirror the speaker's thoughts and feelings. Repeat or rephrase what the speaker has said to show that you are listening. Show empathy.
- Avoid interrupting the speaker, but ask questions when appropriate.

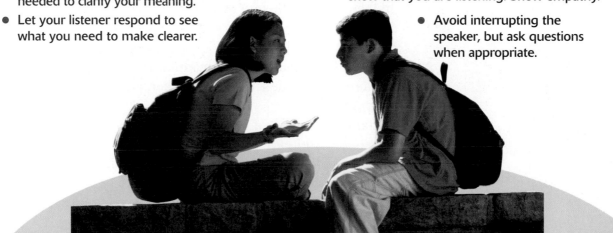

Lesson 1 Review

Using complete sentences, answer the following questions on a sheet of paper.

Reviewing Terms and Facts

1. **Vocabulary** Define *communication.*
2. **Recall** What three elements are necessary for communication?
3. **Distinguish** Explain the difference between verbal and nonverbal communication.
4. **Restate** In what ways can a listener demonstrate good communication skills?

Thinking Critically

5. **Explain** What body language might convey that someone is not listening?

6. **Depict** In a small group, pantomime realistic body language to show an emotion. Ask the others in your group to identify the emotion. Determine which gestures or movements show which emotions.

Applying Health Skills

7. **Communication Skills** Using tact effectively is an important skill. Imagine that a friend came to school with a bad haircut. What would you say to this friend when he asked what you thought of it? In a paragraph, write a tactful but honest response to your friend.

Understanding Family Relationships

Being Part of a Family

Name all of the groups you belong to—classes, clubs, teams, and circles of friends. Did you include your family among the groups? It is the first and most important group in your life. The **family**, in fact, is *the basic unit of society*. Different types of families are described below.

- A couple family is made up of two adults living together.
- Nuclear families include a mother, a father, and one child or two or more children.
- Blended families consist of a parent, a stepparent, and one child or two or more children.
- Single-parent families are made up of a parent and one child or two or more children.
- Extended families are any of the above types of families that also includes other relatives.

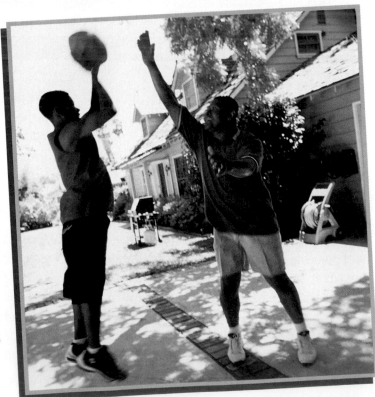

Spending quality time with parents is important. *What do you do when you spend time with relatives?*

Your Family and Your Health

One role of the family is to nurture its members. To **nurture** means *to provide for physical, mental, emotional, and social needs.* The ways in which your family fulfills these needs influence all aspects of your health. Look at **Figure 8.2** to find some specific ways in which families support their members.

Your family also helps you develop your values as you grow into adulthood. The values you learn from family members may be based on family history, traditions, and religious beliefs. They will become the basis of your decision making in the real world. The values that people learn through family life have an enormous influence on the health of a community.

Reading Check
Discover what you know about *nurturing*. List ways you nurture members of your family.

FIGURE 8.2

HOW FAMILIES MEET THE NEEDS OF THEIR MEMBERS

Families help meet the physical, mental/emotional, and social needs of their members.

Meeting Physical Needs
Families provide the basic needs for survival: food, clothing, and shelter. They care for family members during illness and protect each other. Families practice health-promoting behaviors and encourage younger family members to practice these positive behaviors as well.

Meeting Mental Needs
Families teach children everyday tasks, from tying shoes to speaking languages. Families promote intellectual development by reading, helping with schoolwork, and answering questions. Eventually children and adults share their knowledge, skills, and experiences.

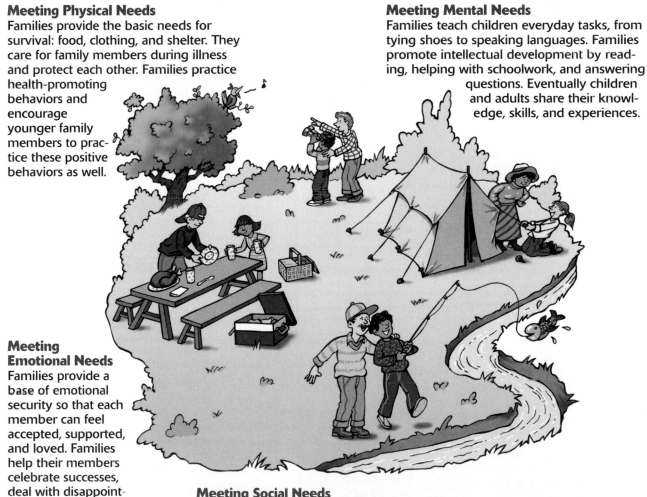

Meeting Emotional Needs
Families provide a base of emotional security so that each member can feel accepted, supported, and loved. Families help their members celebrate successes, deal with disappointments, and face life's challenges.

Meeting Social Needs
Families teach the skills their members need to get along with others and be productive members of the community. Family members learn to take turns, to share, to accept responsibilities, and to respect one another.

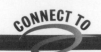

Language Arts

Coping with Changes and Challenges

Family life involves changes and challenges. A new brother or sister may join the family. Older siblings might move away from home. Parents may divorce or remarry. Some changes are happy occasions, but at times families have to cope with difficult situations. These changes may cause stress, which can have a negative effect on family health. Sometimes serious family situations require outside help. Substance abuse and physical abuse are examples of these types of problems. Families may turn to counselors, religious leaders, or medical or law enforcement workers for help. Here are some common family challenges and a few ways to cope with them:

- **Moving.** Before your family moves, find out as much as you can about the new neighborhood and the school. Once you're in your new school, look for clubs or activities that interest you, and get involved as soon as you can. Above all, keep a positive attitude. Try to help other family members adjust. Spend more time with your family as you learn your way around your new neighborhood and make new friends.

- **Job loss.** Avoid blaming or criticizing the adult who is faced with finding a new job or managing a budget with less income. Instead, be supportive. Look for ways in which you could help out with family expenses, such as cutting back on spending or contributing earnings from a part-time job.

- **Separation and divorce.** Although you may be having a difficult time understanding what is going on, show your parents that you care for them. Talk to them about your feelings if you can. If your parents are unable to give you the support you need, share your feelings with a school counselor or some other trusted adult. Try to help younger brothers and sisters understand and cope. Let them know that the divorce is not their fault.

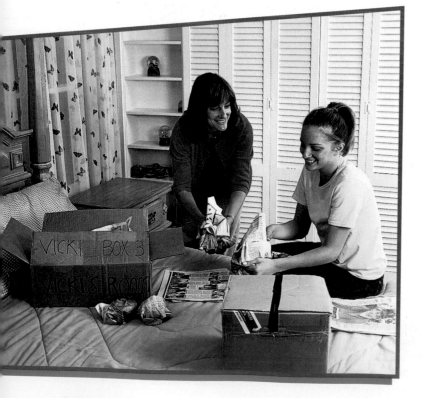

- **Illness or injury.** Take responsibility for tasks you can do, both in the care of the sick or injured family member and in everyday family chores. Demonstrate care and concern toward the ill or injured family member.

If you're faced with a family move, focus on its positive aspects. Exploring a new community and making new friends could be exciting. *What strategies could you demonstrate to cope with the stress of moving?*

- **Death, grieving, and loss.** Accept and talk about emotions such as sadness, fear, or anger. Recognize that it is natural for your grief to last for a while. Do not be critical of family members who show their grief in ways that are different from yours. Many people hide sadness behind forced cheerfulness or what seems like a lack of emotion. Pay special attention to younger members of the family. Offer them as much comfort and security as you can, and help them look toward the future. Seek help from others, such as school counselors or religious leaders.

Hands-On Health

TIPS FOR TEEN TALKERS

Good communication at home can help build healthy relationships. In a small group, design a pamphlet that offers tips to help teens communicate with family members. Keep in mind that a successful pamphlet is easy to read, has a simple design, and does not have too many words on a page.

WHAT YOU WILL NEED
- writing paper and pens/pencils
- construction or art paper
- crayons or markers

WHAT YOU WILL DO
1. In small groups, brainstorm a list of situations in which teens might have trouble communicating with family members. How could teens communicate more effectively in these situations? Discuss your ideas with your group.
2. Organize your ideas. What will your pamphlet's main message be? What information will you include as details?
3. Plan your pamphlet. You might include role-play scenarios, straight information, or questions and answers in your pamphlet.

4. Create your pamphlet using the materials listed. Write the text as neatly as you can.

IN CONCLUSION
Present your group's pamphlet to the class. Discuss which aspects of the pamphlets seem to be the most effective and why.

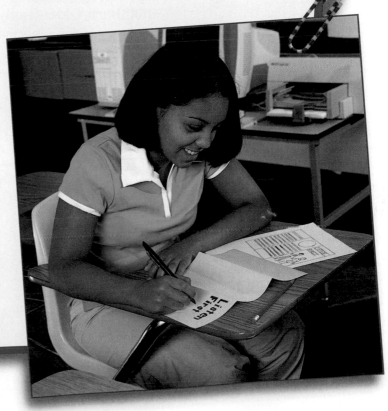

Respect

Showing respect for family members builds trust within the family. How can you show respect for members of your family? Be considerate— ask before you borrow their possessions. Include family members in discussions or decisions. Make an effort to speak kindly and politely. *How do these actions show that you value your family members?*

Strengthening Family Relationships

Think about the roles you have in your family. You may be a son or daughter, a sibling, a cousin, and a baby-sitter. Balancing various roles and responsibilities can cause some stress. When family members work together, however, they can manage stress and keep family bonds strong. Respect, understanding, and humor are good qualities to start with. Here are some specific strategies and characteristics of healthy families.

- **Show appreciation.** After you've done a household task, such as washing the dishes or doing the laundry, you know that it feels good when someone thanks you or compliments you on a job well done. Other family members feel the same way. Remember to say thank you to show your appreciation to anyone who prepares meals or does an errand for you. Show support for family members who are struggling. Offer to help if someone in your family seems stressed.

- **Communicate ideas, information, and feelings.** Share your thoughts and feelings. Talk openly with family members on a regular basis, not only when a problem arises. Be a good listener when a family member shares feelings with you.

- **Spend quality time together.** As often as possible, spend time with your family. While you are together, share your experiences and talk about family interests. Eating meals together, playing games, and going on family outings can be good ways to enjoy quality time as a family.

- **Appreciate your grandparents and other extended family members.** Older family members have lived through the history you are learning in school. Ask them to tell you about their experiences and opinions. They may be able to help you to better understand yourself and your family.

Your grandparents and other relatives are part of your family. *List some ways you can become closer to extended family members. How can you show respect for older relatives?*

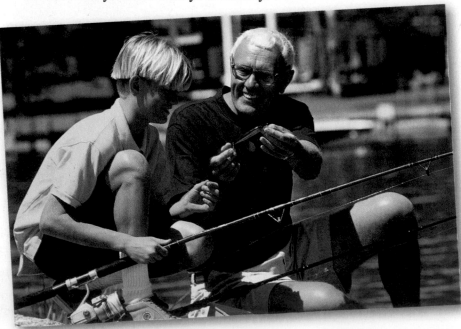

- **Respect family members' privacy.** Your belongings and your privacy are important to you. You want other family members to respect them. Remember this, and respect their belongings and privacy, too. Don't borrow from others or intrude on them without asking. Be careful with others' possessions.
- **Show responsibility.** Do assigned chores and pitch in with other family tasks. For example, clean your room or wash the dishes without being asked.
- **Share family resources.** Various members of your family may have to share the bathroom, computer, telephone, television, and other possessions. Agree to reasonable limits on their use, and stick to them.
- **Follow family guidelines.** Your parents or guardians are responsible for the family's health and safety. Therefore, they have the authority to set and enforce rules. Follow their rules. If you have reasonable concerns about these rules, communicate them clearly and respectfully. These guidelines are meant to protect and educate you.

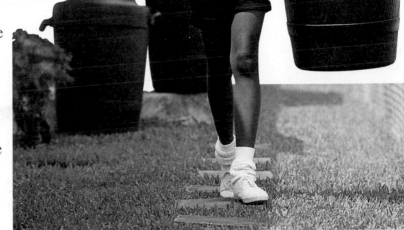

Families are stronger when all family members take responsibility for necessary tasks. *How is this teen showing responsibility?*

Lesson 2 Review

Using complete sentences, answer the following questions on a sheet of paper.

Reviewing Terms and Facts

1. **Vocabulary** Define the term *nurture*.
2. **Restate** What are three changes and challenges that may occur in families?
3. **Recall** List two ways in which you might show appreciation to other family members.

Thinking Critically

4. **Analyze** How can positive family relationships influence health?

5. **Infer** How can strong families strengthen the community around them?

Applying Health Skills

6. **Analyzing Influences** Choose a TV show that features a family. Do its members communicate effectively? How much time do they spend together? Do they show respect for one another? How do they handle family challenges? Write a brief review of the show's family. Explain whether or not you think the program presents a realistic and healthy family. How might this show influence individual and community health?

Friendships and Peer Pressure

Quick Write

Write a paragraph describing a situation in which your friends or classmates tried to influence your ideas or behavior. Did they influence you in a positive way or a negative way? Explain your answer.

LEARN ABOUT...

- qualities of good friends.
- recognizing peer pressure.
- how to deal with negative peer pressure.

VOCABULARY

- friendship
- compromise
- peers
- peer pressure

The Importance of Friends

Your relationships with friends become especially important during the teen years. **Friendships** are *relationships between people who like each other and who have similar interests and values.* Good friendships generally begin when people realize that they have common experiences, goals, and values. Each person must also show a willingness to reach out, to listen, and to care about the needs of the other person.

Forming strong friendships is an important part of social health. To make new friends, get involved in activities at school or in the community. For example, join a school club or volunteer at a local youth group. When you participate in activities that you enjoy, you're likely to meet others who share your interests.

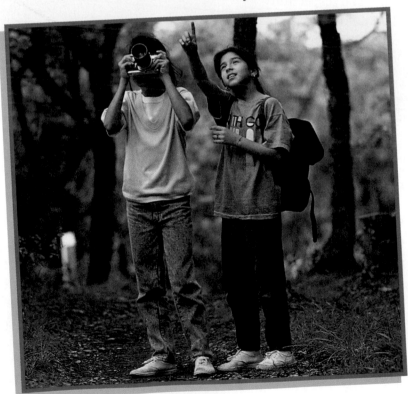

Friends spend time together in activities they both enjoy. *Why is it important to have friends and be a part of other social groups?*

How Can You Be a Good Friend?

A friend is much more than an acquaintance, someone you see occasionally or know casually. Your relationship with a friend is deeper and means more to you. Although there is no accepted test for friendship, most people whom you call friends will have the following qualities:

✓
Reading Check
Notice italics. Find the phrases on these two pages that are italicized *(slanted)*. Determine the author's reasoning for using italics for these phrases.

- **Trustworthiness.** Good friends are there for you when you need support. They are honest with you, they keep their promises, and they don't reveal your secrets. Good friends live up to your realistic expectations. If necessary, these friends would be willing to make sacrifices for you.

- **Caring.** Good friends listen carefully when you want to talk. They try to understand how you feel. In fact, they empathize with you when you have strong feelings such as joy, sadness, or disappointment. Friends don't just recognize your strengths and talents—they tell you about them and help you develop them. Caring friends might try to help you overcome your weaknesses, but they accept you as you are. They don't hold grudges and can forgive you if you make a mistake.

- **Respect.** Good friends will not ask you to do anything that is wrong or dangerous or pressure you if you refuse. They respect your beliefs because they respect you. They also understand that your opinions may be different from theirs, and they realize that this is healthy. Because you and your good friends usually share similar values, they will not expect you to betray those values. If friends disagree, they are willing to **compromise**, which means *to give up something in order to reach a solution that satisfies everyone.*

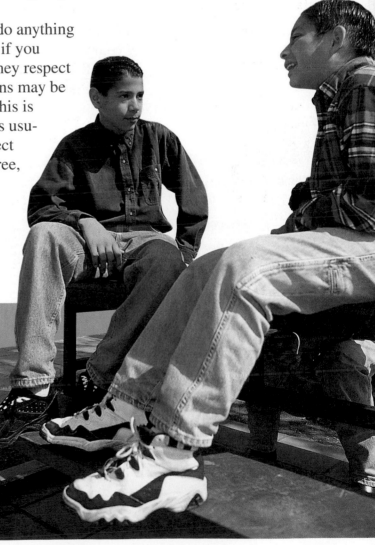

Caring friends listen to each other's concerns. *How can you tell if a friendship is having a positive or negative influence on your health? What strategies can you develop to monitor this influence?*

HEALTH
Online

Topic: Peer pressure

For a link to more information on ways to resist negative peer pressure, to to **health.glencoe.com**.

Activity: Using the information provided at this link, write a short story about a teen who resists peer pressure to engage in an unsafe behavior.

Peer Pressure

Most of your friends are probably your **peers**—*people close to your age who are similar to you in many ways.* You may be concerned about what your peers think of you, how they react to you, and whether they accept you. Their opinions can affect your ideas of how you should think and act. This is called **peer pressure**—*the influence that people your age have on you to think and act like them.* As **Figure 8.3** explains, peer pressure can have either a positive or negative influence on your health.

Resisting Negative Peer Pressure

There may be times when your peers want you to do something that you know is not right. You want to stand your ground, but it's difficult, especially if they are persuasive. You may worry that you will be unpopular or that people will make fun of you if you don't go along. It takes courage to stand up for yourself when others want you to take risks.

As a teen you are developing the ability to think for yourself and make more of your own decisions. Even when you're sure of yourself, however, it can be difficult to stand up to your peers. **Figure 8.4** on the next page gives you some practical tips for resisting negative peer pressure.

FIGURE 8.3

POSITIVE AND NEGATIVE PEER PRESSURE

Peer pressure can be a powerful influence during your teen years. *What are some other examples of positive and negative peer pressure?*

Positive Peer Pressure	Negative Peer Pressure
Examples	**Examples**
Peers can	**Peers can**
• challenge you to work hard on a team project.	• urge you to use tobacco, alcohol, or other drugs.
• encourage you to do your best in school.	• dare you to take unnecessary risks.
• persuade you to work to help others.	• persuade you to break the rules of your family, school, or community.
• inspire you to stay fit and safe.	• encourage you to betray your values.
• urge you to expand your friendships to include those of different backgrounds and cultures.	• expect you to fear or dislike someone who is different.
Results	**Results**
• Self-improvement	• Dangerous or unlawful situations
• Higher self-esteem	• Lower self-esteem
• Health, fitness, and safety	• Health and safety risks

HEALTH SKILLS ACTIVITY

DECISION MAKING

Facing Peer Pressure

While shopping in a department store one Saturday, Alisha sees her friends Miranda and Tina trying on sunglasses. After they look around to see if anyone is watching, they slip several pairs of sunglasses into their pockets. As they turn to leave the store, Miranda and Tina see Alisha. They know by the look on her face that she saw them. "Go ahead," Tina whispers. "Take some free sunglasses. The store is very busy—no one is paying attention." What should Alisha do?

WHAT WOULD YOU DO?

Apply the six steps of the decision-making process to Alisha's situation. In small groups, discuss options that Alisha might choose. What would you have done in her situation? Explain your answer.

1. **STATE THE SITUATION.**
2. **LIST THE OPTIONS.**
3. **WEIGH THE POSSIBLE OUTCOMES.**
4. **CONSIDER VALUES.**
5. **MAKE A DECISION AND ACT.**
6. **EVALUATE THE DECISION.**

FIGURE 8.4

HANDLING NEGATIVE PEER PRESSURE

List two situations in which these tips could come in handy.

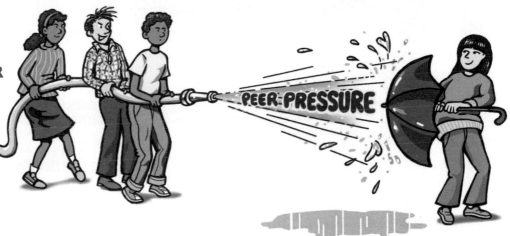

PEER PRESSURE

Avoid the situation.
If you can tell in advance that a situation is potentially unhealthy or dangerous, stay away. For example, if a friend asks you to ride with someone who has been drinking, say no.

Rely on values.
When confronted by peer pressure, remember the H.E.L.P. criteria. Consider whether the action you are being asked to take is **H**ealthful, **E**thical, **L**egal, and acceptable to your **P**arents. If it is not, explain why you do not want to do it. For example, a friend might ask you to shoplift. Point out that you don't want to break the law or betray your values.

Focus on the issue.
If people make fun of you for refusing to go along with them, don't exchange insults with them. Instead, focus on why you are saying no. Suppose that you refuse to go swimming in an unsafe place, and a peer says, "What are you, a baby?" You might say, "No, I just don't think it's safe."

Walk away.
If a peer becomes angry or abusive with you, walk away. Don't let yourself be hurt by a bully. For example, suppose that you refuse to join in when a peer makes hurtful remarks to someone. Your peer then begins insulting you, too. Walk away, and avoid future contact with this abusive person.

Respect from Your Peers

People of all ages want to be well liked by their peers. You, too, probably would like to be popular. Remember, however, that just being popular isn't enough. You also want your peers to respect you—to hold you in high regard because of your responsible behavior.

The respect of others is important, whether or not you're part of the popular crowd. *What guidelines might you use to determine whether relationships are healthy or unhealthy?*

Popularity can be based on your possessions or on how you look. What makes a person popular can vary depending on styles and the changing makeup of different groups. Respect, on the other hand, is based on who you are as a complete person. Although it's natural to want to be popular, you may face situations in which you discover that preserving your character is worth more than popularity. If other teens pressure you to take drugs, for example, and you give in, you may become part of a popular crowd. However, you will probably also lose some people's respect. Character traits such as trustworthiness, fairness, and responsibility earn the lasting respect of peers and adults.

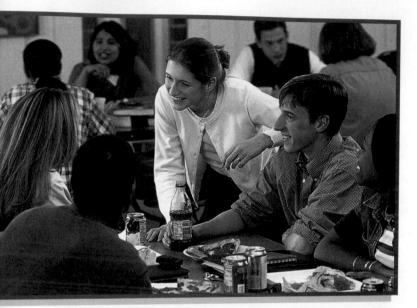

Lesson 3 Review

Using complete sentences, answer the following questions on a sheet of paper.

Reviewing Terms and Facts

1. **Vocabulary** Define the terms *friendship* and *peers*.
2. **List** Identify three qualities of a good friend. Give an example of each quality.
3. **Restate** Differentiate between positive and negative peer pressure. Give an example of each.
4. **Identify** Name two ways to deal with negative peer pressure. Give an example of each.
5. **Define** State the difference between popularity and respect. Which do you think is more important? Why?

Thinking Critically

6. **Compare and Contrast** What makes some people your friends and some just acquaintances? How are they alike? How are they different?
7. **Hypothesize** Imagine that one teen in a group resists negative peer pressure. How could such an action have a positive effect on the other teens in the group?

Applying Health Skills

8. **Communication Skills** Create a poster to explain to young children what a good friend is. Include the qualities to look for in a good friend and tips on how to be such a friend.

Abstinence and Refusal Skills

Acting Responsibly

As you enter your teen years, your parents may no longer spell out all the rules to guide and protect you the way they did when you were younger. They know that you understand right and wrong behavior, and they expect you to take responsibility for many of your own decisions and actions. You're eager to accept the challenge because it carries new freedom along with it. It also carries some risks.

Avoiding Risk Behaviors

As an adolescent, your world is larger and more complicated than it was when you were a child. You may be pressured by your peers to use tobacco, alcohol, or other drugs or to engage in sexual activity. Recognizing that negative social influences can harm your health will help you respond appropriately to peer pressure and avoid risk behaviors.

Quick Write

Compose a brief letter to the editor of your school paper. In your letter, explain one reason teens are better off when they avoid risk behaviors.

LEARN ABOUT...

- why avoiding health risk behaviors is important.
- what you gain by abstaining from tobacco, alcohol, and other drugs.
- the benefits of abstinence from sexual activity.
- effective ways to say no to risk behaviors.

VOCABULARY

- abstinence

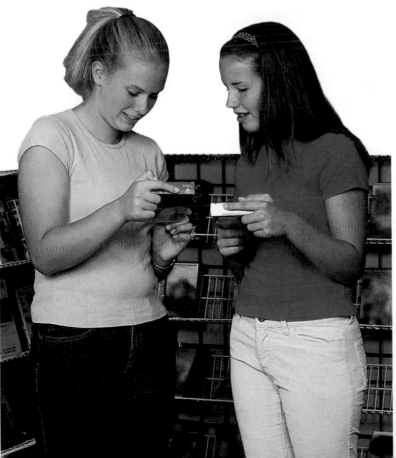

Being free to make more decisions on your own is part of adolescence. However, with this new freedom comes increased responsibility for your actions.

What Is Abstinence?

The only way to stay safe from risk behaviors is to practice abstinence. **Abstinence** is *not participating in unsafe behaviors or activities.* When you abstain from tobacco, alcohol, drugs, and sexual activity, you are showing self-respect.

Abstinence from Tobacco, Alcohol, and Other Drugs

By avoiding tobacco, alcohol, and other drugs, you protect yourself against the many dangers associated with the use of these substances. (See **Figure 8.5**.) These dangers include

- **poor physical health.** Smoking decreases breathing capacity. It is also linked to heart and lung diseases and certain cancers. Using alcohol or other drugs can seriously damage the nervous system and liver.
- **dependence.** Once you start using tobacco, alcohol, or other drugs, you may not be able to quit without professional help.
- **trouble with the law.** Only adults can legally use tobacco or alcohol. The use of certain other drugs is illegal for everyone. There are serious legal consequences of possessing or using these substances.
- **inability to reach your goals.** Using alcohol or other drugs can lower your performance in school. It can also weaken your commitment to abstain from sexual activity. Both of these situations can interfere with your goals.

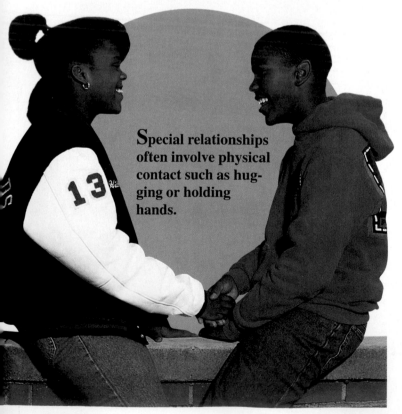

Special relationships often involve physical contact such as hugging or holding hands.

The Benefits of Abstinence from Sexual Activity

Abstinence from sexual activity before marriage is the standard that is expected of all teens. Teens who abstain from sexual activity

- never have to worry about unplanned pregnancy.
- will not be faced with difficult decisions that are associated with unplanned pregnancy, such as teen marriage or adoption.
- do not have to worry about sexually transmitted diseases (STDs).
- are making a choice that is always legal. It is illegal for unmarried minors to engage in sexual activity.
- do not have to deal with the emotional consequences of sexual activity, which can include guilt, regret, and rejection.

- can establish nonsexual closeness with members of the opposite gender and can develop genuine feelings of love and trust.
- can focus on setting and achieving their life goals and dreams.

Abstinence from sexual activity before marriage is the only method that is 100 percent effective in preventing pregnancy, STDs, the sexual transmission of HIV, and emotional trauma associated with adolescent sexual activity. Making a commitment to abstain from sexual activity before marriage will protect your health.

FIGURE 8.5

CHOOSING ABSTINENCE

Abstaining from risk behaviors protects your physical, mental/emotional, and social health. *What are some other reasons to choose abstinence?*

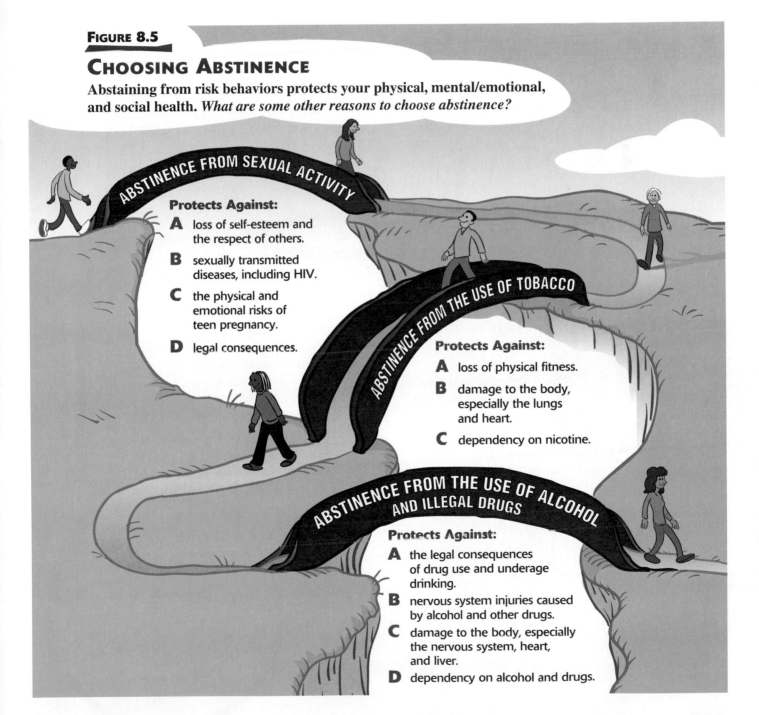

ABSTINENCE FROM SEXUAL ACTIVITY

Protects Against:

A loss of self-esteem and the respect of others.

B sexually transmitted diseases, including HIV.

C the physical and emotional risks of teen pregnancy.

D legal consequences.

ABSTINENCE FROM THE USE OF TOBACCO

Protects Against:

A loss of physical fitness.

B damage to the body, especially the lungs and heart.

C dependency on nicotine.

ABSTINENCE FROM THE USE OF ALCOHOL AND ILLEGAL DRUGS

Protects Against:

A the legal consequences of drug use and underage drinking.

B nervous system injuries caused by alcohol and other drugs.

C damage to the body, especially the nervous system, heart, and liver.

D dependency on alcohol and drugs.

Effective Refusal Skills

In Lesson 3 you learned ways to resist negative peer pressure. You will find more tips on these pages. S.T.O.P. is an easy way to remember how to use refusal skills.

- **S**ay no in a firm voice.
- **T**ell why not.
- **O**ffer another idea.
- **P**romptly leave.

Choosing friends who share your values and standards is a good place to start. Friends who think and feel the same way you do will not ask you to do anything unhealthful or unsafe. In fact, they will depend on you to support them if others pressure them.

Changing the subject is sometimes a good approach. It can often get you out of a potentially dangerous situation. If peers pressure you to do something that violates your values, simply suggest an alternative activity. You might say that playing video games sounds like more fun. Sometimes putting off any kind of answer works, especially with people you don't expect to see again.

HEALTH SKILLS ACTIVITY

REFUSAL SKILLS

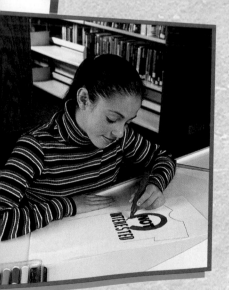

Ways to Say No

It is important to practice behaviors that support the decision to abstain from tobacco, alcohol, and other drugs and sexual activity. Using refusal skills can protect you from these risk behaviors. To refuse, you can

- say no over and over until the other person gets the message.
- give a reason for refusing. If you think that your peers will see your point, tell them exactly why you're not interested. You could

say, "Hey, we're all minors. We could get into trouble for drinking." If you think that they won't accept your reason, make up a convincing excuse or just leave.
- reverse the pressure. If you're talking to friends, tell them: "A good friend would respect my decision."
- avoid the question or change the subject.
- suggest a healthful alternative.
- be direct. Make it clear that your mind is made up.

WITH A GROUP
Create a design for a T-shirt that uses words and images to illustrate one way to say no. As a class, vote on the T-shirt design that is the most appealing and that presents the most convincing message.

Evaluate every situation carefully. Does it sound dangerous? Suspicious? Just plain wrong? Say no, and avoid the situation. It is much easier to avoid a bad situation completely than to try to get out of one once you're already in it. If someone threatens you or urges you to do something that makes you feel uncomfortable, walk away. This may be difficult, but getting involved in a risky situation could turn out far worse. If someone whom you consider a friend is pressuring you to compromise your values or place your safety at risk, you may need to take another look at that relationship. This person may not be a good friend if your values are so different.

Talking about refusal skills with adults you trust can help you develop the strength and confidence you need. Their experiences may be helpful to you.

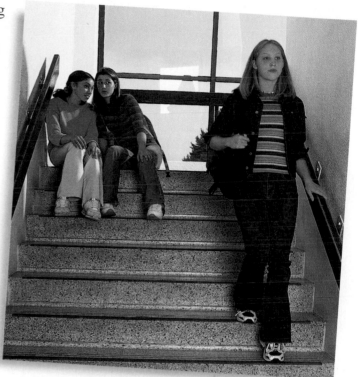

It takes courage to walk away when peers pressure you to engage in a risk behavior. *How do you feel after you have resisted such pressure?*

Lesson 4 Review

Using complete sentences, answer the following questions on a sheet of paper.

Reviewing Terms and Facts
1. **Vocabulary** Define *abstinence*.
2. **List** Name two negative results of using tobacco, alcohol, or other drugs.
3. **Recall** State three benefits of sexual abstinence for teens.
4. **Identify** List five of the refusal tips mentioned in this lesson.

Thinking Critically
5. **Apply** How can you promote positive health behaviors among your peers?

6. **Apply** Think of a risk behavior that could have long-term negative effects for a teen. Explain what these effects might be.

Applying Health Skills
7. **Practicing Healthful Behaviors** In a few paragraphs, discuss negative peer pressure and the effectiveness of refusal skills. Your title should be "How Well Do Refusal Skills Work?" Explain when you think the skills would work best and when they would be hard to use. Which tips seem to you to be the most useful? What mistakes do your peers commonly make when they try to use refusal skills?

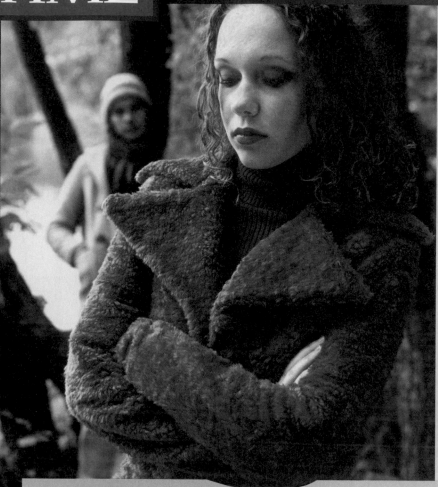

What happens when friendships don't work out? We interviewed Patty and Anne— two teens who were once best friends—to get both sides of the story.

WHEN Friendships Hurt

When did you two become friends?

PATTY: In sixth grade, Susie, Jasmine, Anne, and I were a group of popular girls. I was really close with Anne. We went to the mall a lot, and we also went to the movies. We called boys and giggled about it.

ANNE: I'm pretty sure we were all in the same homeroom, and that's how we became friends. I was better friends with Patty than Susie and Jasmine were. But we weren't the most popular girls.

How did the friendship end?

PATTY: I remember clearly the day Anne stopped talking to me. I sat down with her and our other friends at lunch, tried to add to the conversation, and no one responded. So I moved down to the other end of the table. The next day still no one would talk to me. They just abandoned me completely.

ANNE: We didn't get into a big fight. That winter Susie and I started hanging out more with the popular girls, and maybe that's where the break was. Patty didn't really fit into that group. I don't think she was really into clothes and stuff like we were.

How did things change?

PATTY: Everything changed. After they stopped talking to me, Susie came up to me in the cafeteria and asked me if wanted to come over to her house after school. When I said yes, she said, "Never mind, just kidding," laughed, and walked away. Everyone was watching.

How To End an Unhealthy Friendship

Do you have a friendship that doesn't seem to be working anymore, or feels "out of control"? A friend who pressures you to do things you don't want to do? A friend who insults other people—or you?

Try to work things out. If your attempts fail, however, here are a few tips on how to end an unhealthy friendship:

Avoid Fireworks

You've already tried everything to get your friend to act differently, right? The only reason to confront your friend again is to get something off your chest—which creates more drama. Instead, says Erika Lutz, author of *The Complete Idiot's Guide to Friendship for Teens,* let them know it's over by calling them less often and "don't spend time with them alone."

Hold Your Ground

Your friend might confront you about the way you're fading out the friendship. Christine Wickert Koubek, author of *Friends, Cliques and Peer Pressure,* suggests responding with something like, "It's hard to tell you this because we've been such good friends, but I just don't feel the same about our friendship anymore." Avoid criticizing your friend's behavior.

Minimize Your Losses

You may be tempted to backstab your old friend. Wrong move. "No matter what the other person says, don't bad-mouth them back," says Kristen Kemp, author of *What a Friend.* "If people ask, just say you wish things could have worked out."

Trust Your Decision

If you're losing a close friend, you'll naturally be very hurt by what's happening. You might even want to reconnect with your old pal. Be strong and stay positive during the painful period after a friendship ends. This will allow you to concentrate on forming friendships that make your life better, not worse.

ANNE: I don't remember that. I don't remember teasing Patty. We weren't mean to her.

Do you have different friends now?
PATTY: I wondered every day what really happened with Anne. What did I do wrong? Then, I realized that it might have nothing to do with me. Sometimes, two people are just different—and don't have to be best friends. I see Anne around school and now we smile and say hi, but I have a new group of friends who are great.
ANNE: Susie and Jasmine and I are still really close. I think about how much fun Patty and I had sometimes, but I know that things are better this way. ■

TIME TO THINK...

About Friendships

In small groups, brainstorm a list of specific situations that could have a negative effect on friendships—for example, a teen who pressures a friend to do something unhealthy or dangerous. Choose one of the situations on your list and create a skit that shows how this situation might impact a friendship. Role-play your skit for the rest of the class. After groups have had a chance to perform their skits, discuss the specific issues presented in each one, as well as other situations in which a friendship might need to end.

PRACTICING GOOD COMMUNICATION

Model

Gabriella has been practicing her speaking and listening skills. Here is part of a conversation she had with her father.

DAD: **Gabriella, I have a favor to ask. I need you to watch your little brother again tonight. I'm sorry to ask three nights in a row.**

GABRIELLA: **I can see you are upset.** *Show empathy.* **Is everything okay?** *Ask questions.*

DAD: **Everything's okay, but I really need to get some of this extra paperwork done.**

GABRIELLA: **I'm sorry you are so stressed.** *Use an "I" message and show empathy.* (Gabriella pauses.) *Think before you speak.* **I had plans with Kiara, but I can do it if you need me to. I'll call her now.** *Use "I" messages.*

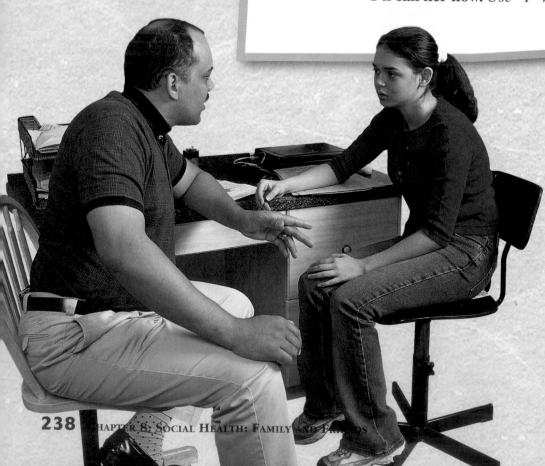

Practice

Here's a chance to become a better communicator. Work with a partner to have a five-minute conversation on paper. One of you will begin by writing a greeting to the other. Then the partner will respond. Here's the tricky part: You have to use one of the communication skills from this chapter every time you add to the conversation. You can include nonverbal communication in parentheses. Don't plan your conversation ahead. If you're stuck for ideas, try one of these:

- My responsibilities at home
- Activities or holidays my family enjoys
- A funny family story

After everyone's done, paired students should take turns reading their conversations to the class. Identify the skills that were used in each conversation. Why are good communication skills important?

Apply/Assess

Think of a situation that would require good communication skills. It might involve telling a friend a secret, consoling someone, or encouraging a peer. Write your situation on a slip of paper, and place it in a container provided by your teacher.

With a partner, draw one of the slips out of the container. Using good communication skills, start a conversation based on the situation described. Don't plan your conversation ahead of time. Have your classmates identify the speaking and listening skills that you and your partner use.

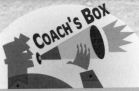

COACH'S BOX

Communication Skills

Speaking skills
- Think before you speak.
- Use "I" messages.
- Be direct, but avoid being rude or insulting.
- Make eye contact and use appropriate body language.

Listening skills
- Use conversation encouragers.
- Pay attention.
- Show empathy.
- Avoid interrupting but ask questions when appropriate.

Self-√Check
- Did we use good speaking and listening skills in our conversation?
- Could I identify the speaking and listening skills in others' conversations?

After You Read

Use your completed Foldable to review the information on verbal and nonverbal communication.

FOLDABLES™
Study Organizer

Reviewing Vocabulary and Concepts

On a sheet of paper, write the numbers 1–8. After each number, write the term from the list that best completes each statement.

- listener
- verbal communication
- tact
- mental
- attitude
- body language
- blended
- society

Lesson 1

1. An e-mail message is a form of _____.
2. A smile is an example of _____.
3. Using _____ when expressing your opinions or thoughts ensures that you will not offend others.
4. Using phrases such as "Really?" or "Go on," is the mark of a good _____.

Lesson 2

5. The basic unit of _____ is the family.
6. A family that consists of a parent, step-parent, and one child or two or more children is a _____ family.
7. As children and adults in a family share their knowledge, skills, and experiences, they meet each other's _____ needs.
8. By being supportive and having a positive _____, you will be better able to deal with family challenges.

On a sheet of paper, write the numbers 9–16. Write *True* or *False* for each statement below. If the statement is false, change the underlined word or phrase to make it true.

Lesson 3

9. <u>Advocacy</u> occurs when two people each give up something to reach a solution that satisfies both of them.
10. The influence that your friends have on you to think and act like them is called <u>peer pressure</u>.
11. Avoiding a potentially risky situation is one way to handle <u>positive</u> peer pressure.
12. <u>Popularity</u> is based on who you are as a complete person.

Lesson 4

13. You choose <u>abstinence</u> when you don't participate in unsafe behaviors and activities.
14. <u>Engaging in</u> risk behaviors shows that you respect yourself.
15. Teens who abstain from <u>sexual activity</u> before marriage can focus on achieving their goals.
16. Making it clear that your mind is made up can be an effective <u>refusal</u> skill.

Thinking Critically

Using complete sentences, answer the following questions on a sheet of paper.

17. **Contrast** Write a sentence that uses a "you" message to express an opinion or idea. Then rewrite the same sentence to express the same idea using an "I" message. Which sentence do you think would get a better response from a listener, and why?
18. **Compare** How are your relationships with family members similar to your relationships with friends? How are they different?

19. **Solve** Review the ways in which a family might deal with a particular challenge. With a classmate, brainstorm other strategies that families could use to cope with this problem and the stress that this challenge may cause.

20. **Analyze** Describe some ways of handling negative peer pressure and situations in which you might use them.

21. **Apply** Explain the effects of peer pressure on decision making.

Career Corner

Family Counselor Do you like to help others solve problems? Are you a good listener and communicator? If so, a career as a family counselor may be for you. These professionals teach family members how to listen to one another effectively and to work together to find solutions. To become a family counselor, you'll need four years of college and a two-year advanced degree in counseling. Find out more about this and other health careers by visiting Career Corner at health.glencoe.com.

Standardized Test Practice

Reading & Writing

Read the paragraphs below and then answer the questions.

Janine sighed as she heard her parents unlock the apartment door. Now she'd have to tell them.

"Honey, we're home," said Mom. "What's wrong? You look upset."

Janine looked down at her feet. "I got a D on my math test. I guess I didn't understand the concepts that well, but I didn't want to ask for help."

"Why not, sweetie? You know we would have helped you study," said Dad.

"I thought I should be able to get it on my own," Janine admitted.

"Tell you what," said Mom, "Let's go over the test right now so we can help you do better next time."

"Thanks, Mom and Dad. I'm so glad you guys aren't mad," said Janine.

1. The tone of the conversation can best be described as
   (A) amusing.
   (B) concerned.
   (C) informative.
   (D) angry.

2. Which of the following statements best summarizes this conversation?
   (A) Janine is upset that she did poorly on her test, but her parents aren't angry about this and offer to help her.
   (B) Janine doesn't care that she did poorly on her test.
   (C) Janine's parents expected that she would do poorly on her test.
   (D) Janine's parents are angry with her because she did poorly on her test.

3. Write a paragraph using dialogue to tell about an event.

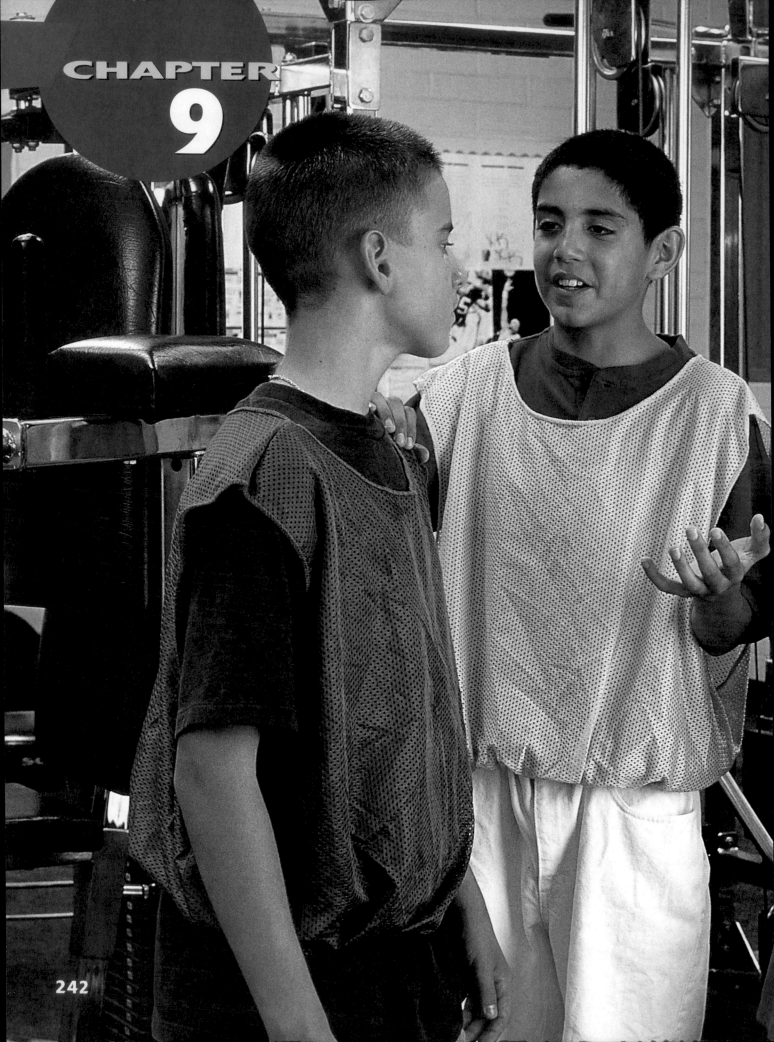

Resolving Conflicts and Preventing Violence

HEALTH *Online*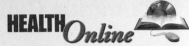

To discover how much you know about resolving conflicts and preventing violence, go to health.glencoe.com and take the Health Inventory for Chapter 9.

FOLDABLES™
Study Organizer

Before You Read

Make this Foldable to help you organize what you learn in Lesson 1 about conflict at home and at school. Begin with a plain sheet of 11″ × 17″ paper.

Step 1

Fold the sheet of paper into thirds along the short axis. This forms three columns.

Step 2

Open the paper and refold into thirds along the long axis, then fold in half again lengthwise. This forms six rows.

Step 3

Unfold and draw lines along the folds.

Step 4

Label the chart as shown.

Cause	Escalation	De-escalation
Argument		
Peer Pressure		
Revenge		
Prejudice		
Additional Notes		

As You Read

In the appropriate column, fill in what you learn about the causes of conflict. Then give an example of a behavior that might escalate and de-escalate that type of conflict.

243

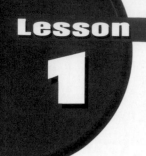

Conflicts at Home and at School

Common Causes of Conflict

In the course of a day, you may see or be involved in conflict. A **conflict** is *a disagreement between people with opposing viewpoints.* Conflicts happen for many reasons. They often occur when one person has not met the expectation of another. The reason for a conflict may seem unimportant, but small quarrels can turn into serious—even deadly—fights. Disagreements do not have to end in violence. People should always look for a nonviolent solution to conflict.

Arguments

Disagreements are a part of life, but they can intensify into arguments. When arguments get out of hand, fights may result. Here are some of the most common reasons teens argue:

- **Property.** Teens may not respect one another's property. They may use others' possessions without asking permission.
- **Hurt feelings.** Jealousy and hurt pride often lead to arguments. Teens may feel jealous when they are left out of activities or

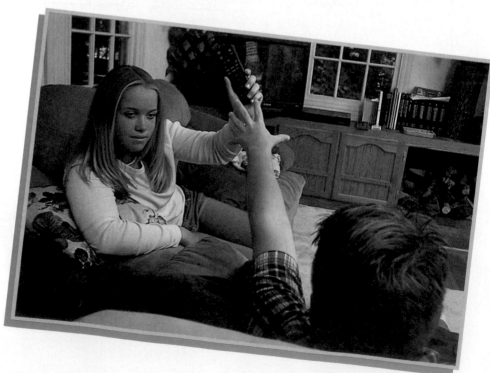

When people live in the same space, conflicts may occur over items that need to be shared, such as the television. *What are some issues that start conflicts between siblings?*

when a friend pays attention to someone else. Hurt pride may result from insults, gossip, or teasing.

- **Values.** Teens may refuse to do something that goes against their values, such as lying, cheating, or stealing.
- **Territory.** Teens may feel that someone is trespassing on territory that they consider theirs. An outsider could be talking to their friends or hanging out in their neighborhood.

Peer Pressure

Peers may urge others to "fight it out." Once a group gathers to cheer on or tease the fighters, it becomes much harder to solve the problem peacefully.

Revenge

If someone insults you or your family, your first instinct may be to get even. If you give in to this instinct, the other person may decide to retaliate. This can set off a chain of events that spirals out of control. Acts of revenge are common among rival gangs and can lead to violence, such as a stabbing or a shoot-out. This obviously has negative effects on both individual and community health.

Prejudice

People may refuse to accept others who are different from themselves. Their feelings may be based on **prejudice** (PRE·juh·dis), *a negative and unjustly formed opinion, usually against people of a different racial, religious, or cultural group.* People who are prejudiced may single out a person to harass, intimidate, or threaten. If that person strikes back, fights or even gang warfare may result.

MEDIA○WATCH

CONFLICTS ON TELEVISION

Television shows often focus on a conflict between characters. Watch your favorite TV program and identify any conflicts that occur in the story. *What caused the conflicts? How were they resolved? Do you think that the characters dealt with the conflict in a healthful way? Why or why not?*

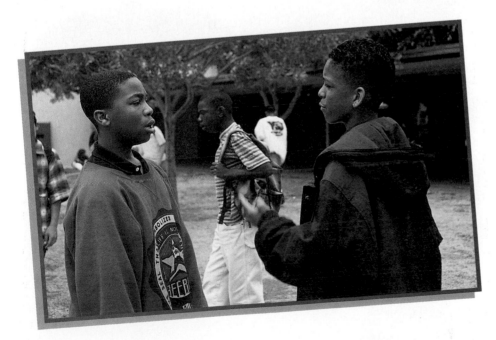

A conflict in values can lead to an argument. *What situations might cause an argument about values?*

CONNECT TO

Language Arts

THE MEANING OF
DEMEANING
**The verb *demean*
means to lower in
character, dignity, or
value. Demeaning
statements are those
that are intended to
hurt others' feelings.
To prevent conflict and
enhance social health,
avoid directing de-
meaning statements
toward others. Every-
one deserves to be
treated with dignity
and respect. *Think of
three antonyms for the
adjective demeaning.***

How Conflicts Build

If conflicts are allowed to escalate, or grow, they can result in violence. Conflicts can escalate if the people involved have never learned how to resolve their differences peacefully. However, you may be able to stop a conflict from getting worse if you notice the warning signs. **Figure 9.1** lists some of these "red flags." Remember, it's easier to resolve a conflict peacefully when you're still in control of your emotions.

Preventing Conflict

It is not always easy to avoid conflicts, but it is possible. Here are some suggestions for preventing serious conflicts.

- **Practice good communication.** When you disagree with some-one, use "I" messages. Good communication can prevent the hurt feelings that may turn a simple disagreement into a fight.
- **Ignore some conflicts.** Show self-control by choosing your bat-tles. Some issues are not worth your time and effort.
- **Don't take sides.** Avoid getting involved in a conflict between other people. Never speak on someone else's behalf.
- **Show disapproval of fighting.** Don't add fuel to the fire of con-flict or urge others to fight as a solution. Refuse to spread rumors, and do your best to ignore people who talk badly about others.

FIGURE 9.1

Spotting the Red Flags

These behaviors may signal that a conflict is escalating.
What might you do if you notice one of these signs?

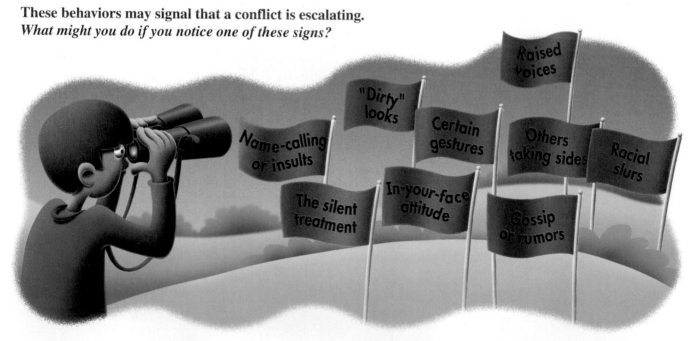

PRACTICING HEALTHFUL BEHAVIORS

Managing Anger

Anger can turn a simple disagreement into something more serious. Be alert for the physical signs of anger: increased heart and breathing rates, sweaty palms, a flushed face, and stuttering or speaking in a high-pitched voice. If you are able to practice self-control, you're more likely to resolve the conflict peacefully. Here are some healthful ways to manage your anger.

- Walk, jog, swim, or shoot some baskets.
- Listen to music.
- Pound a pillow.

- Talk the problem out with a good friend or family member.
- Sit quietly for half an hour or so.
- Find a school counselor or health care professional who can help you manage your anger.

ON YOUR OWN

Write a poem or song that creatively describes several healthful ways to manage anger. You can use the tips listed here and/or incorporate your own ideas.

Lesson 1 Review

Using complete sentences, answer the following questions on a sheet of paper.

Reviewing Terms and Facts

1. **Vocabulary** Define the term *conflict*.
2. **Identify** List and explain three causes of arguments among teens.
3. **Explain** Name four warning signs that conflict may be escalating.
4. **Summarize** In your own words, explain how you can avoid serious conflicts.

Thinking Critically

5. **Synthesize** Explain how mutual respect can help to prevent each of the common causes of arguments among teens.

6. **Apply** Which anger management techniques do you think would work best for you? Why?

Applying Health Skills

7. **Accessing Information** Use Internet and library resources to research the lives of Mohandas Gandhi and Martin Luther King, Jr., two individuals who were committed to nonviolent solutions to conflict. Write a paragraph on your findings and share it with the class. As a class, discuss how these two individuals served as role models. How did their work positively influence community health?

Conflict Resolution Skills

Resolving Conflicts Peacefully

Nobody wins in a violent situation. That is why **nonviolent confrontation**, *resolving a conflict by peaceful methods,* should be the approach you take to deal with unavoidable conflicts. Nonviolent confrontation will allow you to settle matters without angry words or looks, threats, punches, or weapons. This method makes it more likely that everyone will walk away satisfied.

Sometimes, in order to resolve a conflict peacefully, both sides must compromise, or give up something to reach a solution that suits everyone. For example, you may want to go out with your friends when your parents want you to stay home. You agree on a solution: you'll go out but come home early. In this case you and your parents have compromised. Compromise is an essential element of healthy and mature relationships. It works in everyday situations when you and a family member, friend, or peer disagree on common matters. On the other hand, some situations do not allow compromise. Never compromise your deepest values; your sense of right and wrong; or the rules of your parents, school, and community.

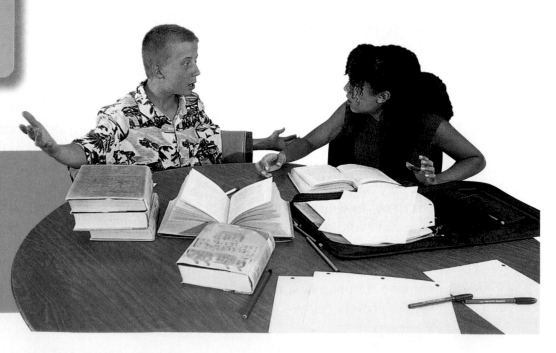

These teens need to work together on a class project, but they cannot agree on the best approach to complete the assignment. *How might they compromise?*

Resolving Conflicts Through Negotiation

A key factor in conflict resolution is negotiation. **Negotiation** (ni·goh·shee·AY·shuhn) is *the process of discussing problems face-to-face in order to reach a solution.* Effective negotiation includes talking, listening, considering other points of view, and compromising. The T.A.L.K. strategy, illustrated in **Figure 9.2,** can help you remember how to negotiate by using the steps of conflict resolution.

- **T**ake time out before you confront the other person— at least 30 minutes.
- **A**llow each person to tell his or her side of the story uninterrupted.
- **L**et each person ask questions of the other.
- **K**eep brainstorming to find a good solution for both parties.

When you negotiate, be sure that you know what you want to say, and stay calm. Try to talk to the other person privately and avoid accusing, insulting, or threatening the other person. Pay attention to body language. Never stay around to negotiate if there is a weapon present or if you are threatened with physical harm.

☑
Reading Check
Understand word parts. The prefixes *com-* and *con-* both mean "together." The root *-flict* means "strike." Write your own definitions for the words *compromise* and *conflict.*

FIGURE 9.2

THE NEGOTIATION PROCESS

By using the process of negotiation, you can find your way through the maze of disagreement. *How could you use these steps to resolve conflicts in your life?*

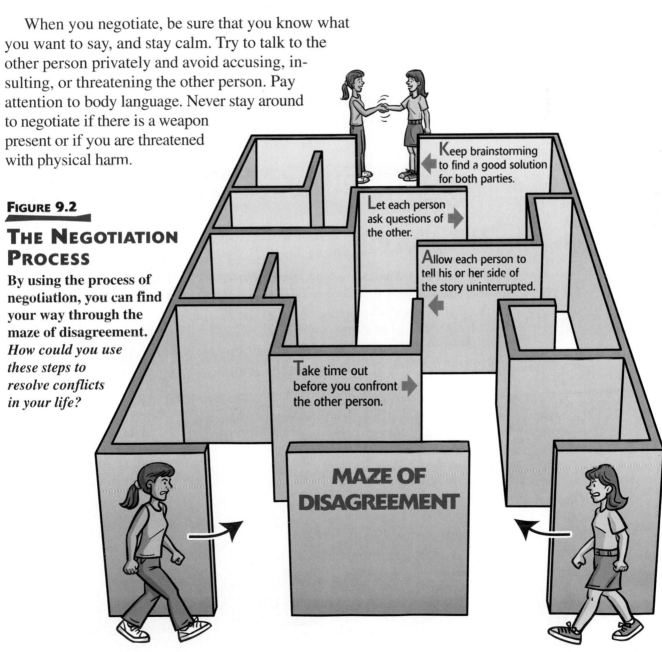

Keep brainstorming to find a good solution for both parties.

Let each person ask questions of the other.

Allow each person to tell his or her side of the story uninterrupted.

Take time out before you confront the other person.

MAZE OF DISAGREEMENT

Peer Mediation

Mediation is another way to solve conflicts. **Mediation** (mee·dee·AY·shuhn) is *resolving conflicts by using another person or persons to help reach a solution that is acceptable to both sides.* The mediator must be neutral. **Neutrality** (noo·TRA·luh·tee) is *a promise not to take sides.* Some schools use peer mediation to resolve conflicts caused by such behavior as name-calling, bullying, or gossiping. A student or a pair of students mediates a discussion between the teens who are in conflict.

Achieving a Win-Win Situation

Some people approach conflict resolution with the belief that someone must win and someone else must lose. This view can make the disagreement worse. One person is likely to feel angry or cheated. It's healthier to think of conflict resolution as a win-win situation. Negotiation and mediation can make this possible.

When people seek to work out their conflicts together, they don't give up until they've reached an agreement. When the solution to a

HEALTH SKILLS ACTIVITY

CONFLICT RESOLUTION

Disagreements with Friends

Dai and Greg have been friends for a long time. Lately, however, Greg has started to spend more time with Shari, a girl he likes. Dai has been looking forward to Saturday, when he and Greg are supposed to go to a baseball game together. However, Greg just told Dai that he is going to the movies with Shari instead. Dai shouted, "If you're going to put Shari ahead of me, you can just spend all your time with her from now on!"

What Would You Do?

Apply the steps of conflict resolution to Dai and Greg's problem. Write a script that shows how Dai and Greg arrive at an acceptable solution.

TAKE A TIME OUT, AT LEAST **30** MINUTES.
ALLOW EACH PERSON TO TELL HIS OR HER SIDE UNINTERRUPTED.
LET EACH PERSON ASK QUESTIONS.
KEEP BRAINSTORMING TO FIND A GOOD SOLUTION.

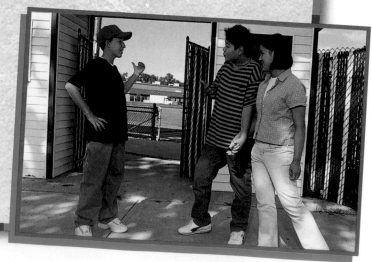

problem is acceptable to each person, everybody wins. By discussing the conflict, they may come up with solutions that make matters better than they were before the conflict. Families, schools, and communities win as well. Negotiation and mediation help to keep conflicts from getting out of hand.

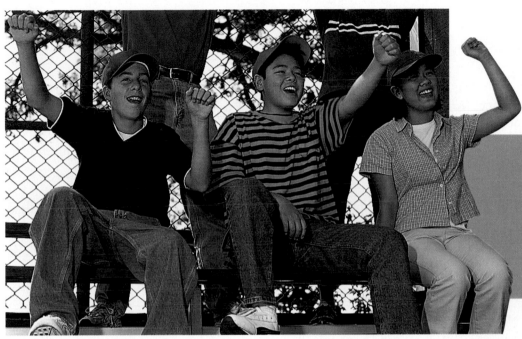

Conflicts don't have to result in winners and losers. *How did Dai and Greg from the Health Skills Activity achieve a win-win situation?*

Lesson Review

Using complete sentences, answer the following questions on a sheet of paper.

Reviewing Terms and Facts

1. **Vocabulary** Define the term *nonviolent confrontation.*
2. **Explain** How can compromise be a part of resolving conflicts peacefully?
3. **Recall** What are the steps of conflict resolution?
4. **Describe** Explain the role of a peer mediator in a disagreement.

Thinking Critically

5. **Categorize** Give an example of a conflict that might be solved by compromise. Then give an example of a conflict in which you should not compromise. Explain why these situations should be handled differently.
6. **Predict** How might conflict-resolution and mediation skills help you in your life?

Applying Health Skills

7. **Advocacy** If your school has a peer mediation program, write an open letter to the editor of your local newspaper. Explain the program to your community. If your school does not have such a program, write a letter to your principal. Ask for a peer mediation program in your school. Either kind of letter should list the benefits of peer mediation. Explain what kinds of conflicts could be solved with peer mediation. Then outline how the program would work.

Preventing Violence

Quick Write

List three ways to protect yourself from violence and the deliberate injuries that can result.

LEARN ABOUT...

- how violence affects teens.
- the causes of violence in society.
- what you can do to avoid becoming a victim of violence.
- what is being done to prevent violence in schools and communities.

VOCABULARY

- assault
- rape
- homicide
- deliberate injury
- hate crime
- gang
- bully
- Neighborhood Watch

Violence in Society

Images of violence are all around you. Grim stories of beatings, stabbings, gang wars, and abuse within families are reported on the news and featured in movies. Violence is a major public health problem in the United States. **Figure 9.3** gives information on how frequently violent crimes are committed in the nation.

Some people blame much of this violence on the media. Because some TV programs, movies, and song lyrics glamorize violence, they may lead people to believe that violence is an acceptable way to settle disagreements. Others feel that violence has increased because of the breakdown of families, a decline in moral values, and the increased availability of weapons.

FIGURE 9.3

VIOLENT CRIME IN THE UNITED STATES

Hundreds of violent crimes take place every day in the United States. Many types of violent crime lead to deliberate injuries.

The Daily News

Assault is *a physical attack or a threat of an attack for the purpose of inflicting bodily injury.* About 2,510 aggravated assaults (assaults that involve weapons or cause serious physical harm) take place each day.

Homicide (HAH-muh-syd) is *a violent crime that results in the death of another individual.* Murder is a form of homicide. Approximately 43 people die in homicides each day.

Rape is *forced sexual intercourse.* Approximately 224 rapes are committed each day.

Robbery is *a completed or attempted theft of property or cash by force or threat of force with a weapon.* About 1,122 armed robberies occur each day.

FIGURE 9.4

VIOLENT VICTIMIZATION RATES BY AGE, 1999

This graph refers to victims of assault, rape, homicide, and robbery in 1999. The bars show how many people in 1,000 have been victims in each age group.

Age of victim

12–15	16–19	20–24	25–34	35–49	50–64	65+
74.5	77.6	68.7	36.4	25.2	14.4	3.9

Source: Bureau of Justice

Teens and Violence

The majority of teens are not violent and do not commit crimes. Nevertheless, about one-fourth of all violent crime in the United States is committed by people under the age of 18. As **Figure 9.4** shows, teens are also more than twice as likely as people age 25 and older to be victims of violence. In fact, the second leading cause of death for all people between the ages of 15 and 24 is homicide. Violent crime often leads to **deliberate injury**, *injury that results when one person intentionally harms another*.

Causes of Violence

People who commit violent acts may not have learned how to cope with feelings such as anger in healthful ways. Other factors that contribute to violence in the community include:

- **Prejudice.** A negative and unjustly formed opinion of a particular group can lead to hate crimes. A **hate crime** is *an illegal act against someone just because he or she is a member of a particular group.*
- **Weapons.** The rise in crime and deliberate injuries may be related to easier access to a variety of weapons, including guns.
- **Peer pressure.** Teens may become involved in violence because they want to show loyalty to or be accepted by a group. Pressure from the group may cause teens to go against their values.
- **Alcohol and other drugs.** People who are under the influence of alcohol or other drugs commit almost half of all violent crimes.

Gangs

A **gang** is *a group of people who associate with one another to take part in criminal activity.* For example, gang members may attack members of other gangs or threaten other people. They may be involved in drive-by shootings, robbery, illegal drugs, and rape. Criminal gangs have strict rules. Members hang out only with each other. They use their own signals, nicknames, and terms. They may wear gang tattoos or colors.

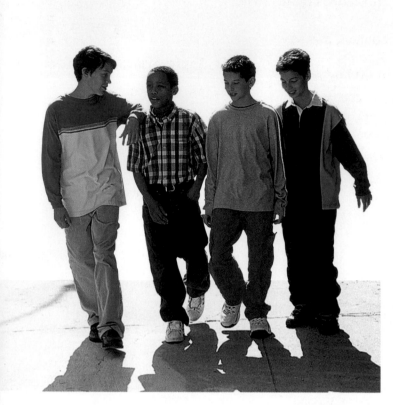

Resist gangs by refusing to hang out with gang members and by encouraging your peers to do the same. *What are some other strategies for avoiding gang violence?*

Why do some teens join gangs? Teens who join gangs may feel lonely, bored, or isolated. Many become part of a gang due to peer pressure. Some think that they will gain respect, power, and friends. Other teens hope that a gang will offer them protection. Still others might want to be with people of their own racial or ethnic group. Here are some ways to stay clear of gangs.

- Use refusal skills to avoid getting involved with gangs.
- Don't hang out with gang members. You might get blamed for what they do or gradually be drawn into the group.
- Resist all pressure to do anything illegal.
- Apply strategies for avoiding weapons.

If gang members threaten you, stay calm and don't overreact. Even if you are afraid, try not to show fear. Walk away calmly. Get help from police, school officials, or other trusted adults.

Violence Prevention

You can help keep yourself safe from violence. You and your peers can also work to stop violence in your school and community.

Protecting Yourself

People who commit violent crimes seek out those who look vulnerable and weak. Reduce the chances of becoming a victim of violent crime by learning to protect yourself. The tips on the next page and in **Figure 9.5** will help you to stay safe.

- Do not look like an easy target. Stand up straight, and walk with a confident stride. If you can, walk with a group or at least one other person.

- Do not use alcohol or other drugs. These substances reduce your ability to protect yourself.
- If someone bothers you, make direct eye contact, and say "Leave me alone" in a firm voice.
- If you are in real physical danger, shout "Fire!" to get other people's attention. Use this approach only if you need help fast—not if someone is simply bothering you.
- If someone attacks you, get away in any way that you can.
- If someone demands your money or jewelry, throw it away from you. Then run in the opposite direction.

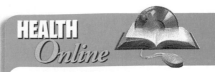

HEALTH *Online*

Topic: Avoiding violence

For a link to more information on avoiding violence, go to **health.glencoe.com**.

Activity: Using the information provided at this link, list ways to prevent violence.

FIGURE 9.5

Safety on the Street and at Home

These safety tips can keep you from becoming a victim of violence. *What other precautions might you take?*

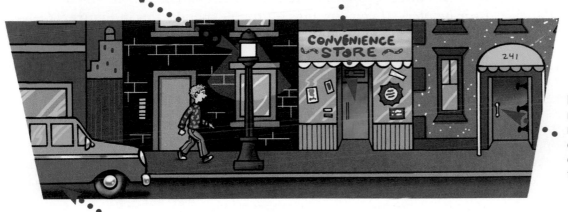

At night, walk in lighted areas, and avoid dark alleyways. Avoid walking alone if possible.

If you think that someone is following you, go into a store or other public place.

Have your keys ready when you reach your front door so that you do not have to fumble for them.

Do not hitchhike or accept rides from strangers.

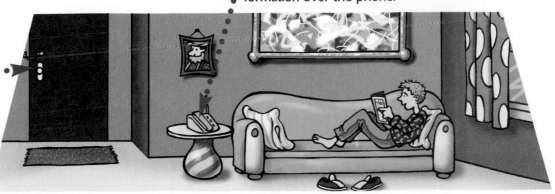

Do not tell unknown callers that you are home alone or give out any personal information over the phone.

At home, keep doors and windows locked. Do not open the door for someone you do not know.

Reading Check
Identify causes and effects. Write sentences using *If..., then...* statements.

Stopping Violence in Schools

Conflict-resolution programs, dress codes, and security measures are making many schools safer. You can support your school's health and safety efforts by understanding and following rules prohibiting possession of weapons at school.

Conflict-resolution programs help teens to understand alternatives to violence and teach them to act responsibly in social situations. Peer mediation helps students to work out problems. Some schools have established dress codes as one way to reduce violence. Dress codes can help to play down the economic differences among students and make it harder for gang members to wear special identifiers.

Some schools keep their students safe by using security systems. Metal detectors, security cameras, and guards help keep weapons out of schools. Under certain conditions, lockers may be searched. Trained dogs can be used to sniff out drugs and weapons.

What to Do if Someone Wants to Fight

You may be in control of your emotions, but when someone else is looking for a fight, you need to think fast. The person may be angry with you or may simply be a bully. A **bully** is *someone who uses threats, taunts, or violence to intimidate people who appear helpless.* If you see signs of trouble, put the tips in **Figure 9.6** to use. You can stop a conflict before it becomes a fight, possibly leading to deliberate injuries. If you are ever hurt or feel threatened, it is important to tell a trusted adult.

FIGURE 9.6

WHAT TO DO IF SOMEONE WANTS TO FIGHT

Stopping a conflict before it begins is the best solution to any problem. *How can these strategies help prevent deliberate injuries?*

Do exercise self-control: Stay calm and speak in a low voice. Apologize or walk away if necessary.

Do something unexpected to divert the other person's attention.

Do use humor.

Do give the other person a way out. Make it possible for her or him to leave and save face without fighting.

Do try to understand what the other person thinks, feels, or needs.

Don't let the other person force you to fight.

Don't let your emotions throw you off balance.

Don't try to even the score.

Don't tease or be hostile, threatening, insulting, rude, or sarcastic.

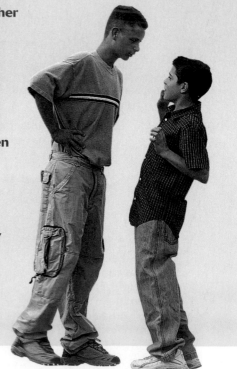

Stopping Violence in Communities

Communities may use the strategies listed below to make their neighborhoods safer:

- **More police on the streets.** Some communities have made an effort to put their law officers on foot, bicycle, or horseback patrols.
- **Neighborhood Watch programs.** A street or block may start a **Neighborhood Watch**, *a widespread crime-prevention effort undertaken by residents of a particular segment of the community.* People are trained to look for signs of trouble around their neighborhood and to help each other.
- **After-school programs.** Many communities offer academic, recreational, or cultural after-school programs for teens. These programs help teens to feel safe and use their time productively.
- **Improved lighting in parks and playgrounds.** Added light can discourage crime by making it more difficult to commit crimes without being seen.
- **Tougher laws.** Because of the Brady Law, people can no longer purchase guns legally without undergoing a background check. Most violent crimes lead to much longer prison sentences than they did 20 years ago.

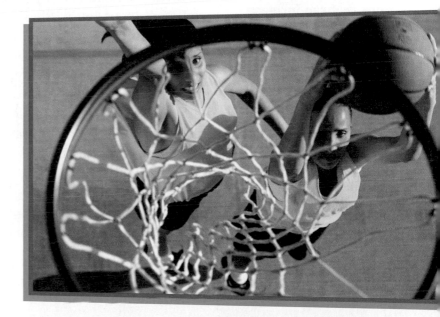

After-school programs give young people a safe place to be with friends. *What kinds of after-school programs does your community offer?*

Lesson 3 Review

Using complete sentences, answer the following questions on a sheet of paper.

Reviewing Terms and Facts

1. **Vocabulary** Define the terms *assault, rape, homicide,* and *hate crime.* Use each word in a complete sentence.
2. **List** What are four factors that may contribute to violence in society?
3. **Recall** Give two reasons a teen might join a gang.
4. **Identify** Name two actions a community might take to reduce violence.

Thinking Critically

5. **Apply** If you were walking home in the evening, what precautions would you take?
6. **Analyze** What two measures would be most effective in preventing school violence? Why?

Applying Health Skills

7. **Practicing Healthful Behaviors** With a partner, write and perform a skit in which you demonstrate strategies for the prevention of and response to deliberate injuries caused by violence.

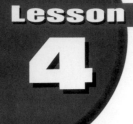

Lesson 4

Dealing with Abuse and Finding Help

Quick Write

What are some situations that can increase the risk that a teen may be abused? What steps can a teen take to avoid these situations?

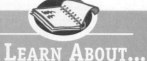

LEARN ABOUT...

- what abuse is and why it happens.
- the signs, causes, and effects of abuse.
- what can be done to prevent and stop abuse.

VOCABULARY

- abuse
- battery
- sexual abuse
- neglect

What Is Abuse?

Abuse (uh·BYOOS) is the *physical, emotional, or mental mistreatment of another person.* **Figure 9.7** reveals some shocking statistics about abuse. Physical signs of abuse, such as bruises, scratches, or broken bones, are clearly visible. Other signs, such as sadness, fear, and anger, are not as easy to see. People can be victims of abuse no matter who they are.

Any kind of abuse does long-lasting damage. Abuse is a serious crime. Physicians and teachers are required by law to report suspected cases of abuse. Abuse is never the fault of the victim.

Types of Abuse

Figure 9.8 on the next page gives some of the warning signs of possible abuse. There are four major types of abuse:

- **Physical abuse.** This category includes any type of abuse that causes physical injury. The most common form of physical

FIGURE 9.7

ABUSE STATISTICS

These figures show the rate of abuse in families for a single year. This information shows only cases that have been reported in the United States. *How does abuse negatively affect family and community health?*

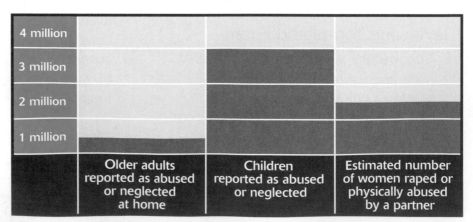

Sources: American Humane Association, National Center on Elder Abuse at the American Public Human Services Association, U.S. Department of Justice

abuse is battery. **Battery** is *the beating, hitting, or kicking of another person.* Signs of physical abuse include bruises, burns, and broken bones. Severe physical abuse may kill a person. Physical abuse has emotional effects as well.

- **Emotional abuse.** The use of words and gestures to hurt someone is called emotional abuse. Insults, repeated threats, constant teasing, and harsh criticism are examples. People who have been abused emotionally may feel worthless and helpless.

- **Sexual abuse.** *Sexual contact that is forced upon another person* is called **sexual abuse**. The abuser may be a parent, stepparent, older brother or sister, or family friend. It is often someone whom the abused person knows and trusts. People who have been sexually abused may feel guilty or responsible for what has happened. However, sexual abuse is *always* the abuser's fault. Anyone who commits sexual abuse needs professional help. The way to stop the abuse and get help for everyone involved is for the person who has been abused to talk to a trusted adult.

- **Neglect.** *The failure to meet the basic physical and emotional needs of a person* is known as **neglect**. Many people depend on others for food, clothing, shelter, health care, and emotional support. If parents or caregivers do not provide for their dependents' needs, they are demonstrating neglect.

Developing Good Character

Respect

Sexual harassment (huh·RAS·muhnt) is any unwanted sexual comment, contact, or behavior. It may include jokes, looks, notes, touching, or gestures. Sexual harassment shows a lack of respect for the other person. It is also a type of sexual abuse. *What is your school's policy for dealing with sexual harassment?*

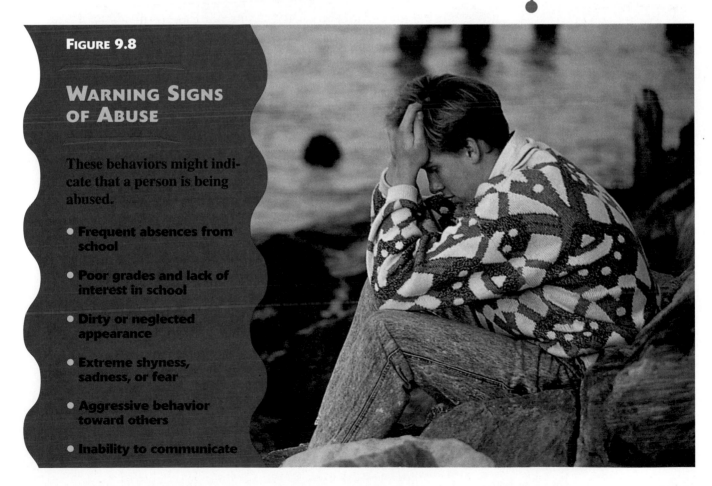

FIGURE 9.8

WARNING SIGNS OF ABUSE

These behaviors might indicate that a person is being abused.

- **Frequent absences from school**

- **Poor grades and lack of interest in school**

- **Dirty or neglected appearance**

- **Extreme shyness, sadness, or fear**

- **Aggressive behavior toward others**

- **Inability to communicate**

Causes and Effects of Abuse

All families experience problems from time to time. Healthy families can solve these problems through good communication. However, there may be an increased risk of abuse in families that don't know how to handle problems in a healthful way. **Figure 9.9** lists some common factors that may increase the risk of abuse. Some situations that increase the risk of abuse can be avoided. Doing so is crucial to health and safety.

FIGURE 9.9

COMMON CAUSES OF ABUSE

These factors can increase the risk that a person will become abusive. *How can identifying and working to improve these situations help prevent abuse?*

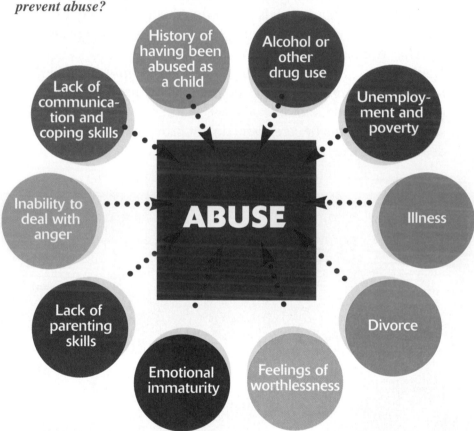

History of having been abused as a child

Alcohol or other drug use

Lack of communication and coping skills

Unemployment and poverty

Inability to deal with anger

ABUSE

Illness

Lack of parenting skills

Divorce

Emotional immaturity

Feelings of worthlessness

Teens who are being abused may try to escape the problem by running away. They may turn to crime to support themselves, or become victims of crime. Many people who have been abused experience low self-esteem, a high level of stress, and emotional problems. These feelings may lead them into relationships in which they are abused as adults. Some may even become abusers themselves.

Why Victims Stay Silent

Victims often do not tell anyone about the abuse. Some of the most common reasons victims stay silent are listed on the next page.

- **Victims may feel that nobody will believe them.** Those who experience or witness abuse, especially children, may not report it because they fear that people will think that they are lying or exaggerating. If you're in danger and tell someone who doesn't believe you, tell someone else.
- **People may think that abuse is a private issue.** Many victims feel uncomfortable sharing something that affects them so personally. However, silence only allows the abuser to do more damage.
- **Males may feel that they cannot or should not be victims.** Some boys and men may feel that reporting abuse is a sign of weakness. They may believe that they should be able to protect themselves. Abusers, however, always have an advantage over their victims. They may not always be physically stronger, but they are usually older or in a position of authority or trust.
- **Victims may be afraid of their abusers.** Many victims are afraid to report abuse because they fear that their abusers will seek revenge. Abusers often convince children that they will be punished if they tell. However, victims must confide in a trusted adult to get help.

Reading Check

Make connections. Find "Inability to deal with anger" in Figure 9.9. Then look back at Lesson 1 to find ways to prevent this possible cause of abuse.

Breaking the Cycle of Abuse

To prevent further abuse, the cycle needs to break. The key to breaking the cycle of abuse is to report it and talk about it. A person who is being abused should seek help and support from a trusted adult, such as a parent, teacher, or school nurse.

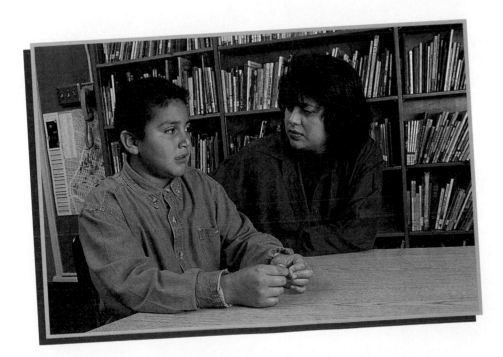

If you or someone you know is being abused, seek help from a trusted adult. *Who are some of the people who could help you?*

Where to Find Help

A crisis hot line is a valuable resource for anyone who is dealing with abuse. Crisis hot lines are telephone services that people can call to get help. They can put victims in touch with other resources, such as the police department and hospitals. Family counseling centers, family violence shelters, and support groups can also help.

If someone is in immediate danger, the safest way to intervene may be to call the police. In many places you can reach the local police department by calling 911. If you are not sure how to reach the police, you can dial 0 to ask the operator.

Many types of counseling can help people deal with abuse. Counseling programs help family members to identify and solve their problems. School guidance counselors, youth counselors, social workers, and religious leaders can provide support to family members. These services help family members improve their relationships with one another.

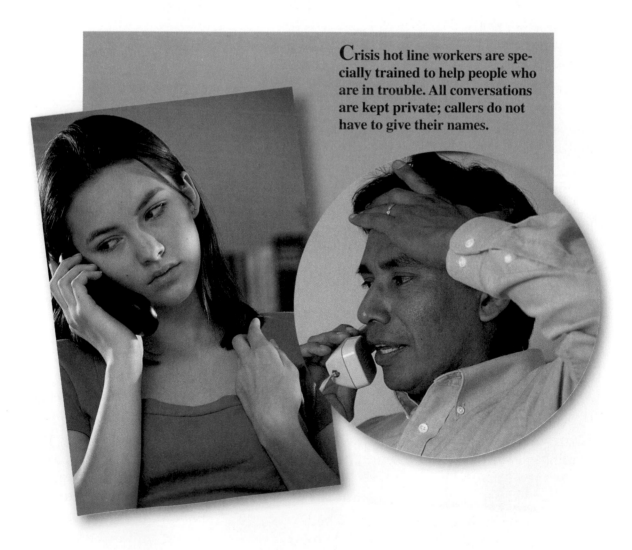

Crisis hot line workers are specially trained to help people who are in trouble. All conversations are kept private; callers do not have to give their names.

Support or self-help groups give people a chance to talk with and listen to others who have similar problems. Some support groups are for victims of abuse; others are for abusers. For example, Parents Anonymous helps parents who have abused their children or are afraid that they might begin to do so. Members help one another to understand and change their behavior. They offer encouragement to overcome obstacles.

Some families in abusive situations go to family violence shelters. These shelters give families a safe place to live while they get their lives in order. Counselors at the shelters help family members find solutions to their problems.

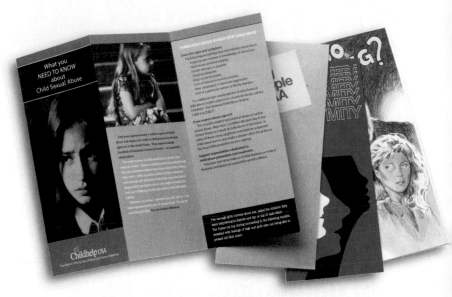

Different programs meet the different needs of victims and abusers. *Where could you go for help if you knew that a peer was being abused?*

Lesson 4 Review

Using complete sentences, answer the following questions on a sheet of paper.

Reviewing Terms and Facts

1. **Vocabulary** Define the term *abuse* and use it in an original sentence.
2. **Describe** Explain the differences between the four types of abuse.
3. **Identify** List two examples of emotional abuse.
4. **List** What are some warning signs of possible abuse?
5. **Restate** Why might victims be afraid to tell someone that they are being abused?

Thinking Critically

6. **Infer** One of the effects of abuse on a victim is a feeling of worthlessness. This is also a common trait of abusers. Why might someone who felt worthless abuse someone else?
7. **Apply** What are two reasons that you might give to convince a peer to call a crisis hot line?

Applying Health Skills

8. **Accessing Information** Do some research to find out where teens in your community can go for help if they are being abused. Then draw a map of your community that shows where these places are located. If possible, display your maps around your school or community. As part of your research, identify strategies for intervention and prevention of abuse.

A Win-Win Situation

In mediation, kids solve their own conflicts.

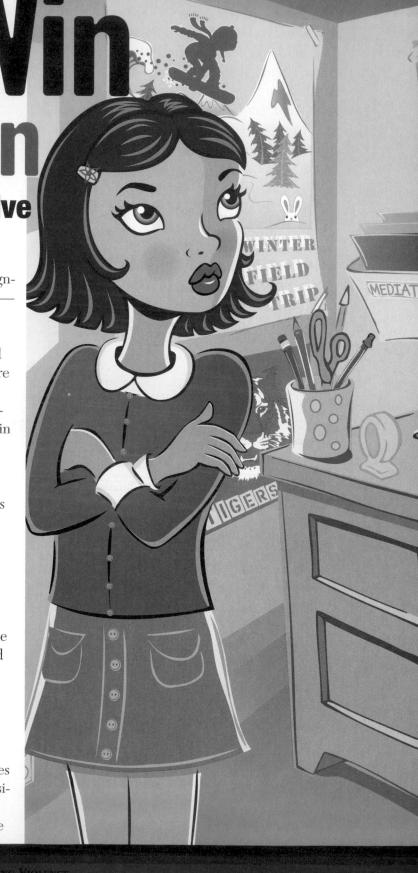

Ivory Kelly was finishing up an English assignment at the blackboard when—Ping! Ping!—he felt staples pelting his head. Suspecting who the culprit was, Ivory spun around and shouted at DeAngela Byrd. DeAngela claimed she was innocent. Within seconds, the two were angrily trading insults.

Their teacher didn't send them to the principal. Instead, she sent them to work things out in a small storage room in this Nashville, Tennessee, school. The room is Glengarry Elementary's mediation center.

Mediation in school is a way to solve disputes without having teachers punish students. Kids called mediators are trained to listen to classmates accused of misbehaving or fighting. Without taking sides, the mediators help troubled kids come up with their own solutions. It usually takes no more than 15 minutes.

At Glengarry, 30 students are trained to settle disputes. Ivory and DeAngela calmly discussed the staple attack and name calling with two mediators. Then they signed a pledge "not to mess with each other."

No Detention, No Time Out

Many elementary schools in the United States are starting to give young people more responsibility for discipline. In the past few years, one tenth of the nation's 86,000 public schools have

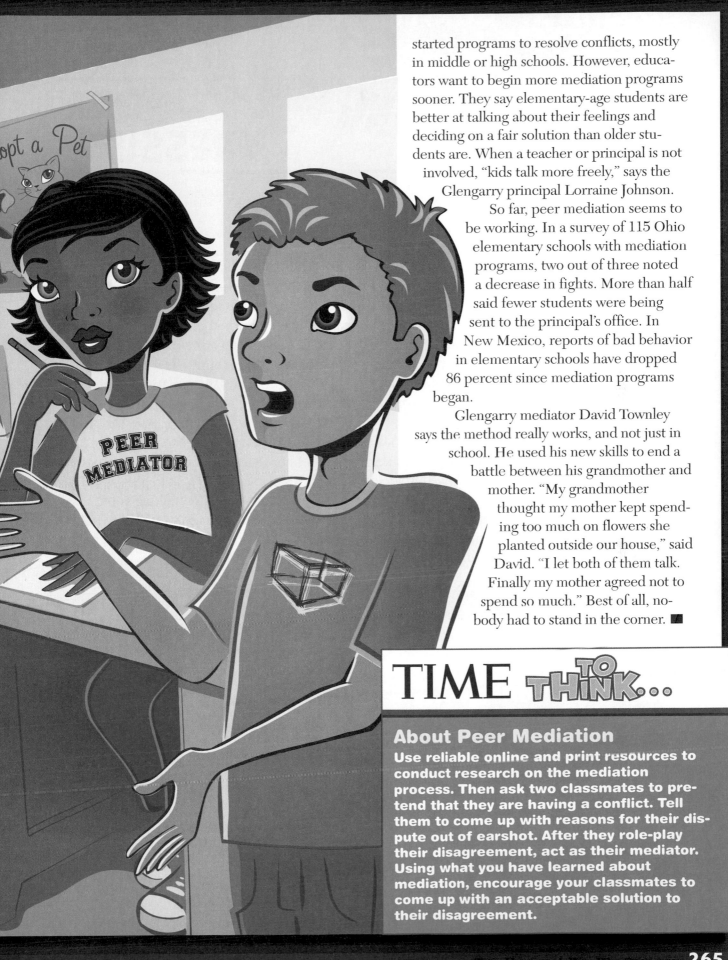

started programs to resolve conflicts, mostly in middle or high schools. However, educators want to begin more mediation programs sooner. They say elementary-age students are better at talking about their feelings and deciding on a fair solution than older students are. When a teacher or principal is not involved, "kids talk more freely," says the Glengarry principal Lorraine Johnson.

So far, peer mediation seems to be working. In a survey of 115 Ohio elementary schools with mediation programs, two out of three noted a decrease in fights. More than half said fewer students were being sent to the principal's office. In New Mexico, reports of bad behavior in elementary schools have dropped 86 percent since mediation programs began.

Glengarry mediator David Townley says the method really works, and not just in school. He used his new skills to end a battle between his grandmother and mother. "My grandmother thought my mother kept spending too much on flowers she planted outside our house," said David. "I let both of them talk. Finally my mother agreed not to spend so much." Best of all, nobody had to stand in the corner. ◢

TIME TO THINK...

About Peer Mediation

Use reliable online and print resources to conduct research on the mediation process. Then ask two classmates to pretend that they are having a conflict. Tell them to come up with reasons for their dispute out of earshot. After they role-play their disagreement, act as their mediator. Using what you have learned about mediation, encourage your classmates to come up with an acceptable solution to their disagreement.

KEEPING COOL UNDER PRESSURE

Model

Kami and Madeline are both trying out for a spot on the swim team. When the race began, Madeline was in the lead. However, Kami saw that Madeline did not touch the wall with both hands when she reached the end of the pool. This should disqualify her from the race. Unfortunately, the coach did not see what had happened and declared Madeline the winner. Kami was very angry, but she approached the situation using the skills of conflict resolution.

First, Kami took time to calm down and think about what she would say. Then she told Madeline what she believed she had seen and allowed Madeline to tell her side of the story. Both girls asked questions to clarify the other's point of view. After talking about the situation, they decided that the best thing to do would be to talk to the coach and ask her opinion. Madeline said that she would be willing to swim the race again.

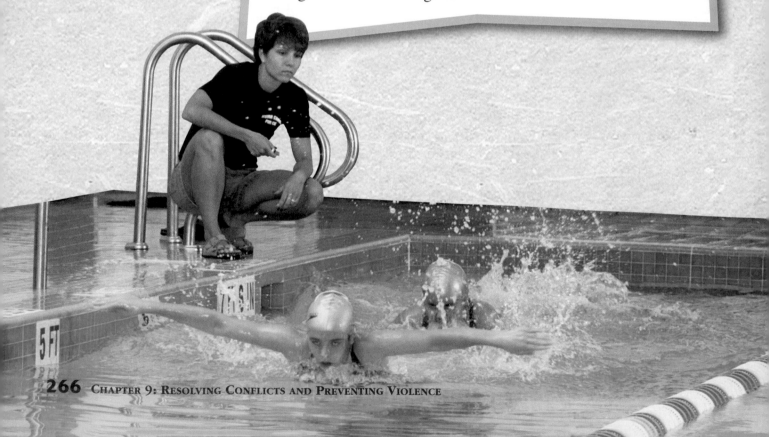

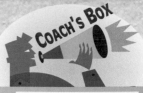

Practice

Taylor and Claire usually get along well, but not tonight! Claire is trying to do her homework while Taylor is practicing on her keyboard. Claire can't concentrate on her math problems while Taylor works on a new piece of music. Tomorrow Claire has a math test, and Taylor has orchestra practice. On a piece of paper, write a dialogue between the two sisters in which they use the T.A.L.K steps to resolve their conflict. Give yourself extra credit if you can think of more than one solution for this situation. Share your conversation with other students in your class. How many different solutions did you develop?

Conflict Resolution

T Take a time out, at least 30 minutes.

A Allow each person to tell his or her side uninterrupted.

L Let each person ask questions.

K Keep brainstorming to find a good solution.

Apply/Assess

With a partner, use the skills of conflict resolution to write a script for a skit about a conflict. In your script, include a reason for the conflict. Show each character's point of view, have the characters ask questions, and suggest at least one solution. Choose one of the following situations or develop your own.

- You and a classmate are working together on a report. Your classmate thinks that you aren't doing your fair share.
- Your brother or sister does not want to share something that belongs to the whole family.

With another team, take turns practicing your scripts. Identify the T.A.L.K. steps in the other team's skit.

Self-√Check

- Did the characters in our script use the T.A.L.K. steps?
- Can I identify the steps in others' scripts?

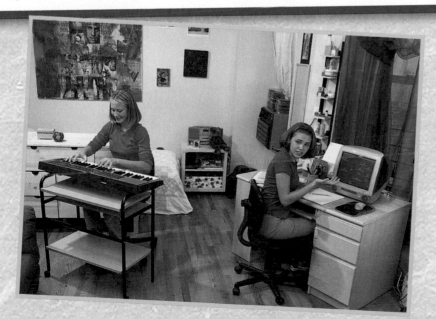

After You Read

Use your completed Foldable to review the information on causes of conflict and the factors that can affect conflict.

FOLDABLES™
Study Organizer

Reviewing Vocabulary and Concepts

On a sheet of paper, write the numbers 1–6. After each number, write the term from the list that best completes each sentence.

- negotiation
- revenge
- prejudice
- neutrality
- compromise
- anger

Lesson 1

1. A common cause of conflict is _____, or "getting even" with someone.

2. _____ is an unjustly formed, negative opinion of a group.

3. Managing _____ when you disagree with someone can help prevent the conflict from turning into a fight.

Lesson 2

4. Disagreements on everyday matters may be resolved by _____.

5. In the process of _____, people discuss problems face-to-face in order to come up with a solution.

6. An important element of peer mediation is _____, which is a promise not to take sides.

Lesson 3

On a sheet of paper, write the numbers 7–10. After each number, write the letter of the answer that best completes each statement.

7. Prejudice may lead to
   a. compromise.
   b. hate crimes.
   c. mediation.
   d. conflict resolution.

8. If gang members threaten you, you should
   a. stay calm and try not to show fear.
   b. start fighting with them.
   c. not tell anybody about the incident.
   d. be willing to compromise.

9. You can protect yourself from becoming a victim of violent crime by
   a. not making eye contact with anyone.
   b. walking by yourself at night.
   c. staying in well-lit areas when walking at night.
   d. confronting someone who's following you.

10. A person who wants to frighten or hurt someone who is smaller or weaker is a
   a. mediator.
   b. bully.
   c. peer.
   d. victim.

Lesson 4

On a sheet of paper, write the numbers 11–14. Write *True* or *False* for each statement below. If the statement is false, change the underlined word or phrase to make it true.

11. Beating, hitting, or kicking another person is known as <u>battery</u>.

12. Harsh criticism is an example of <u>emotional abuse</u>.

13. In cases of sexual abuse, the abuser is often someone <u>unknown</u> to the victim.

14. An older adult whose caregiver fails to provide her or him with enough food is a victim of <u>sexual abuse</u>.

Thinking Critically

Using complete sentences, answer the following questions on a sheet of paper.

15. Analyze How can positive peer pressure be a factor in effective conflict resolution?

16. Apply How do good communication skills play a role in nonviolent confrontation?

17. Evaluate How do you think violence in the media affects people? Explain.

18. Analyze Give three examples of how peers might help each other avoid and cope with potentially dangerous situations in healthy ways.

Career Corner

Professional Mediator Are you often called upon to solve your friends' disagreements? Are you a good listener and able to see both sides of a conflict? These are some of the skills used by professional mediators. These professionals work in corporations, government agencies, and schools. Professional mediators help people work together to solve problems peacefully.

To enter this career, you'll need a four-year college degree and training in mediation. Read more about it in Career Corner at health.glencoe.com.

Standardized Test Practice

Math

Read the paragraph below and then answer the questions.

Violence is a serious problem in our society. Young people may be the victims of violent crime, which includes child abuse and gang violence. They may also commit such crimes. Factors that may contribute to violence include living in a high-crime area and being a victim of abuse.

1. One study found that one-third of all youths aged 11 to 18 have been involved in at least one serious fight in the last year. According to these figures, if a school contains 642 students, how many of them have had a violent fight in the last year?
- **A** 36 students
- **B** 58 students
- **C** 214 students
- **D** 428 students

2. About 33 percent of all sexual assaults that are reported to the police involve victims that are between the ages of 12 and 17. If 57 cases were reported to a city police department, how many victims were not in this age range?
- **A** 19 victims
- **B** 25 victims
- **C** 38 victims
- **D** 50 victims

3. Twenty percent of the more than 30 million American students who use the Internet regularly reported that they have been sexually harassed online at least once over the past year. According to these figures, how many students does this problem involve? Show your work.

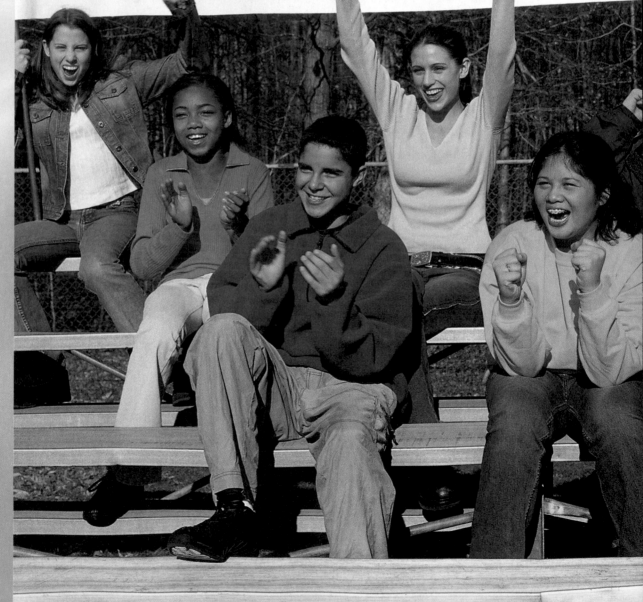

DRUG-FREE W

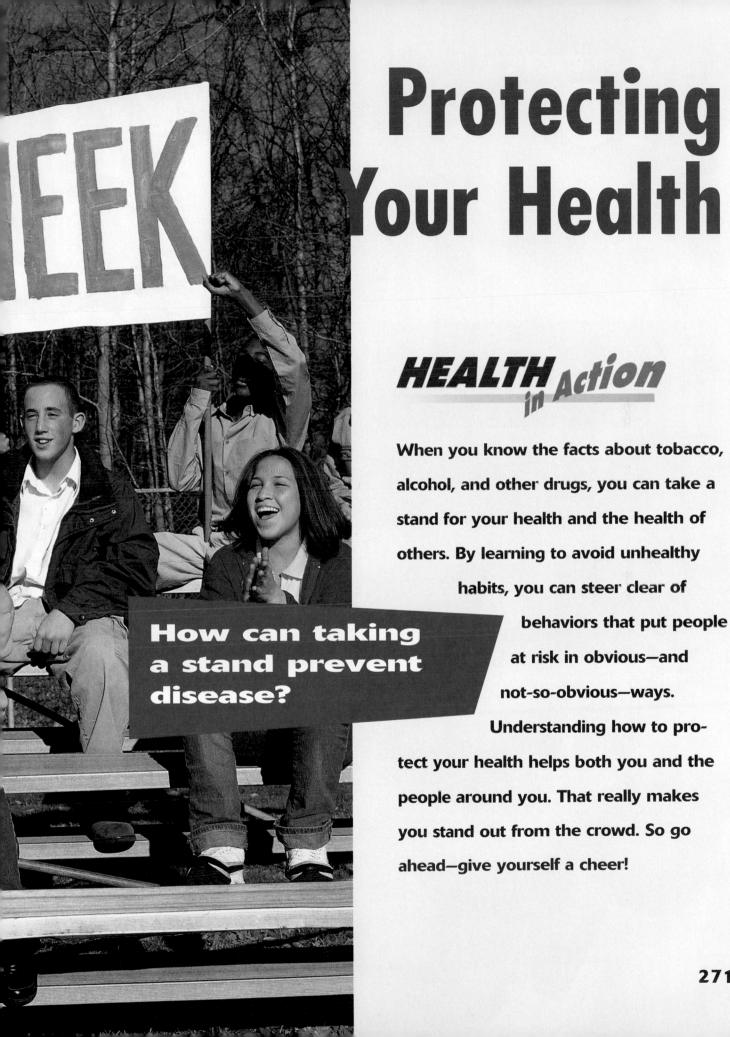

Protecting Your Health

HEALTH *in Action*

When you know the facts about tobacco, alcohol, and other drugs, you can take a stand for your health and the health of others. By learning to avoid unhealthy habits, you can steer clear of behaviors that put people at risk in obvious—and not-so-obvious—ways. Understanding how to protect your health helps both you and the people around you. That really makes you stand out from the crowd. So go ahead—give yourself a cheer!

How can taking a stand prevent disease?

CHAPTER 10

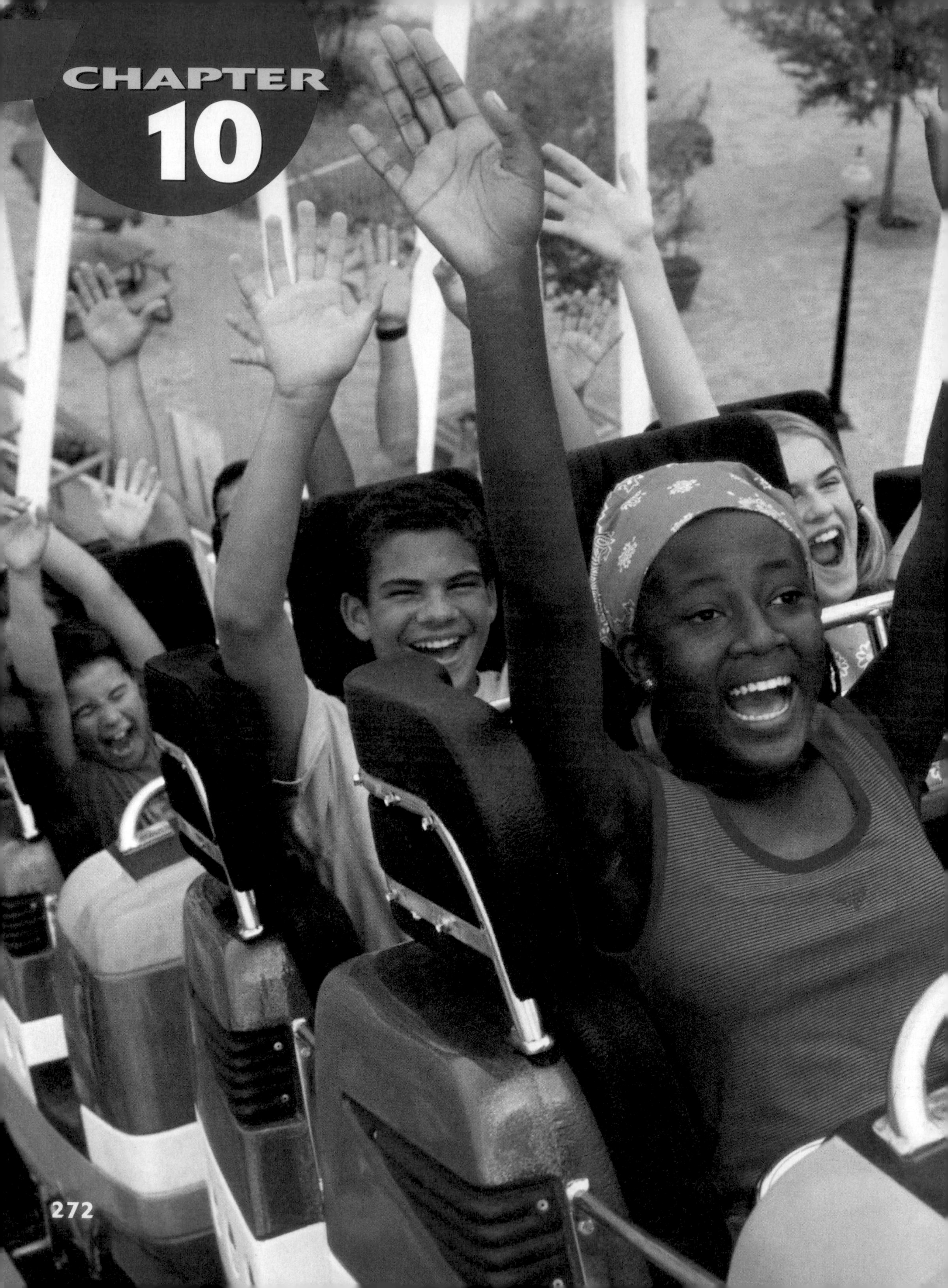

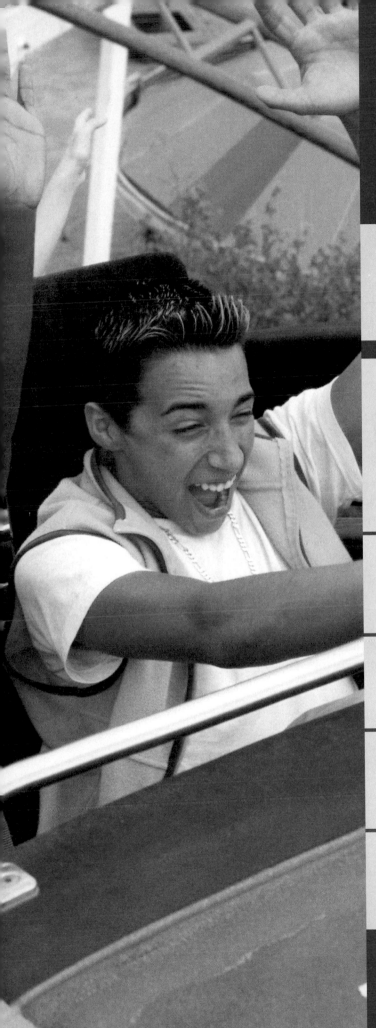

Tobacco

HEALTH *Online*

Can you separate the facts about tobacco from the myths? To find out, take the Health Inventory for Chapter 10 at health.glencoe.com.

FOLDABLES™ Study Organizer

Before You Read

Make this Foldable to help you record what you learn in Lesson 1 about tobacco's effects on the respiratory system. Begin with a sheet of notebook paper.

Step 1

Fold the sheet of notebook paper in half along the long axis.

Step 2

On the top layer, cut every third line. This will form 10 tabs.

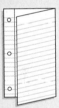

Step 3

Label the tabs as shown.

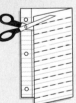

As You Read

Define key terms and record facts about tobacco's effects on the body.

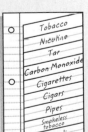

Tobacco
Nicotine
Tar
Carbon Monoxide
Cigarettes
Cigars
Pipes
Smokeless tobacco
Alveoli
Emphysema

What Tobacco Does to the Body

LEARN ABOUT...

- the substances in tobacco that cause health problems.
- why all forms of tobacco are harmful to health.
- how tobacco affects various parts of the body.

VOCABULARY

- nicotine
- tar
- carbon monoxide
- alveoli
- emphysema

The Facts About Tobacco

A single puff of tobacco smoke contains more than 4,000 chemicals. Almost all of these chemicals prevent the body from functioning the way it should. At least 43 of them cause cancer in smokers. In the United States more than 400,000 people die each year as a result of smoking-related illnesses. Smoke also harms the health of nonsmokers. Even smokeless tobacco causes health problems for its users.

What Is in Tobacco?

Tobacco contains three substances that are especially harmful to health. **Nicotine** (NIK·uh·teen) is *an addictive drug found in tobacco.* Nicotine makes tobacco users crave even more nicotine. **Tar** is *a thick, dark liquid that forms when tobacco burns.* This liquid coats the lining of the lungs and causes diseases. **Carbon monoxide** (KAR·buhn muh·NAHK·syd) is *a colorless, odorless, poisonous gas produced when tobacco burns.* Tobacco smoke from a cigarette, cigar, or pipe contains all of these substances. **Figure 10.1** on the next page shows the harmful substances in tobacco.

Here are several forms of tobacco products. *What harmful substances do all tobacco products contain?*

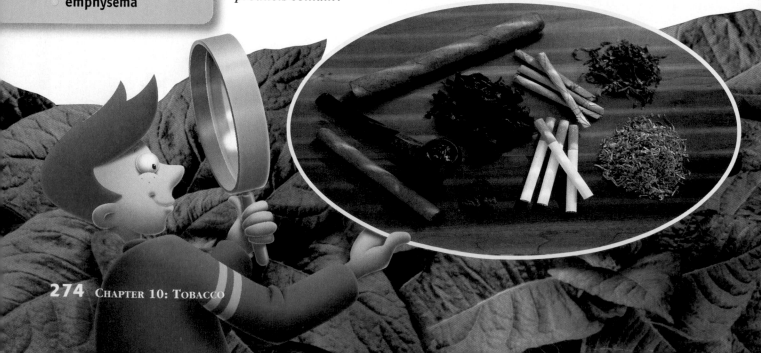

Forms of Tobacco

Tobacco products come in several forms. They can be smoked, chewed, or inhaled. The most commonly used form is a cigarette.

Cigarettes

Cigarettes are made from shredded tobacco leaves. Some cigarettes contain filters, which reduce the amount of nicotine and tar in cigarette smoke. However, filters do not decrease the amount of harmful chemicals that pass through a smoker's lungs. Flavored cigarettes taste and smell sweet, but they produce even more nicotine, tar, and carbon monoxide than regular cigarettes do.

Cigars and Pipes

Shredded tobacco leaves are also used in cigars and pipes. Cigar smoke contains 25 times more carbon monoxide and up to 400 times more nicotine than cigarette smoke. People who smoke cigars or pipes are more likely to develop cancers of the lip, mouth, and tongue than nonsmokers are.

Smokeless Tobacco

Chewing tobacco and snuff are placed in the mouth rather than smoked. Snuff may also be inhaled. The nicotine in smokeless tobacco is just as harmful and addictive as that in cigarettes. Users of smokeless tobacco face a higher risk of cancers of the mouth, esophagus, larynx, and pancreas. They can also develop gum disease and stomach ulcers.

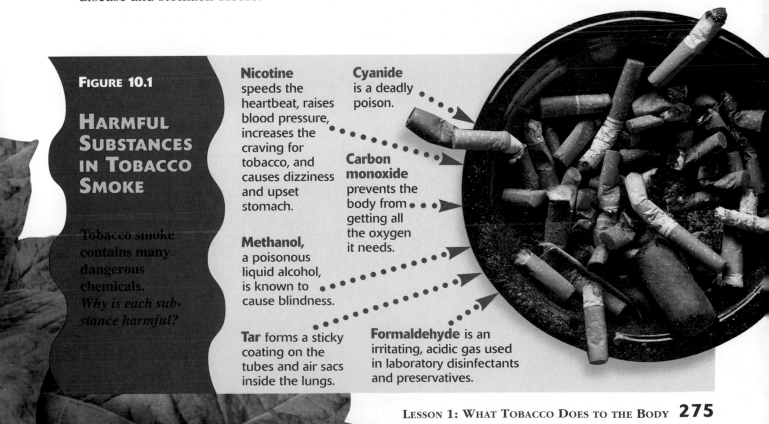

FIGURE 10.1

HARMFUL SUBSTANCES IN TOBACCO SMOKE

Tobacco smoke contains many dangerous chemicals. *Why is each substance harmful?*

Nicotine speeds the heartbeat, raises blood pressure, increases the craving for tobacco, and causes dizziness and upset stomach.

Cyanide is a deadly poison.

Carbon monoxide prevents the body from getting all the oxygen it needs.

Methanol, a poisonous liquid alcohol, is known to cause blindness.

Tar forms a sticky coating on the tubes and air sacs inside the lungs.

Formaldehyde is an irritating, acidic gas used in laboratory disinfectants and preservatives.

Reading Check
Create your own chart. Design and complete a chart about what tobacco does to the body.

Tobacco's Effects on the Body

Tobacco poses a great risk to the normal functioning of the body. Besides causing problems in the mouth and lungs, tobacco damages the body in many other ways. **Figure 10.2** lists the effects tobacco has on five body systems.

Regulating the Tobacco Industry

The federal government has developed regulations to protect the public from the health hazards of tobacco use. Cigarette packs must have warnings on the health risks of smoking. Cigarette advertisements are banned from radio and television. It is illegal to sell tobacco products to anyone under age 18; in some states, the age is even higher. Clothing and other souvenir items cannot feature the name or logo of a tobacco brand. Tobacco companies cannot sponsor sporting events and teams.

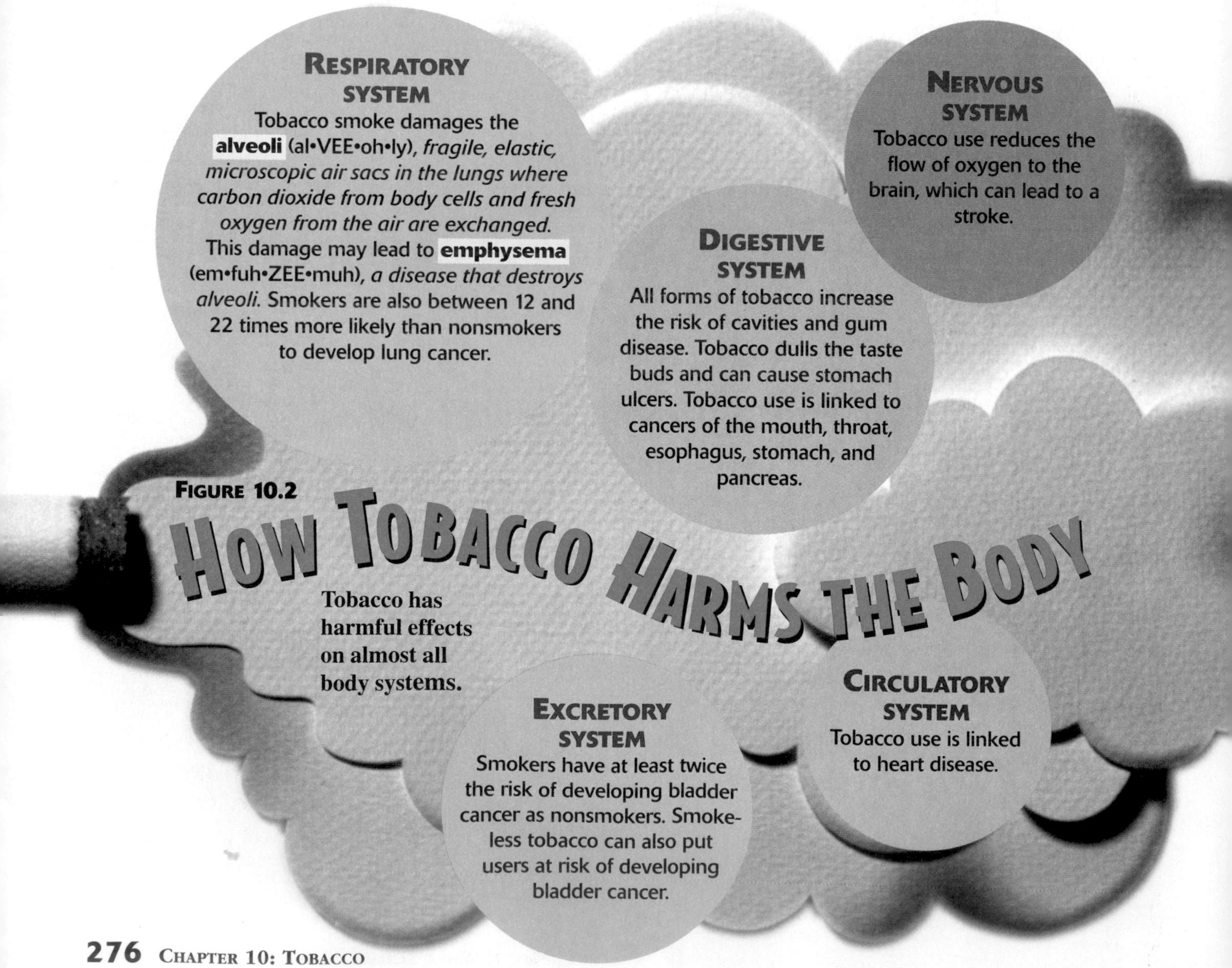

RESPIRATORY SYSTEM
Tobacco smoke damages the **alveoli** (al•VEE•oh•ly), *fragile, elastic, microscopic air sacs in the lungs where carbon dioxide from body cells and fresh oxygen from the air are exchanged.* This damage may lead to **emphysema** (em•fuh•ZEE•muh), *a disease that destroys alveoli.* Smokers are also between 12 and 22 times more likely than nonsmokers to develop lung cancer.

NERVOUS SYSTEM
Tobacco use reduces the flow of oxygen to the brain, which can lead to a stroke.

DIGESTIVE SYSTEM
All forms of tobacco increase the risk of cavities and gum disease. Tobacco dulls the taste buds and can cause stomach ulcers. Tobacco use is linked to cancers of the mouth, throat, esophagus, stomach, and pancreas.

FIGURE 10.2

HOW TOBACCO HARMS THE BODY

Tobacco has harmful effects on almost all body systems.

EXCRETORY SYSTEM
Smokers have at least twice the risk of developing bladder cancer as nonsmokers. Smokeless tobacco can also put users at risk of developing bladder cancer.

CIRCULATORY SYSTEM
Tobacco use is linked to heart disease.

DECISION MAKING

Asking Others Not to Smoke

After school Marisa runs into her friend Eileen, who offers to give her a ride home. When Eileen's older brother, Zachary, arrives to pick them up, he lights up a cigarette in the car. Marisa has asthma and wants to ask Zachary to put out the cigarette. She feels uncertain about saying anything to him, though, because it is his car and he is being nice enough to drive her home.

What Would You Do?

Apply the six steps of the decision-making process to Marisa's problem. Explain your decision to your class and have a group discussion about the risks and benefits of decision making about personal health.

1. STATE THE SITUATION.
2. LIST THE OPTIONS.
3. WEIGH THE POSSIBLE OUTCOMES.
4. CONSIDER VALUES.
5. MAKE A DECISION AND ACT.
6. EVALUATE YOUR DECISION.

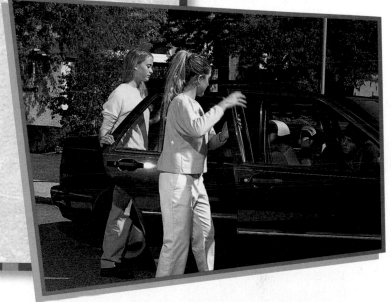

Lesson 1 Review

Using complete sentences, answer the following questions on a sheet of paper.

Reviewing Terms and Facts

1. **Vocabulary** Define the term *nicotine.*
2. **Identify** Name four substances in tobacco smoke that are harmful to the body.
3. **Recall** List three forms of tobacco.
4. **Explain** Describe four ways in which smoking and chewing tobacco harm the body.

Thinking Critically

5. **Hypothesize** What might you say to persuade a friend to quit chewing tobacco?
6. **Explain** Why do you think tobacco companies are prohibited from putting their names and logos on clothing?

Applying Health Skills

7. **Advocacy** Collect newspaper and magazine articles about the unhealthful effects of tobacco. Use the articles to make a pamphlet that encourages others to remain tobacco free.

Lesson 2

The Respiratory System

Quick Write

Although you breathe all the time, you probably don't think about it very often. Describe the activities or conditions that make you aware of your breathing.

Oxygen for Life

Take a deep breath. Now let the air out. These two motions, inhaling and exhaling, are the basic actions of your respiratory system. Your **respiratory system** is *the set of organs that supplies your body with oxygen and rids your body of carbon dioxide.* Your body cannot survive without the oxygen you take in every time you take a breath.

Parts of the Respiratory System

All the parts of the respiratory system work together to help you breathe. **Figure 10.3** lists and describes the functions of many of the body parts that make breathing possible.

LEARN ABOUT...

- the parts of the respiratory system.
- how the breathing process works.
- illnesses that can damage the respiratory system.

VOCABULARY

- respiratory system
- trachea
- bronchi
- diaphragm

FIGURE 10.3

PARTS OF THE RESPIRATORY SYSTEM

All of these structures work together to help you breathe. ***Why do you think you have a hard time breathing when you have a cold?***

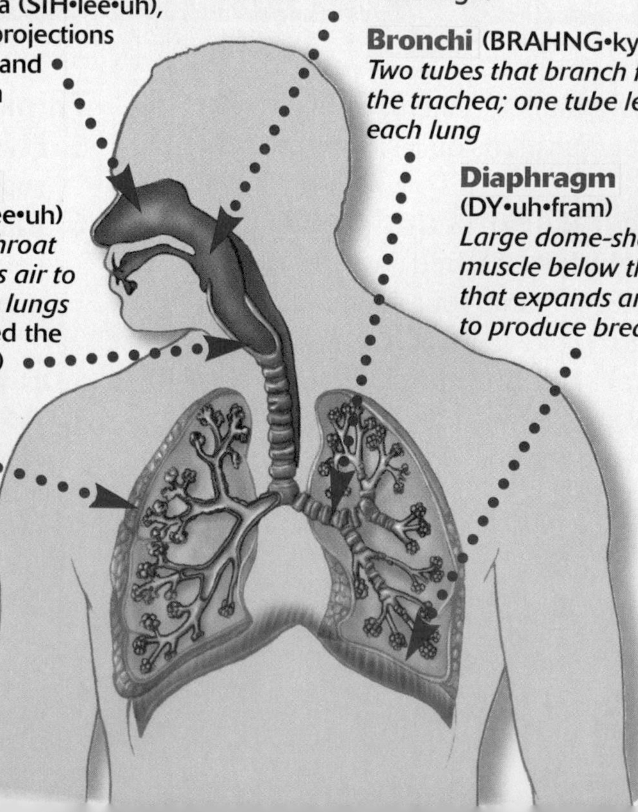

Epiglottis (eh•pi•GLAH•tis)
Flap of tissue in back of mouth that covers the trachea to prevent food from entering it
Nose/Mouth
Passages for air; nose lined with cilia (SIH•lee•uh), tiny hairlike projections that trap dirt and particles from the air
Bronchi (BRAHNG•ky)
Two tubes that branch from the trachea; one tube leads to each lung
Trachea
(TRAY•kee•uh)
Tube in throat that takes air to and from lungs (also called the windpipe)
Diaphragm
(DY•uh•fram)
Large dome-shaped muscle below the lungs that expands and relaxes to produce breathing
Lungs
Two large organs that exchange oxygen and carbon dioxide

How Breathing Works

Breathing consists of three main stages. When you inhale, you take air into your lungs. There oxygen from the air enters the bloodstream and replaces the carbon dioxide that must leave your body. When you exhale, you breathe out the carbon dioxide. These three stages repeat in a cycle. **Figure 10.4** shows the steps in the breathing process.

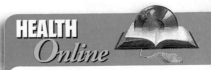

HEALTH Online

Topic: Respiration

For a link to more information on respiration, go to **health.glencoe.com**.

Activity: Using the information provided at this link, summarize the breathing process.

FIGURE 10.4

THE BREATHING PROCESS

Every day you take about 25,000 breaths of air. *How do you think smoking affects a smoker's breathing?*

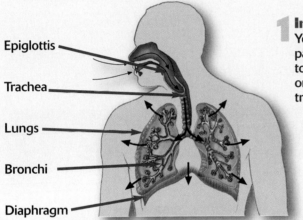

Epiglottis

Trachea

Lungs

Bronchi

Diaphragm

1 Inhaling
Your diaphragm moves down and your rib cage expands, creating more room in your chest. This causes air to rush into your body. The air enters through the nose or mouth, then moves past the epiglottis and into the trachea and bronchi.

2 Inside the Lungs
The bronchi divide into smaller passages called bronchioles (BRAHNG·kee·ohlz). Air passes through the bronchioles into the alveoli, which are surrounded by capillaries. Here the oxygen in the air moves into your bloodstream, and carbon dioxide from the blood enters the alveoli.

3 Exhaling
Your diaphragm pushes up, and your ribs move in and down, forcing air out of your lungs. The air, now containing carbon dioxide, moves back through the bronchioles and bronchi, up the trachea, and out through the nose or mouth.

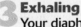

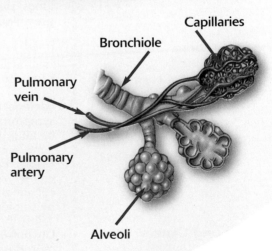

Capillaries

Bronchiole

Pulmonary vein

Pulmonary artery

Alveoli

Reading Check

Investigate word parts. Investigate the word *tuberculosis*. What is the root of the word? What does the root mean? What is the suffix? What does the suffix mean?

Problems of the Respiratory System

Germs, tobacco smoke, inhaled chemicals, and environmental pollution can easily damage the many complex parts of the respiratory system. **Figure 10.5** describes some of the illnesses that can harm your respiratory system.

Caring for Your Respiratory System

You know how uncomfortable you are when you have a cold and can't breathe freely. Your whole body depends on a healthy respiratory system and on the air you breathe. It is important to take good care of your respiratory system—here are some simple tips to follow:

- Don't smoke.
- Avoid people and situations that would expose you to tobacco smoke in the air.
- Take care of your body when you have a cold, flu, or any other respiratory illness.

FIGURE 10.5

PROBLEMS OF THE RESPIRATORY SYSTEM

Respiratory problems can be dangerous if they are not treated quickly and properly. *Which respiratory illnesses can you help prevent by remaining tobacco free?*

Disease or Disorder	Description	Treatment
Cold/Flu	Diseases caused by viruses; symptoms include runny nose, cough, fever, aches	Bed rest and fluids; vaccines can prevent some types of flu
Pneumonia	Bacterial or viral disease that affects the lungs; symptoms include fever, chest pain, breathing difficulty	Antibiotics for bacterial type; bed rest for viral type
Asthma	Disease in which airways narrow; symptoms include wheezing, shortness of breath, coughing	Medication to relieve symptoms; avoiding activities or substances that trigger attacks
Tuberculosis	Bacterial disease that affects the lungs; symptoms include cough, fatigue; can be fatal	Antibiotics
Emphysema	Disease in which alveoli harden and disintegrate; symptoms include extreme difficulty in breathing; almost entirely caused by smoking	No known cure; pure oxygen can make breathing easier
Lung Cancer	Uncontrolled growth of cells that reproduce abnormally in lungs; often caused by smoking	Surgery, radiation, and medications; survival rates are very low

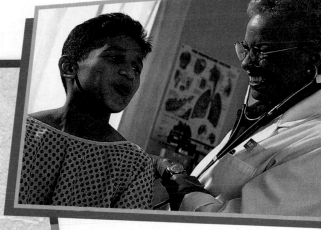

HEALTH SKILLS ACTIVITY

PRACTICING HEALTHFUL BEHAVIORS

Every Breath You Take

Here are some additional guidelines for keeping your respiratory system healthy:

- Participate in regular physical activity that makes you breathe deeply. Giving your lungs a good workout makes them stronger and helps them work more efficiently.
- Avoid areas where the air is polluted. Exercise away from streets where there is heavy traffic.
- If you know that you are allergic to a substance that affects your respiratory system, avoid it as much as possible. If you have asthma, avoid irritants that could trigger an attack.
- See a doctor right away if you have any trouble breathing.
- Do not intentionally inhale fumes of any kind.

ON YOUR OWN
List ways that you could put these tips to use. For example, how can you avoid smoke and air pollution? What activities will give your lungs a good workout? Compare your list with a classmate's to find more ideas.

Lesson 2 Review

Using complete sentences, answer the following questions on a sheet of paper.

Reviewing Terms and Facts

1. **Vocabulary** Define the term *respiratory system*.
2. **Recall** List the parts of the respiratory system through which air passes when you inhale.
3. **Identify** What two gases are exchanged in your lungs when you breathe?
4. **List** Name three ways to care for the respiratory system.
5. **Recall** List three problems of the respiratory system. Describe the effects of one of these illnesses.

Thinking Critically

6. **Describe** How do cilia and the epiglottis protect the respiratory system?
7. **Analyze** How might the rest of the body be affected when a respiratory illness remains untreated?

Applying Health Skills

8. **Communication Skills** Write a letter to a movie studio, asking the company to prohibit smoking scenes in films that feature teen actors. Using facts from this lesson, explain why it is important for movies to send out an antismoking message to teens.

Teens and Tobacco Addiction

Tobacco Addiction

You may wonder why people get "hooked" on tobacco products. The answer is nicotine. The tobacco user forms an **addiction** (uh·DIK·shuhn), *a psychological or physical need for a drug or other substance.* Nicotine is as addictive a drug as alcohol, cocaine, or heroin. Nicotine addiction leads to more diseases and deaths than all other addictions combined.

A person who is addicted to nicotine finds it difficult to stop using tobacco. Reducing or cutting off the supply of nicotine causes withdrawal. **Withdrawal** is *the unpleasant symptoms that someone experiences when he or she stops using an addictive substance.* People who are going through withdrawal usually feel anxious, irritable, hungry, depressed, and tired.

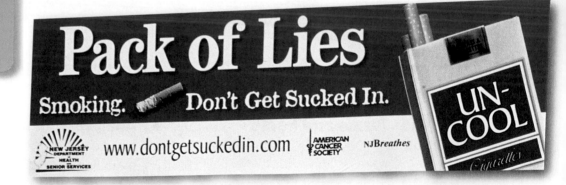

In April of 1999, tobacco advertisements were banned from billboards. In many states, these ads were replaced with antismoking messages like the one shown here. *How can antismoking messages in the media positively influence individual and community health?*

Psychological Dependence

A tobacco user first becomes psychologically dependent on the tobacco habit. **Psychological** (sy·kuh·LAH·ji·kuhl) **dependence** is *an addiction in which a person believes that he or she needs a drug in order to feel good or function normally.* The user may feel that the tobacco habit is a necessary part of his or her daily routine, and associate it with pleasurable activities such as talking on the phone or taking a break from work. To break a psychological dependence on tobacco, users need to change their habits. For example, a smoker could drink herbal tea or chew sugarless gum instead of reaching for a cigarette.

Physical Dependence

Physical dependence is *an addiction in which the body develops a chemical need for a drug.* Physical addiction to a chemical or drug is also called chemical dependency. Physical dependence on tobacco is directly related to nicotine. A tobacco user's need for nicotine is very strong. Users crave tobacco when their bodies are low on nicotine. They do not feel comfortable until they have another dose of the drug. When they get it, the relief does not last long—they soon feel the need to use tobacco again.

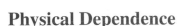

✓

Reading Check

Learn about the term *addiction.* Create a concept map for the term as it relates to tobacco.

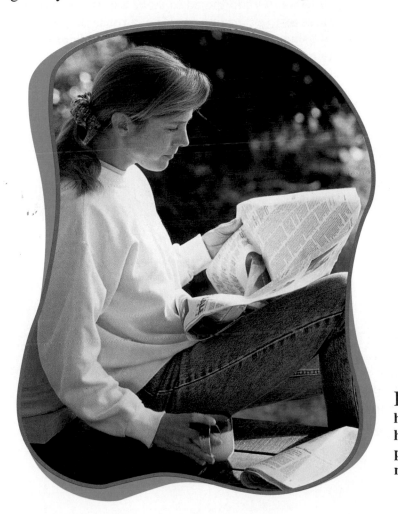

Replacing tobacco use with a healthful activity such as drinking herbal tea is one way to break a psychological dependence on nicotine.

As a person continues to use tobacco, the body's tolerance for nicotine increases. **Tolerance** is *the body's need for larger and larger doses of a drug to produce the same effect.* For example, someone might smoke half a pack of cigarettes a day. After a while that person will need to smoke more cigarettes in order to feel the effects of the nicotine. Soon he or she could be smoking a pack a day, and the increase won't stop there. The smoker will always feel an urge to smoke more.

Hands-On Health

ANALYZING A MEDIA MESSAGE

What flashes through your mind when you see a tobacco ad that shows smokers having fun? Does the ad make you think that using tobacco is a way to make friends and share good times? This is the hidden message that tobacco companies want you to receive. They show appealing pictures to make you feel good about the idea of using tobacco and to try to persuade you to use it. However, they don't tell you the truth about its harmful effects.

WHAT YOU WILL NEED
- paper
- pencil or pen
- poster board
- crayons, colored pencils, or markers

WHAT YOU WILL DO
1. Divide a sheet of paper into two columns. Label the first column *Images* and the second column *Messages*.
2. Look carefully at the tobacco ad on this page. In the first column list the kinds of images used in the ad, including words, setting, people, and activities. Describe the overall mood or tone of the ad. In the second column record the ad's hidden messages about the use of tobacco.
3. Use some of the techniques you noticed in the ad to make a poster showing teens having fun. The purpose of your ad is to sell a tobacco-free attitude or product.
4. Present your poster to the class.

IN CONCLUSION
1. In what ways was the ad on this page inaccurate or misleading?
2. How does your poster promote a healthy idea or product?

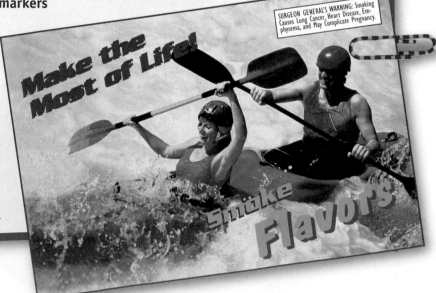

SURGEON GENERAL'S WARNING: Smoking Causes Lung Cancer, Heart Disease, Emphysema, and May Complicate Pregnancy.

Make the Most of Life!

Smoke Flavors

Why Teens Begin Using Tobacco

Why do teens start to use tobacco products? One of the main reasons is that their friends smoke or use smokeless tobacco. Many teens think that using tobacco products will make them appear "cool," adult, or sophisticated, and will give them confidence in social situations. Some teens are just curious and want to experience it for themselves. Others may try tobacco because they've been told not to use it—they are attempting to rebel. See **Figure 10.6** for other reasons that teens use tobacco.

Tobacco advertising is another major influence. The advertisements associate having fun or being "cool" with tobacco use. Teens may think that the negative consequences they have heard mentioned about tobacco just happen to people who are much older and who have used it for many years. In reality, the negative effects of tobacco begin the very first time a person uses it.

FIGURE 10.6

REASONS FOR TOBACCO USE AMONG TEENS

Although schools and media warn teens about the health risks of tobacco use, every day more than 4,800 American young people (ages 11–17) smoke their first cigarette. *For each of the reasons listed here for using tobacco, state a reason for avoiding it.*

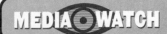

MEDIA WATCH

BANNING TOBACCO ADS

The U.S. government has taken action to reduce the appeal of tobacco to teens. It has prohibited outdoor ads for tobacco products within 1,000 feet of schools and playgrounds. Tobacco companies are also forbidden to use color in many of their ads. *What impact do you think this law has had on young people's health?*

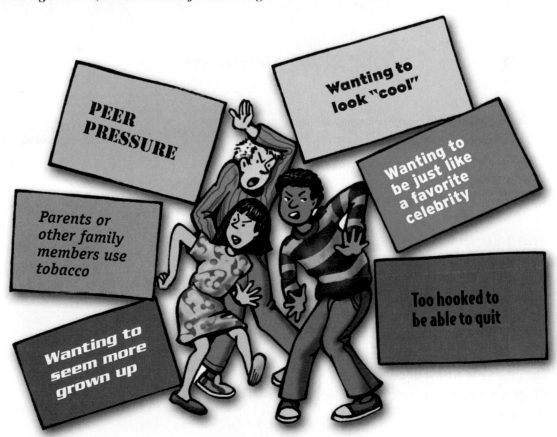

Most young tobacco users think that they can quit at any time. According to the American Lung Association, most teens who have smoked at least 100 cigarettes would like to quit, but they may not be able to do so. Also, of all teens who smoke a first cigarette, 42 percent will become regular smokers. Approximately one-third of these smokers will die from a tobacco-related illness. Of the 12 to 14 million Americans who use smokeless tobacco, one third are under the age of 21, and more than half of those developed the habit before they were 13 years old. The earlier in life people start using tobacco, the more likely they are to develop a chemical dependency, or physical addiction to nicotine.

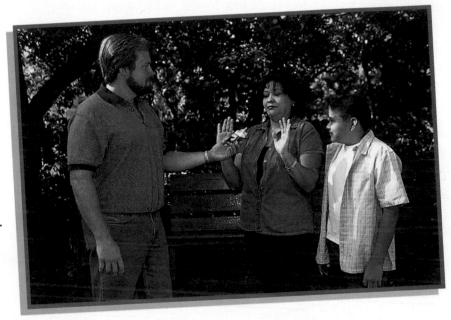

Nonsmokers serve as positive role models to others. *How might you influence other people to avoid using tobacco?*

Lesson 3 Review

Using complete sentences, answer the following questions on a sheet of paper.

Reviewing Terms and Facts
1. **Vocabulary** Define the terms *addiction* and *withdrawal.*
2. **Differentiate** Describe the difference between psychological dependence and physical dependence.
3. **Explain** Why will a tobacco user crave greater amounts of tobacco?
4. **Identify** List three factors that influence a teen's decision to use tobacco.

Thinking Critically
5. **Analyze** Explain the impact of chemical dependency and addiction to tobacco.
6. **Apply** Select a magazine ad for cigarettes. Analyze how the images and words in the ad encourage tobacco use.

Applying Health Skills
7. **Refusal Skills** With a classmate, write a skit that shows a teen using S.T.O.P. to say no to a person offering a cigarette.

Avoiding Tobacco

Tobacco Free: The Best Choice

The decision to avoid tobacco is the healthiest choice you can make. Other people might want to convince you that tobacco use is safe. If you're unprepared, the pressure you may feel might seem difficult to resist. Practice your refusal skills ahead of time. Find and take part in tobacco-free events in your community; this can strengthen your decision to avoid tobacco products.

Figure 10.7 features some great reasons to say no to tobacco use. One way to resist the pressure to use tobacco is to choose friends who also want to stay tobacco free.

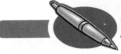

Quick Write

Briefly explain why you think staying tobacco free is good for your health.

LEARN ABOUT...

- the benefits of avoiding tobacco use.
- ways to help others break the tobacco habit.
- how tobacco smoke affects nonsmokers.
- how to defend your rights as a non-smoker.

VOCABULARY

- secondhand smoke
- mainstream smoke
- sidestream smoke
- passive smoker

FIGURE 10.7

THE BENEFITS OF SAYING NO TO TOBACCO

You give yourself all these gifts by deciding not to use tobacco. *What are some other reasons to remain tobacco free?*

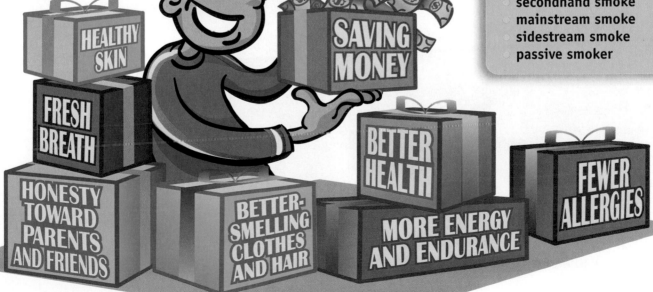

HEALTHY SKIN
SAVING MONEY
FRESH BREATH
BETTER HEALTH
FEWER ALLERGIES
HONESTY TOWARD PARENTS AND FRIENDS
BETTER-SMELLING CLOTHES AND HAIR
MORE ENERGY AND ENDURANCE

It isn't easy to beat an addiction. If you know someone who is trying to quit, provide encouragement and help the person avoid situations that might bring on the urge to use tobacco. *What would you include in a care package for someone trying to quit using tobacco? Why?*

Kicking the Tobacco Habit

The nicotine in tobacco makes it hard to kick the habit, but it can be done. A person who wants to quit using tobacco has several options. There are many ways to stop and numerous organizations that can help tobacco users break the habit and improve their health.

People who quit using tobacco may experience withdrawal symptoms. These symptoms include nervousness, moodiness, difficulty sleeping, hunger, and cravings for nicotine. Some symptoms may last for months. If someone you know is trying to quit, share the following tips.

- **Make a list of the reasons to quit using tobacco.** Read the list whenever the urge to use tobacco arises.
- **Set small goals.** Try quitting one day at a time. Every year the American Cancer Society sponsors the "Great American Smokeout," a campaign that calls for all smokers to stop smoking for one day.
- **Avoid being with people who use tobacco.** For example, stay away from places where you know that smokers gather. Participate in positive alternative activities, such as tobacco-free events.
- **Change any habits that are linked to using tobacco.** For example, eat a healthful snack instead of smoking between meals.
- **Learn stress-relieving techniques.** Try stretching or taking deep breaths.
- **Engage in physical activity.** When a craving for tobacco occurs, take a bike ride, go for a walk, or jog.

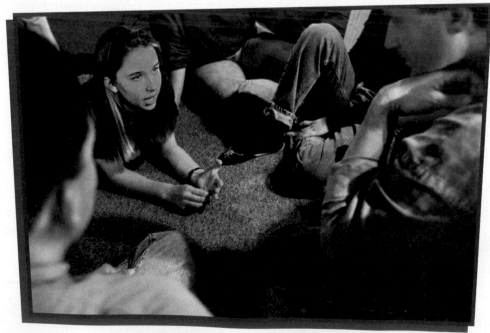

People who are trying to stop using tobacco need support and encouragement from tobacco-free friends.

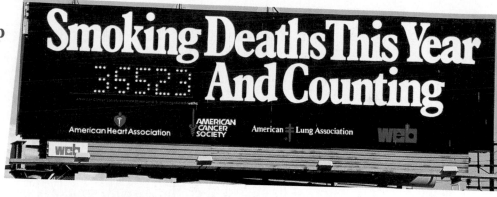

Smoking Deaths This Year And Counting
36523

American Heart Association · AMERICAN CANCER SOCIETY · American Lung Association · web

Programs That Help

The "cold turkey" method of quitting tobacco use is popular, and many experts recommend it. In this method the user simply stops all use of tobacco products. The user's body will be nicotine free three or four days later, although withdrawal symptoms may last longer. Books and recordings, often available at local libraries, can help people quit using tobacco on their own.

Some people need support or assistance to quit. Groups such as the American Lung Association, the American Heart Association, and the American Cancer Society offer information and programs to help people kick the smoking habit. Most counties have local chapters of these national groups.

Some people who quit need help to overcome withdrawal symptoms. For these people, doctors might recommend a nicotine gum or patch. These options will supply the body with small amounts of nicotine to help lessen the severity of withdrawal symptoms. There is also a non-nicotine medication that reduces a person's urge to smoke.

Getting the word out that tobacco is dangerous will help people decide not to smoke, or to quit. *How effective are antismoking messages? Which type of antismoking messages do you think are the most effective? Why?*

HEALTH SKILLS ACTIVITY

ACCESSING INFORMATION

Helping Others Quit

If you are close to someone who wants to kick the tobacco habit, help him or her learn about programs designed to help people stop using tobacco. Start with the following places and organizations:

- A local chapter of the American Cancer Society, the American Lung Association, or the American Heart Association
- Your school
- Your local health department
- Community health care providers, such as hospitals and clinics

ON YOUR OWN
Use one of the resources listed here to gather information about how to quit using tobacco. Put the materials you collect in a large envelope. Ask if you can keep it in the school library, so that students can check out the material.

How Tobacco Affects Nonsmokers

Even if you do not smoke, breathing in secondhand smoke can harm your health. **Secondhand smoke**, or environmental tobacco smoke, is *air that has been contaminated by tobacco smoke.* When someone smokes, two kinds of smoke fill the air: mainstream smoke and sidestream smoke. **Mainstream smoke** is *the smoke that a smoker inhales and then exhales.* It becomes environmental smoke after it passes through the smoker's lungs and, in some cases, through a filter. **Sidestream smoke** is *smoke that comes from the burning end of a cigarette, pipe, or cigar.* Sidestream smoke contains twice as much tar and nicotine as mainstream smoke because sidestream smoke enters the air directly from the burning tobacco.

Exposure to secondhand smoke causes people to become passive smokers. **Passive smokers** are *nonsmokers who breathe secondhand smoke.* Passive smoking is harmful because, just like any other kind of smoking, it contributes to respiratory problems, including lung cancer. Passive smoking irritates the nose and throat and causes itchy and watery eyes, headaches, and coughing.

A smoke-filled room contains high levels of nicotine, carbon monoxide, and other pollutants. In such a room a nonsmoker can inhale as much nicotine and carbon monoxide in one hour as if he or she had smoked a cigarette. People who have long-term exposure to secondhand smoke risk getting the same illnesses that affect smokers, including heart and lung diseases and respiratory problems. According to the U.S. Environmental Protection Agency, secondhand smoke is a human carcinogen, or cancer-causing substance. Each year 53,000 people die in the United States as a result of passive smoking.

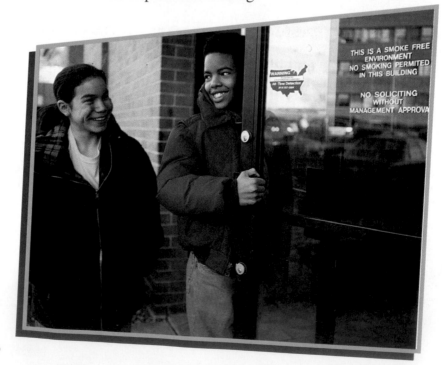

Smoking is not permitted in many buildings because of the dangers of secondhand smoke.

Children and Unborn Babies

A woman who uses tobacco during pregnancy seriously endangers the health of her unborn child. Tobacco use during pregnancy is associated with increased chances of miscarriage, stillbirth, and low birth weight. The lower a baby's birth weight, the higher the risk of complications in the baby's development. Infants whose mothers smoke during and after pregnancy are three times more likely to die from a condition known as Sudden Infant Death Syndrome than are infants whose mothers do not smoke. Children of smokers experience higher rates of allergies, asthma, chronic bronchitis, ear infections, and heart problems.

Rights of Nonsmokers

As a nonsmoker you have the right to breathe air that is free of tobacco smoke. You also have the right to express your preference that people not smoke around you. Starting in the late 1980s, the federal government passed laws to help reduce people's exposure to secondhand smoke. In 1989 the government banned smoking on all domestic airplane flights. Almost every state government has put restrictions on smoking. Employers now have a legal right to restrict smoking in the workplace, and many have banned smoking. It has become common for restaurants to ban smoking completely instead of creating nonsmoking sections. Support school and local efforts to reduce smoking and encourage others to become involved as well.

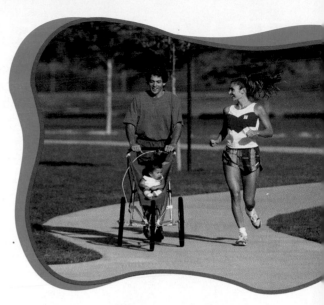

Parents who choose a tobacco-free lifestyle and stay active give their children a healthy start in life.

Lesson 4 Review

Using complete sentences, answer the following questions on a sheet of paper.

Reviewing Terms and Facts

1. **List** Name five benefits of saying no to tobacco use.
2. **Identify** What does it mean when a person quits using tobacco "cold turkey"?
3. **Vocabulary** Define *secondhand smoke*.
4. **Distinguish** What is the difference between mainstream smoke and sidestream smoke?

Thinking Critically

5. **Analyze** How have the laws passed to reduce people's exposure to secondhand smoke had a positive impact on health?

6. **Decide** Imagine that you and your family are sitting in the nonsmoking section of a restaurant. What would you do if the smoke from the smoking section bothered you?

Applying Health Skills

7. **Goal Setting** Make a plan to help someone quit using tobacco. Include alternative activities the tobacco user can do when he or she experiences the urge to use tobacco.

Spittin' Image

Using smokeless tobacco is just as deadly as smoking cigarettes.

Smokeless tobacco users are 50 times more likely to develop oral cancer than nonusers. Half the people who get cancer from using smokeless tobacco die within five years of being diagnosed. Yet many major league baseball players and other professional athletes keep chewing, despite the very real dangers.

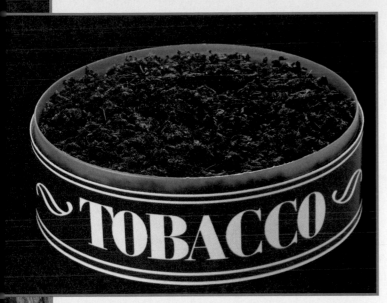

Tobacco leaves, shown drying in a barn (left), are used to make chewing tobacco (above). It is often sold in cans.

Consider this: A baseball player is not allowed to smoke on the field or in the dugout. Yet he can chew or "dip" (place a wad of tobacco between the lip and teeth) during the game, even though using smokeless tobacco for 30 minutes delivers the same amount of nicotine to the body as four cigarettes.

The problem isn't limited to major league baseball. Golfers on the PGA Tour are using smokeless tobacco. Rodeo riders will forget their horse before their chewing tobacco. Female athletes are taking up this dangerous habit, too.

Smokeless tobacco is banned on the college and minor league levels of baseball, but in the major leagues it is not only accepted, it's often encouraged by other players.

Tobacco's Terrible Toll

People who think using smokeless tobacco is cool should consider former major league outfielder Bill Tuttle. He chewed until he lost his teeth, his taste buds, his right cheekbone, his hearing, and, finally, his life.

Umpire Doug Harvey worked the big leagues with a cheek full of chew for 31 years. He retired with a lump in his throat—caused by chewing tobacco. He had developed cancer and had to undergo 60 radiation treatments. Harvey dropped from 205 to 145 pounds and fed himself liquid meals through a straw-sized hole in his breastbone just to stay alive. Recovered, he's now told about 156,000 school kids to stay away from chewing tobacco.

People who've been through both say quitting smokeless tobacco is twice as hard as quitting cigarettes. Ask Arizona Diamondbacks righthander Curt Schilling, co-MVP of a World Series. A few years ago doctors operated on a lesion, or open wound, on the inside of his lower lip. Caused by chewing tobacco, the lesion was precancerous, which means that it could have become cancerous. Despite the operation, Schilling can't quit chewing tobacco. "It's so unbelievably hard," says Schilling, who has tried sunflower seeds, gum, nicotine patches, hypnosis, and counseling. "I've got to quit—I want to see my kids grow up, and I want them to see me with a full face—but I haven't been able to."

A Hard-to-Kick Habit

Schilling's teammate Greg Colbrunn can't stop either. "I've tried," he says. "I wish I'd never started." His teammate Brian Anderson, who also chews tobacco, says, "It's dirty, it's filthy, and your breath reeks."

The baseball players' association allows its members to use smokeless tobacco in front of millions of young people. You've heard of National Smoke Out Day. Somebody needs to start a National Chew Out Day. Anybody using smokeless tobacco in front of young people should get chewed out! ◼

TIME TO THINK...

About the Dangers of Smokeless Tobacco

Make a poster that will persuade young people not to use smokeless tobacco. Come up with an eye-catching headline, and include a short list of facts that details how harmful the habit is. Display posters in the classroom, and discuss how each one gets its message across.

CHOOSING TO STAY TOBACCO FREE

Model

Analyzing influences means that you recognize the ways in which internal and external factors affect your health choices. Read about the factors that influence this teen to remain tobacco free.

Janna's teacher asked for volunteers to help put together an antitobacco program for elementary school students. Janna signed up immediately because she believes that it is important to remain tobacco free. Janna thinks about what influenced her decision not to smoke. Look at the factors that influenced Janna's choice.

Internal Influences

I want to do my best in sports.

I don't want my breath to stink.

I'd rather spend my money on something else.

External Influences

My parents would be very disappointed in me if I smoked.

My religion teaches me to respect my body and to avoid harmful substances that could endanger my health.

My friends think that tobacco is for losers.

Tobacco is illegal for people my age.

I like to hang out with Olivia and Cindy, and they don't like the smell of smoke.

Practice

Below you will find a list of factors that might influence a teen to be tobacco free. Which influences are internal, and which are external? What other influences could you add to this list?

1. Cigarettes are a waste of my money.
2. I don't want to damage my health.
3. I don't want to get into trouble with my family or the law.
4. Other people have a bad opinion of smokers.
5. No one in my family smokes.
6. I don't like polluting the air.
7. I might become addicted to nicotine.

Apply/Assess

On a separate sheet of paper, list the factors that have influenced you to be tobacco free. Then, on a sheet of light-colored construction paper, use a pencil to draw the shape of an object that symbolizes an aspect of your personality. For example, if you enjoy in-line skating, you might draw a skate. Make a jigsaw puzzle of this shape. On each piece, use a marker to write one of the influences you have listed. Then cut the pieces, and switch puzzles with a classmate. Glue your classmate's puzzle back together on poster board. Display the completed puzzles in your classroom. Walk around the classroom with your original list, and record how many of your classmates listed similar influences about tobacco.

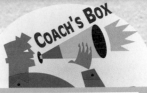

COACH'S BOX

Analyzing Influences

Both internal and external influences affect your choices. These influences may include:

Internal
- Interests
- Likes/dislikes
- Fears
- Curiosity

External
- Family
- Friends
- Media
- Culture

Self-√Check
- Did I think of factors that influenced me to be tobacco free?
- Did I create a jigsaw puzzle based on an aspect of my personality?
- Does each puzzle piece contain a factor that has influenced my decision to be tobacco free?

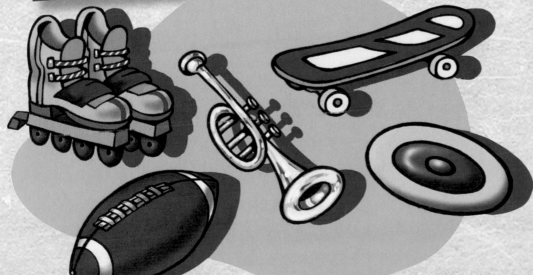

After You Read

Use your completed Foldable to review terms and recall information on tobacco's harmful effects.

FOLDABLES™
Study Organizer

Reviewing Vocabulary and Concepts

On a sheet of paper, write the numbers 1–7. After each number, write the term from the list that best completes each sentence.

- alveoli
- bronchi
- carbon monoxide
- diaphragm
- emphysema
- tar
- trachea

Lesson 1

1. _____ is a thick, dark liquid that forms when tobacco burns.
2. The colorless, odorless, poisonous gas produced when tobacco burns is called _____.
3. The exchange of oxygen and carbon dioxide takes place in the _____ of the lungs.
4. A serious lung disease that damages the alveoli is _____.

Lesson 2

5. The _____ is a tube in the throat that takes air to and from the lungs.
6. When you inhale, the air enters your nose and mouth and then moves past the epiglottis into the trachea and _____ before it reaches the alveoli.
7. The _____ is a large, dome-shaped muscle below the lungs that draws air in and pushes air out.

Lesson 3

On a sheet of paper, write the numbers 8–10. Write *True* or *False* for each statement below. If the statement is false, change the underlined word or phrase to make it true.

8. People experiencing <u>withdrawal</u> are often anxious, depressed, and irritable.
9. <u>Physical dependence</u> is when a person believes that he or she needs a drug to function normally.
10. A person who develops a tolerance for nicotine needs <u>less</u> of the drug to feel its effect.

Lesson 4

On a sheet of paper, write the numbers 11–13. After each number, write the letter of the answer that best completes each of the following statements.

11. Mainstream smoke
    a. is smoke coming from the burning end of a cigarette, pipe, or cigar.
    b. is air that has been contaminated by tobacco smoke.
    c. is the smoke that a smoker inhales and exhales.
    d. contains twice as much tar and nicotine as sidestream smoke.

12. Sidestream smoke
    a. is safer than mainstream smoke.
    b. is smoke that has passed through a smoker's lungs.
    c. contains twice as much tar and nicotine as mainstream smoke.
    d. cannot cause lung cancer.

13. A passive smoker
    a. is a smoker who does not inhale smoke.
    b. is a smoker who smokes less than one pack of cigarettes a day.
    c. is not in danger of getting a tobacco-related illness.
    d. is a nonsmoker who breathes second-hand smoke.

Thinking Critically

Using complete sentences, answer the following questions on a sheet of paper.

14. **Assess** Some brands of cigarettes contain very little tar. Do you think that these brands are safe to smoke? Explain.

15. **Apply** How can you support your school as a tobacco-free environment and encourage your classmates to do so as well?

16. **Compare and Contrast** Do you think that adults who start using tobacco do so for the same reasons as teens? What reasons do you think they have in common? How might their reasons differ?

Career Corner

Dentist Would you like to help improve people's smiles? If so, you might consider a career as a dentist. Dentists help people maintain healthy teeth and gums. These professionals complete four years of dental school and may have advanced training. Dentists come in contact with a lot of people. They also work with a variety of precision tools and new technology. Learn more about this and other health careers by clicking on Career Corner at health.glencoe.com.

Standardized Test Practice

Reading & Writing

Read the paragraphs below and then answer the questions.

A practice called visualization can be a beneficial tool for people who want to break an unhealthy habit, such as smoking.

Visualization often involves repeating positive statements aloud. These statements should be in the present tense, so that it sounds as though the desired result has already been achieved. For example, a smoker who wants to quit might repeat, "I am enjoying a tobacco-free lifestyle." The smoker should then enter a state of deep relaxation by sitting quietly, closing his or her eyes, and breathing deeply. Once this state is has been reached, a smoker can focus on the positive statements he or she has made and the goal to quit.

1. In the first paragraph, the word *beneficial* means
   - **A** harmful.
   - **B** helpful.
   - **C** useless.
   - **D** ineffective.

2. What is the second paragraph mainly about?
   - **A** the process of visualization
   - **B** the history of visualization
   - **C** the reasons that visualization works
   - **D** the problems of visualization

3. Write a paragraph explaining why you think a person might use visualization to stop smoking.

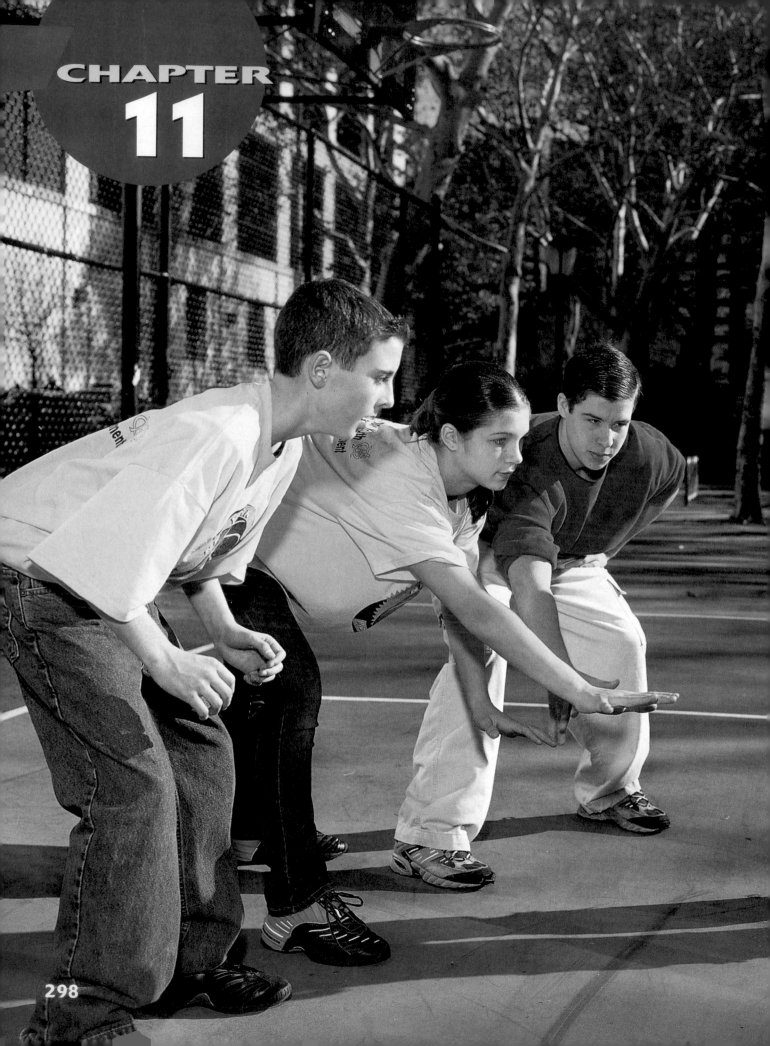

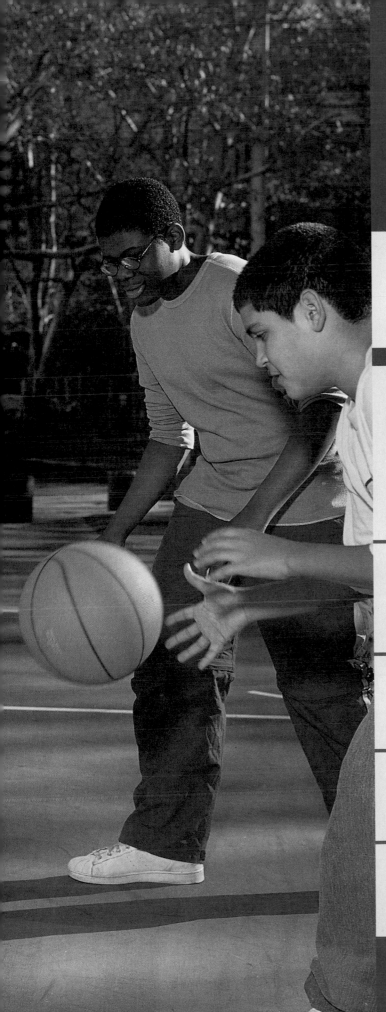

Drugs and Alcohol

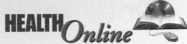

HEALTH *Online*

Rate what you know about medicines, alcohol, and drugs by taking the Chapter 11 Health Inventory at health.glencoe.com.

FOLDABLES™
Study Organizer

Before You Read

Make this Foldable to help you organize the main ideas on using medicines safely in Lesson 1. Begin with four circles of paper—one large (8″ across), one medium (7″ across), and two small (each 2½″ across).

Step 1

Fold the medium circle in half. Glue the top half onto the large circle, making sure that the bottoms of the two circles are aligned. This will create a tab from the unglued part of the medium circle.

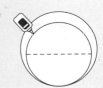

Step 2

Fold the two small circles in half. Glue the top half of each circle onto the bottom half of the medium circle. This will create two more tabs.

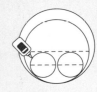

Step 3

Label as shown.

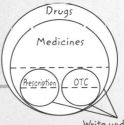

Write under tabs.

As You Read

Under the appropriate tab, define key terms and record information on using medicines safely.

Using Medicines Safely

Quick Write

Do you read the label on an over-the-counter medicine before you take it? Why or why not?

LEARN ABOUT...

- different types of medicines.
- the proper use of medicines.
- how to avoid misusing medicines.

VOCABULARY

- drug
- medicine
- prescription medicine
- over-the-counter (OTC) medicine
- side effect

Drugs and Medicines

People sometimes refer to new medicines as "miracle drugs." However, drugs are also blamed for causing serious problems in society. How can these substances be both helpful and harmful? The effects depend on the type of drug and how it is used. A **drug** is *a substance other than food that changes the structure or function of the body or mind.* A **medicine** is *a drug that prevents or cures illness or eases its symptoms.*

What Medicines Do

Medicines can help your body in many ways. They are generally grouped according to their effect on the body. The various kinds of medicines can do the following:

- **Prevent diseases.** Vaccines (also called immunizations) are medicines that protect against diseases that can spread such as measles and mumps. Vaccines cause the immune system to produce substances that destroy specific germs before they can cause disease. Immunizations are an important part of disease prevention.

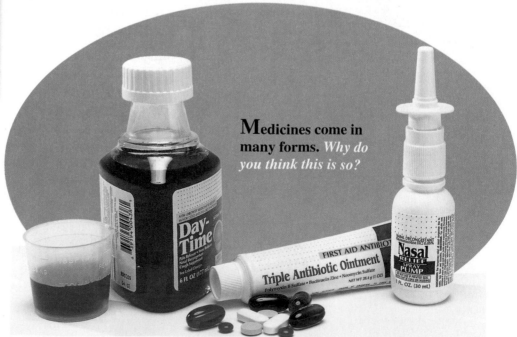

Medicines come in many forms. *Why do you think this is so?*

- **Fight germs.** Antibiotics (an·tee·by·AH·tiks) are a type of medicine used to fight disease-causing germs. They kill harmful bacteria that can cause infections.
- **Relieve pain.** Many medicines, including ibuprofen (EYE·byoo·PROH·fen) and acetaminophen (uh·SEE·tuh·MI·nuh·fen), are used to relieve pain and reduce fever and inflammation.
- **Treat other conditions.** When you have a cold, you can use a decongestant (dee·kuhn·JES·tuhnt) to help you breathe more easily. Medicines containing antihistamines (an·tee·HIS·tuh·meenz) can relieve allergy symptoms. Certain health problems or conditions such as diabetes can be treated or controlled with medicine.

✓ **Reading Check**
Make connections. Reread *What Medicines Do* and find examples of medicines that prevent diseases, fight germs, relieve pain, and treat other conditions.

Types of Medicines

When you are sick, you might take either prescription or over-the-counter medicine. A **prescription medicine** is *a medicine that can be used safely only with a doctor's written permission.* **Over-the-counter (OTC) medicines** are *medicines that you can buy without a doctor's prescription.* Both kinds of medicines can have side effects and should be used with caution.

Prescription Medicines

The doctor's order, or prescription, shows how much of the medicine is needed and how often it should be taken. **Figure 11.1** shows a sample prescription label. Only licensed pharmacists are authorized to fill prescriptions and give you the medicine to take home.

FIGURE 11.1

PRESCRIPTION MEDICINE LABEL

To make sure that you are interpreting the instructions on a medicine label correctly, ask your doctor or pharmacist to explain it to you.

Pharmacy name, address, and telephone number

Name of pharmacist

Prescription number

Date prescription was filled

Name and address of patient

Name of prescribing doctor

Directions from the doctor

Name of the medicine

Strength and/or amount per container

Number of refills allowed

Expiration date

Special instructions

M **McGrath Pharmacy**
123 Main St., Miller, NJ 09009
(609) 555-1122
Pharmacist: T. Lewis

Rx #125690
Date Filled 4/09/05
Dr. Tobe Friedland

Candace Sanchez
1578 Lakeside Lane
Miller, NJ 09009

Take one capsule every six hours, one hour before a meal.

Erythromycin
250 mg capsules
Quantity: 60 capsules
Refills: 0
Drug Expires: 04/09/06

Delayed release capsules— do not crush or break

Take medication on an empty stomach

Finish all medication unless otherwise directed by doctor

Over-the-Counter Medicines

OTC medicines are generally safe when used as directed. When choosing an OTC medicine, check the label to find the product's active ingredients. This will help you select a product that contains only the medicine you need. If you think you need to take more than one OTC medicine at the same time, ask a pharmacist if the medicines can be combined safely.

Guidelines for the Safe Use of Medicines

Medicines may cause **side effects**, *reactions to medicines other than the ones intended.* Make sure that you are aware of any side effects that may lead to injury, such as drowsiness. Here are some other guidelines for using medicines safely.

- **Read the label.** Take all medicine exactly as instructed. Make sure you understand the instructions on prescription and OTC medicine labels. Ask a doctor or pharmacist if you need help interpreting the information or have questions about listed side effects. Check the expiration dates on medicines and discard any that have expired. Some medicines become less effective over time; others can become stronger.

- **Take safety precautions.** Use only medicine that has been prescribed for you. Keep all medicines out of the reach of children. If anyone takes too much medicine (overdoses), or has an allergic reaction to a medicine, get medical help immediately.

HEALTH SKILLS ACTIVITY

DECISION MAKING

Following Doctor's Orders

The antibiotic that Mary's doctor prescribed for her infection worked quickly. After three days of taking the pills every eight hours, Mary feels much better. The doctor told her to keep taking the pills for ten days. The warning label says to finish all medicine. Mary wonders whether she really needs to take the rest of the medicine. The pills make her stomach feel a little upset. What should Mary do?

What Would You Do?

Apply the six steps of the decision-making process to Mary's problem. With a classmate, discuss what you would do if you were Mary. Explain how you came to your decision.

1. **STATE THE SITUATION.**
2. **LIST THE OPTIONS.**
3. **WEIGH THE POSSIBLE OUTCOMES.**
4. **CONSIDER VALUES.**
5. **MAKE A DECISION AND ACT.**
6. **EVALUATE THE DECISION.**

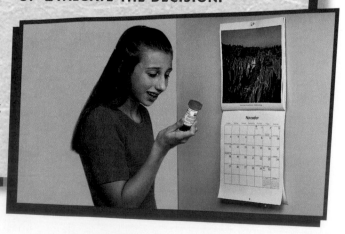

Misusing Medicines

Medicines should be taken only when needed. Remember that medicines are drugs, and drug misuse can cause serious health problems.

Doctors and pharmacists provide detailed instructions and information to help you use medicines properly. Follow their instructions and these tips to avoid misusing medicines.

- Take medicine according to directions.
- Take the recommended or prescribed dosage.
- Take the medicine for the length of time prescribed by a doctor, even if you start to feel better before you've stopped taking it. Don't take an OTC medicine for a longer period of time than is recommended on the label.
- Do not give your prescription medicines to others.
- Don't mix medicines without your doctor's approval.

Inappropriate use of medicine can sometimes lead to health problems later in life, such as liver or kidney failure. Also, certain medicines can harm a developing fetus. Females who are pregnant or who plan to become pregnant should always check with a doctor before taking any medication.

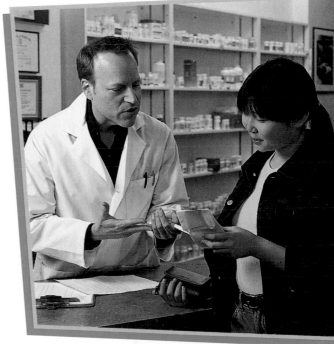

A pharmacist is a reliable source of information on medicines.

![Lesson 1 Review]

Using complete sentences, answer the following questions on a sheet of paper.

Reviewing Terms and Facts

1. **Vocabulary** Define *drug* and *medicine.*
2. **List** What are four ways that medicines can help the body?
3. **Recall** How do prescription medicines differ from over-the-counter medicines?
4. **Restate** What is a *side effect?*

Thinking Critically

5. **Hypothesize** What might happen if you took a medicine after its expiration date had passed?

6. **Describe** Explain the role of immunizations and treatment with medicines in disease prevention.

Applying Health Skills

7. **Accessing Information** Visit a local supermarket or pharmacy and examine the labels of four different types of OTC medicines. On a sheet of paper, write the name of each medicine. Note the purpose of the medicine, any possible dangerous combinations with other medicines, and any possible side effects. Share your findings with the class.

Lesson 2

Alcohol Use and Abuse

Quick Write

What effects do you think using alcohol has on a person's body? Make a list of these effects.

LEARN ABOUT...

- how alcohol affects the body.
- why people's bodies react differently to alcohol.
- what alcoholism is and what can be done about it.

VOCABULARY

- alcohol
- cirrhosis
- intoxicated
- alcoholism

What Is Alcohol?

Alcohol is *a drug created by a chemical reaction in some foods, especially fruits and grains.* Found in beer, wine, whiskey, and other beverages, alcohol affects a person physically and mentally.

In the United States, it is illegal for anyone under the age of 21 to drink alcohol. Many people who start drinking in their early teens become dependent on alcohol; they are also likely to try other drugs. Using alcohol may result in chemical dependency on this substance. Being addicted to alcohol is associated with many serious health problems.

Teens may begin drinking to escape from problems or relieve stress, or because of peer pressure. Learning about alcohol's harmful effects on the body, however, will help you decide not to drink.

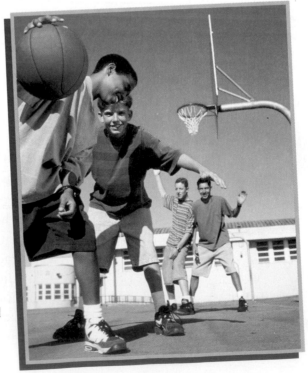

Choose friends who enjoy healthy activities and avoid the use of alcohol and other drugs.

How Alcohol Affects the Body

A person can feel the effects of alcohol just a few minutes after taking the first drink. Alcohol can impair a person's judgment and cause other short-term effects. People who drink large quantities of alcohol also risk serious long-term effects. These include permanent damage to organs and even death. **Figure 11.2** details how the body is damaged by the use of alcohol.

Reading Check
Make your own web. Write *Effects of Alcohol* in the center of your paper inside an oval. Add two ovals connecting to the center oval, titled *Short-term Effects* and *Long-term Effects*. Write examples branching from these ovals.

FIGURE 11.2

HARMFUL EFFECTS OF ALCOHOL

Alcohol has both short- and long-term effects on many different body systems.

Brain
Immediate effects: Impaired judgment, reasoning, memory, and concentration; slowed reaction time, decreased coordination; slurred speech; distorted vision and hearing; reduced inhibitions; alcohol poisoning, causing unconsciousness and even death.

Long-term effects: Brain cell destruction, nervous system disorders, and memory loss.

Heart
Immediate effects: Increased heart rate.

Long-term effects: Irregular heartbeat, heart muscle damage.

Liver
Immediate effects: Processes of the liver, which filters out over 90% of the alcohol in the body, may become unbalanced.

Long-term effects: **Cirrhosis** (suh•ROH•suhs), or *scarring and destruction of liver tissue*, and liver cancer. Both can cause death.

Kidneys
Immediate effects: Increased urination, which can result in dehydration, headache, and dizziness.

Long-term effects: Kidney failure resulting from high blood pressure.

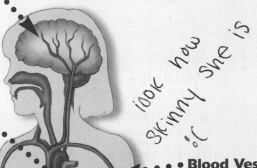

Blood Vessels
Immediate effects: Enlarged blood vessels, creating false sense of warmth.

Long-term effects: High blood pressure; stroke.

Stomach
Immediate effects: Vomiting, which can lead to choking and death.

Long-term effects: Ulcers (open sores) in the stomach lining; stomach cancer.

FIGURE 11.3

DIFFERENT DRINKS = SAME ALCOHOL CONTENT

A typical serving of each of these three alcoholic beverages contains about the same amount of alcohol. *What factors might cause different effects in people who drink the same amount of alcohol?*

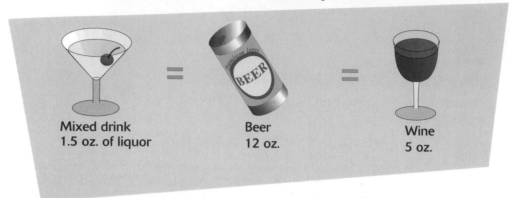

Mixed drink
1.5 oz. of liquor

Beer
12 oz.

Wine
5 oz.

Differing Effects

Figure 11.3 shows three common types of alcoholic beverages. The more alcohol a person drinks, the more he or she will be affected. However, the amount of alcohol is only one factor in determining how drinking affects a person. Below are other factors to consider:

- **Size and gender.** Generally, females can tolerate less alcohol than males. In addition, the less a person weighs, the more easily he or she will be affected by alcohol.
- **Food in the stomach.** The body's absorption of alcohol will be slower if there is food in the stomach.
- **How fast a person drinks.** Gulping down a drink raises the level of alcohol in the blood because the body has less time to process it.
- **Other substances in the body.** Drinking alcohol while taking certain drugs may have dangerous effects and can even be fatal.

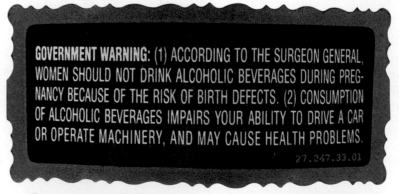

GOVERNMENT WARNING: (1) ACCORDING TO THE SURGEON GENERAL, WOMEN SHOULD NOT DRINK ALCOHOLIC BEVERAGES DURING PREGNANCY BECAUSE OF THE RISK OF BIRTH DEFECTS. (2) CONSUMPTION OF ALCOHOLIC BEVERAGES IMPAIRS YOUR ABILITY TO DRIVE A CAR OR OPERATE MACHINERY, AND MAY CAUSE HEALTH PROBLEMS.

27.247.33.01

In the United States, warnings about the health risks of drinking have been required on alcoholic beverages since late 1989.

Drinking and Driving

Drunk drivers are said to be driving under the influence (DUI) of alcohol or driving while intoxicated (DWI). A person who is **intoxicated** (in·TAHK·suh·kay·tuhd) is *drunk*. Driving drunk is illegal.

Even one alcoholic beverage begins to impair coordination and can make driving unsafe. When a driver has been drinking, the chances that she or he will be involved in an accident are very high. The more alcohol a person drinks, the more dangerous she or he is behind the wheel. Slower reaction times and impaired judgment make drunk drivers dangerous to other drivers and pedestrians. Alcohol use contributes to almost half of all motor-vehicle–related deaths, the most frequent cause of death among Americans ages 15 to 20.

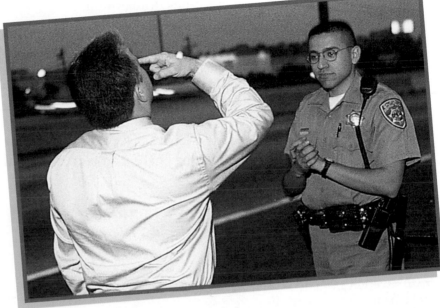

Police officers test drivers to determine whether they are intoxicated. *What behaviors might signal that a person is intoxicated?*

HEALTH SKILLS ACTIVITY

ACCESSING INFORMATION

Helping Someone with a Drinking Problem

You may suspect that someone close to you has a problem with alcohol. Alcohol addiction is an illness, and a person who is drunk sometimes cannot control his or her behavior. Here are some strategies for helping someone with a drinking problem.

- Learn about alcohol addiction and sources of treatment.
- Talk to the person about the problem only when she or he is sober.
- Encourage the person to learn about the damage that drinking does to the body and to seek help from a health care professional or a support group.

- Contact Alcoholics Anonymous and learn about the group's 12-step program.
- Show concern and sympathy.
- Join a support group such as Al-Anon for people who have friends or relatives who are addicted to alcohol.
- Do not cover up or make excuses for the person.

ON YOUR OWN

Find out if your community has a chapter of Alateen or a similar group for teens who have friends or relatives who have problems with alcohol. How does this organization help teens cope with the challenges of this situation?

Alcoholism

Alcoholism is *an illness characterized by a physical and psychological need for alcohol.* People who become addicted to alcohol are not able to limit the amount they drink. Alcoholics develop a tolerance for alcohol. They need to drink more and more alcohol to experience its effects. A person may be an alcoholic if he or she

- becomes drunk often.
- drinks alone.
- stops participating in other activities so that he or she can drink.
- acts like a different person when drinking alcohol.
- makes excuses for drinking.
- promises to quit but does not.
- refuses to admit how much he or she drinks.
- experiences blackouts—periods when he or she cannot remember what he or she said or did while drinking.

If you suspect that a friend or relative has a problem with alcohol, you can seek help from a trusted adult. *Who are some of the people in your community to whom you could turn for help?*

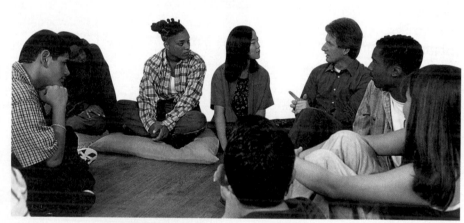

Lesson 2 Review

Using complete sentences, answer the following questions on a sheet of paper.

Reviewing Terms and Facts

1. **Vocabulary** Define the term *alcohol.* Give two examples of beverages that contain alcohol.
2. **Recall** Name three long-term effects of alcohol on the body.
3. **Explain** Why is it dangerous for people to drive when they are intoxicated?
4. **List** What are three signs of alcoholism?

Thinking Critically

5. **Evaluate** Explain how a chemical dependency on alcohol negatively impacts health.
6. **Analyze** Do you think that warning labels on alcohol are necessary? Explain your answer.

Applying Health Skills

7. **Refusal Skills** If someone were pressuring you to use alcohol, how could you use S.T.O.P. to refuse? Would your response to a friend be different from your response to an acquaintance? Predict the consequences of refusing in each situation.

Drug Use and Abuse

What Is Drug Abuse?

Some drugs have no medical use. These **illegal drugs** are *substances it is against the law for people of any age to manufacture, possess, buy, or sell.* Illegal drugs damage the user's mind and body.

Drug abuse is the *use of a drug for nonmedical purposes.* When people use illegal drugs, or when they intentionally misuse legal drugs for nonmedical purposes, they are abusing drugs. When people drink alcohol with the intention to get drunk, they are abusing alcohol.

Marijuana

Marijuana (mar·uh·WAH·nuh) is a drug made from the hemp plant. It is usually smoked, and it is often the first illegal drug that teens use. This mood-altering drug is also called "pot" or "weed." **Figure 11.4** lists some of the effects of marijuana use.

FIGURE 11.4

EFFECTS OF MARIJUANA USE

Marijuana has many immediate and long-term effects on the body.

Immediate Effects of Marijuana Use

- Inability to think or speak clearly
- Difficulty paying attention
- Loss of short-term memory
- Lack of coordination, slowed reaction time
- Increased heart rate and appetite
- Unusual sensitivity to sights and sounds
- Sadness or fearfulness

Long-Term Effects of Marijuana Use

- Problems with normal body development in young users
- Damage to lung tissue and the immune cells that fight cancer
- Feelings of anxiety and panic
- Possible psychological dependence
- Possible inability to have children

Quick Write

Make a list of illegal drugs that you have heard about. Jot down what you have heard about them.

LEARN ABOUT...

- what drug abuse is.
- how different drugs affect the body.

VOCABULARY

- illegal drugs
- drug abuse
- stimulant
- amphetamine
- depressant
- narcotic
- hallucinogen
- inhalant

Reading Check

Analyze word structure.
What is the prefix in *illegal*? What does it mean?
Think of other words with
this prefix. Then, find
words with the prefix *un-*
as you read this page.

Stimulants

Stimulants (STIM·yuh·luhnts) are *drugs that speed up the body's functions.* They cause an increase in heart rate, breathing rate, and blood pressure and provide a false sense of energy and power. As the effects wear off, the user feels exhausted and emotionally unbalanced. Stimulants can affect the body in unpredictable ways and can lead to addiction or even death.

Amphetamines

Amphetamines (am·FE·tuh·meenz) are *strong stimulant drugs that speed up the nervous system.* For this reason amphetamines are commonly called "speed." They come in many forms and can be swallowed, inhaled, smoked, or injected. **Figure 11.5** lists the harmful effects of amphetamine abuse.

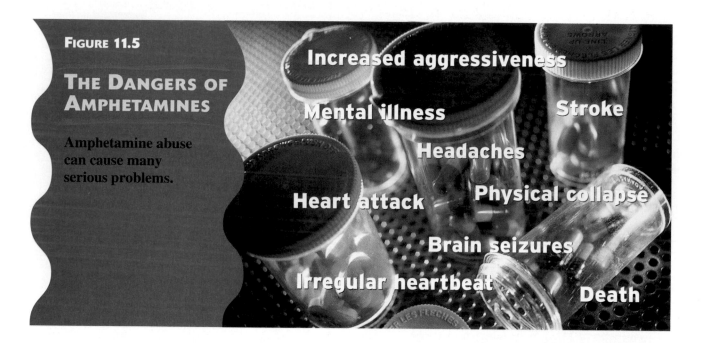

FIGURE 11.5

THE DANGERS OF AMPHETAMINES

Amphetamine abuse can cause many serious problems.

Increased aggressiveness
Mental illness
Stroke
Headaches
Heart attack
Physical collapse
Brain seizures
Irregular heartbeat
Death

Cocaine and Crack Cocaine

Cocaine (koh·KAYN) is an illegal stimulant made from the coca plant. It can be inhaled, smoked, or injected. Street names for cocaine include "blow," "snow," and "coke." At first the user gets a brief, powerful feeling of well-being and confidence. When the feeling wears off, the user becomes anxious and depressed. In a matter of days a cocaine user can become addicted to the drug.

Because cocaine affects the heart rate, even first-time users run the risk of a fatal heart attack. Repeated use can damage nasal membranes and cause lung problems. Users may act aggressively or deny responsibility for their actions.

Crack is a concentrated form of cocaine. After smoking crack, a person may feel more energetic and alert for a few minutes. Then the user feels depressed and craves more of the drug. Crack users can become dependent on the drug even faster than cocaine users. The side effects of crack are similar to those of cocaine, including possible heart attack and death.

Depressants

Depressants (di·PRE·suhnts) are *drugs that slow down the body's functions and reactions, including heart and breathing rates.* Most come in tablet or capsule form and are swallowed. Doctors sometimes prescribe depressants called tranquilizers (TRANG·kwuh·ly·zuhrz) to treat patients who are experiencing anxiety, muscle spasms, or sleeplessness. Other depressants include barbiturates (bar·BI·chuh·ruhts) and hypnotics (hip·NAH·tiks). Alcohol is also a depressant.

Depressants may make users feel relaxed and less anxious. However, depressants can also impair coordination and judgment and cause sleepiness. Depressant users can become physically and psychologically dependent. They may become depressed and experience mood swings. Depressants can cause coma and death if they are combined with alcohol.

HEALTH Online

Topic: Substance abuse

For a link to more information on teens and drug use, go to **health.glencoe.com.**

Activity: Using the information provided at this link, create a poster that features an antidrug message.

FIGURE 11.6

OTHER TYPES OF DRUGS AND SUBSTANCES

There are over 2,000 names for drugs. *Which of the names in this chart are familiar to you?*

Type of Drug or Substance	Examples	Characteristics
Narcotics	heroin, morphine, codeine	**Narcotics** are *drugs that relieve pain and dull the senses.* Heroin is an illegal narcotic. Morphine and codeine may be prescribed for certain conditions; they are carefully controlled because they are highly addictive. Abuse of narcotics damages the lungs, liver, kidneys, and brain.
Hallucinogens	phencyclidine (PCP, angel dust), lysergic acid diethylamide (LSD, acid)	**Hallucinogens** are *drugs that distort moods, thoughts, and senses.* Users may become disoriented, less sensitive to pain, and violent. They may also lose control.
Club Drugs	Ecstasy (X, MDMA), GHB (G, liquid Ecstasy), Rohypnol (Roofie), Ketamine (special K, vitamin K)	Club drugs are illegal drugs that were originally available mostly in nightclubs or at all-night dance parties called raves. They may be used to reduce inhibitions. Because some club drugs are easily slipped into drinks, they are sometimes used in date rape. These drugs can cause disorientation; nausea; unconsciousness; and, at higher doses, even death.
Inhalants	glue, gasoline, spray paint	**Inhalants** (in·HAY·luhnts) are *substances whose fumes are breathed in to produce mind-altering sensations.* Inhaling them can cause nausea, dizziness, mental confusion, and loss of motor skills. Inhaled poisons go directly to the brain, where they can cause permanent damage or even death.

Other Drugs

In addition to marijuana, stimulants, and depressants, many other types of drugs and substances may be abused. **Figure 11.6** on the previous page lists and describes these drugs and substances.

The Dangers of Drug Use

Using drugs is very dangerous. Many drugs can cause brain damage, coma, and death. If users share needles when injecting heroin or other drugs, they may contract hepatitis or HIV. A person under the influence of drugs cannot think clearly, increasing the possiblity of injury, as well as unplanned pregnancy and exposure to sexually transmitted diseases.

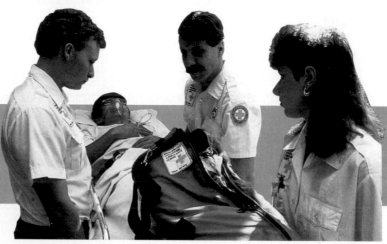

Drug use can destroy lives. *Why do you think some teens experiment with drugs even though they know the dangers of drug use?*

Lesson 3 Review

Using complete sentences, answer the following questions on a sheet of paper.

Reviewing Terms and Facts

1. **Vocabulary** Define the terms *illegal drugs* and *drug abuse.*
2. **Distinguish** How do stimulants differ from depressants?
3. **Recall** What is a *narcotic?*
4. **Restate** Describe the effects of hallucinogens. Give an example of a drug that falls into this category.

Thinking Critically

5. **Analyze** In what ways are inhalants different from the other drugs discussed in this lesson?

6. **Suggest** What advice would you give to a friend who was thinking about taking amphetamines so that she could stay awake to study for a test?
7. **Infer** Explain how chemical dependency on and addiction to drugs and other substances can negatively impact health.

Applying Health Skills

8. **Analyzing Influences** Think about how drugs are referred to in song lyrics, on the radio, on television, and in movies. Do these references make drug use seem fun, cool, or normal? How could these kinds of messages from the media—even as jokes—promote illegal drug use?

The Nervous System

The Body's Control Center

Alcohol and other drugs can permanently damage the nervous system, the body's control center. The nervous system carries messages to and from the brain. It controls the senses, thoughts, movements, and bodily functions.

The cells that make up the nervous system are called **neurons** (NOO·rahnz), or nerve cells. Neurons send and receive information in the form of tiny electrical charges. **Figure 11.7** shows how neurons work.

FIGURE 11.7

HOW NEURONS CARRY MESSAGES

These steps show how neurons help you catch a ball.

1 When the ball hits your gloved hand, the skin's receptor cells receive the message: "The ball has arrived."

2 Sensory neurons send this message in the form of an electrical charge to the spinal cord and brain.

3 In the spinal cord and brain, connecting neurons translate the message "The ball has arrived" into one directed to your muscles: "Squeeze."

4 Motor neurons deliver the "Squeeze" message to your muscles, and your hand grips the ball.

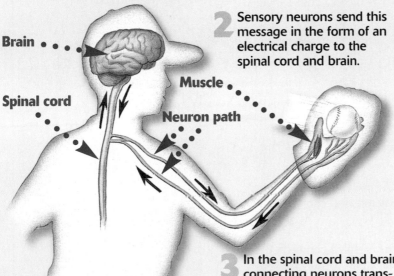

Brain · · · ·
Spinal cord · · ·
Muscle · · · · ·
Neuron path · · ·

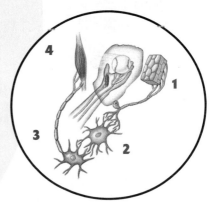

LEARN ABOUT...

- the parts of the nervous system.
- problems of the nervous system
- how you can keep your nervous system healthy.

VOCABULARY

- neuron
- central nervous system (CNS)
- peripheral nervous system (PNS)
- brain
- spinal cord

The Nervous System

The nervous system has two main parts. The **central nervous system (CNS)** consists of *the brain and the spinal cord*. The **peripheral** (puh·RIF·uh·ruhl) **nervous system (PNS)** is made up of *the nerves that connect the central nervous system to all parts of the body.*

The **brain** is *the command center, or coordinator, of the nervous system.* It receives and screens information and sends messages to the other parts of the body. The **spinal cord** is *a long bundle of neurons that relays messages to and from the brain and all parts of the body.* **Figure 11.8** shows the parts of the nervous system and explains how the three main parts of the brain function.

FIGURE 11.8

PARTS OF THE NERVOUS SYSTEM

The brain is the largest organ of the central nervous system. The CNS controls heart rate, breathing, and digestion. The peripheral nervous system, which is shown in green, links the CNS to the skeletal muscles.

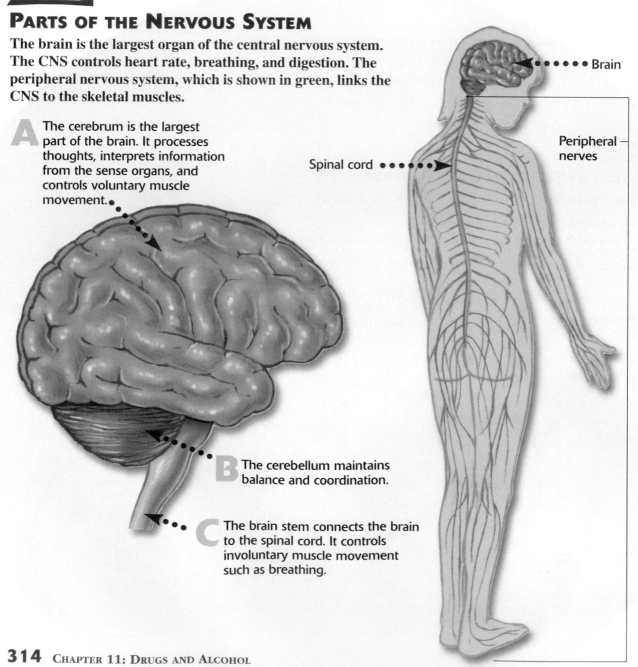

A The cerebrum is the largest part of the brain. It processes thoughts, interprets information from the sense organs, and controls voluntary muscle movement.

B The cerebellum maintains balance and coordination.

C The brain stem connects the brain to the spinal cord. It controls involuntary muscle movement such as breathing.

Brain

Peripheral nerves

Spinal cord

Problems of the Nervous System

Several factors can lead to nervous system disorders:

- **Injuries.** The most common cause of nervous system damage is physical injury. The results of head, neck, and back injuries can be severe. A spinal cord injury, for example, can cause paralysis—the loss of feeling and movement in parts of the body.

- **Disorders.** Multiple sclerosis is a disorder that causes damage to the protective outer coating of some nerves. This condition prevents the nerves from transmitting messages and impulses properly. Cerebral palsy is a group of disorders caused by damage or injury to the brain as it develops. Scientists have yet to find ways to prevent or cure multiple sclerosis or cerebral palsy.

- **Infections.** Certain viruses cause illnesses that affect the nervous system, such as polio, rabies, and meningitis (me·nuhn·JY·tuhs). Vaccines against some of these diseases are available. Others can be treated with medicines.

- **Drug abuse.** Misuse and abuse of drugs can damage the nervous system. Some drugs act directly on the brain stem—the part of the brain that helps control heart rate, breathing, appetite, and sleeping. Some drugs affect the way the nervous system sends and receives messages. Drugs can also alter the nervous system's responses and may cause hallucinations and distorted perceptions of reality.

- **Alcohol use.** Drinking alcohol has an immediate effect on the brain. Alcohol can impair memory, thought processes, perception, judgment, and attention. Prolonged abuse of alcohol can destroy millions of brain cells. Once destroyed, these cells can never be replaced. Women who drink alcohol during pregnancy put their fetuses at risk for fetal alcohol syndrome (FAS). FAS affects several of the fetus's body systems, including the CNS.

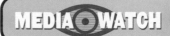
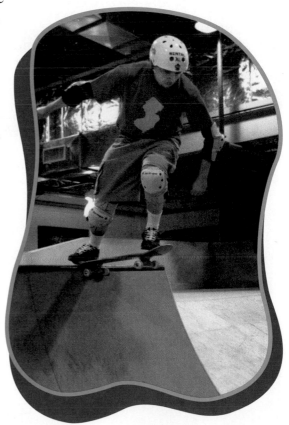

Taking the proper safety precautions can help prevent nervous system injuries. *What safety precautions is this teen taking?*

Caring for Your Nervous System

You can prevent or reduce your risk for developing certain problems of the nervous system by making healthful lifestyle choices such as choosing nutritious foods and getting enough sleep. Here are some tips to keep your nervous system healthy.

- **Protect yourself from disease.** You have already been vaccinated against some diseases that affect the nervous system, such as polio and tetanus. To protect yourself from rabies, avoid contact with strange or wild animals. Good hygiene will help protect you from infections such as meningitis.
- **Wear a helmet.** When you are riding a bike, skateboarding, in-line skating, snowboarding, skiing, or playing a contact sport, wear a helmet to protect your head from injury.

Hands-On Health

NERVOUS SYSTEM TRICKS

An optical illusion tricks your nervous system by making the eyes see something that isn't really there.

WHAT YOU WILL DO

1. Look at the picture of the two circles within squares. Which circle looks larger—the white or the black? Now measure the two circles.
2. Look at the picture of black squares. Focus your eyes on one of the squares. What do you perceive in the intersections of the white bars? Next, focus on one intersection. What happens?

IN CONCLUSION

1. Did the white circle appear to be larger than the black circle? The way your eyes work can make bright objects seem larger than dark ones.

2. Did you see dark spots in the intersections when you were looking at the black squares? Did the spots disappear when you looked directly at the intersections? This happens because the color white appears whiter when it is next to something black. The white bars appear whiter than the intersections because the bars are right next to the black squares. When you look at an intersection, however, you perceive the white as white. Your eye is not comparing it to any other color.
3. How real did these illusions seem?

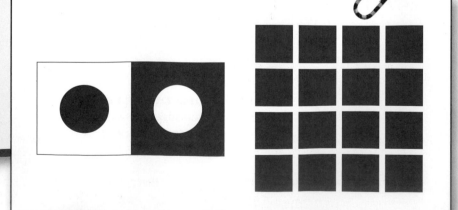

- **Play it safe.** Be careful when you play sports or engage in any physical activity. For example, never dive into shallow water. If you use gymnastics equipment, have spotters watch you.
- **Lift properly.** When lifting heavy objects, use the proper techniques to prevent back injuries. If the object is too heavy, ask someone for help.
- **Observe safety rules.** When you walk or ride a bicycle, follow all traffic safety rules. Always wear a safety belt when riding in a vehicle.
- **Avoid alcohol and other drugs.** Prolonged use of alcohol can permanently damage the central nervous system. Drug use can cause brain damage. Using alcohol or other drugs impairs perception, coordination, judgment, and reaction time. These impairments increase the chances of accidental injury. Avoiding substance abuse will help you protect your nervous system.

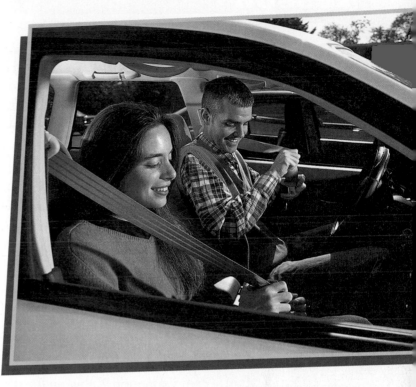

Think about how a safety belt holds you in an upright position when you are riding in a car. *How would a safety belt protect your nervous system if you were in a collision?*

Lesson 4 Review

Using complete sentences, answer the following questions on a sheet of paper.

Reviewing Terms and Facts

1. **Vocabulary** Define the term *neurons*.
2. **Recall** What is the difference between the CNS and the PNS?
3. **Identify** Name the three main parts of the brain, and explain the function of each part.
4. **List** Identify five safety measures you can take to protect your nervous system.

Thinking Critically

5. **Hypothesize** If the peripheral nervous system stopped functioning, what would happen to the central nervous system?

6. **Describe** How would life change for a person who lost the function of all sensory neurons?

Applying Health Skills

7. **Accessing Information** Epilepsy is a disorder of the nervous system in which a person experiences seizures. During a seizure the person may lose consciousness, twitch, and shake. Using library and Internet resources, investigate what happens in the brain of a person who has epilepsy. Prepare a brief report of your findings.

Avoiding Alcohol and Other Drugs

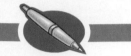

Quick Write

Jot down one physical, mental/emotional, and social risk of using alcohol or other drugs.

LEARN ABOUT...

- how alcohol and drug use poses risks to your physical, mental/emotional, and social health.
- reasons to avoid alcohol and drugs.
- alternatives to using alcohol and drugs.
- ways to say no to alcohol and drugs.

VOCABULARY

- assertive

Understanding the Risks

People who drink alcohol or take other drugs expose themselves to many risks. Most of these risks are serious, and some are even deadly. Alcohol and drugs can be especially dangerous to teens, who are still growing and developing. These substances cause physical, mental/emotional, and social harm.

Being aware of the consequences of alcohol and drug use can help you stay away from risk situations. If you do find yourself in such a situation, knowing the dangers will help you make the right decision. You will feel confident about choosing not to use alcohol or drugs.

Physical Risks

You now know that using alcohol and drugs can have negative effects on physical health. One can never be sure which negative effects might occur. Users can experience short-term effects such as dizziness and vomiting. They may also suffer from long-term effects such as brain damage. Alcohol and drug use may increase the time a teen's body takes to mature physically. Height, weight, and sexual development may be negatively affected. **Figure 11.9** lists some of the physical effects of alcohol and drug use. These effects make it difficult for people to participate in activities they enjoy.

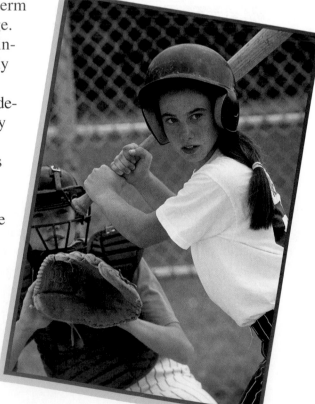

Choosing not to use alcohol or other drugs will help keep you healthy and ready to enjoy the activities you like to do.

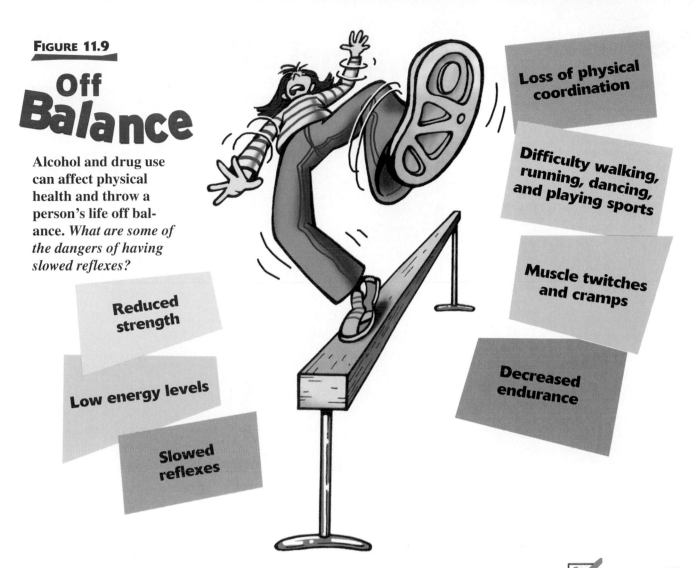

FIGURE 11.9

Off Balance

Alcohol and drug use can affect physical health and throw a person's life off balance. *What are some of the dangers of having slowed reflexes?*

Reduced strength

Low energy levels

Slowed reflexes

Loss of physical coordination

Difficulty walking, running, dancing, and playing sports

Muscle twitches and cramps

Decreased endurance

In addition to health problems, people may face other physical consequences from alcohol and drug use. Use of these substances can be a factor in vehicle crashes, pedestrian accidents, drowning, burns, and falls. Under the influence of alcohol or drugs, a person may take risks that he or she would normally avoid. These risks might include sexual activity, which can lead to pregnancy and sexually transmitted diseases, including HIV.

Risks to the Unborn

Using alcohol or other drugs during pregnancy can cause serious diseases and birth defects in the fetus. Children whose mothers used drugs during pregnancy often experience delays in development and have learning disabilities. Many are born addicted to drugs themselves. A pregnant woman who injects drugs also risks infecting her fetus with HIV. Women who drink alcohol while pregnant may have babies affected by fetal alcohol syndrome. These babies' development will be delayed. They will also experience psychological and behavioral problems throughout life.

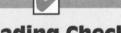

Reading Check
Build vocabulary. Identify synonyms and antonyms for these words: *serious, negative, difficult.*

FIGURE 11.10

Mental and Emotional Effects

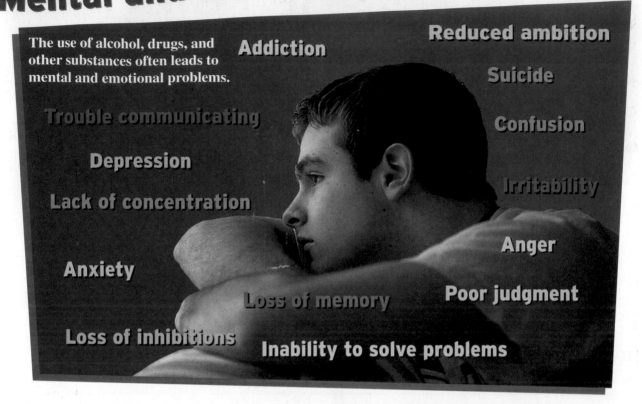

The use of alcohol, drugs, and other substances often leads to mental and emotional problems.

Addiction

Reduced ambition

Suicide

Trouble communicating

Confusion

Depression

Irritability

Lack of concentration

Anger

Anxiety

Poor judgment

Loss of memory

Loss of inhibitions

Inability to solve problems

Mental/Emotional Risks

The changes that you experience during your teen years can be stressful. In trying to relieve this stress, some teens turn to alcohol or drugs. These substances have the opposite effect, making life even more difficult and confusing.

The psychological consequences of alcohol, drug, and substance abuse are very serious. A person's ability to think and learn is impaired. Drug and alcohol users often feel bad about themselves and have trouble relating to others. **Figure 11.10** lists some of the mental and emotional effects of alcohol, drug, and substance abuse.

Social Risks

Drug and alcohol use may cause mood swings and personality changes. Users may lose control of their behavior, which can strain or end relationships.

People who are addicted to a substance become obsessed with it. They may lose interest in family and friends. Some may end friendships or lie to cover up their addiction. Because they push away the people in their lives, those with a chemical dependency on alcohol, drugs, or other substances may be very lonely.

Risks in School

Teens who use alcohol or other drugs cause many problems for themselves—and others—in school. They may

- be late or miss school often.
- do poorly in school because they are unable to pay attention.
- behave in ways that get them suspended or expelled.
- miss the opportunity to be involved in school activities.
- let down classmates or teammates because of poor performance.
- lose chances to learn new skills and develop their abilities.
- fail to meet long-term goals.

Risks to the Family

A family is affected when any member abuses alcohol or other drugs. This family member may

- fail to nurture other family members.
- become violent and hurt other family members.
- spend time away from home and be moody and unpredictable.
- lie or steal to support the habit.
- lose his or her job or fail to fulfill other responsibilities.

Risks with the Law

Teens who use alcohol or other drugs often get into serious trouble with the law. Anyone who buys, sells, or possesses illegal substances can face arrest, fines, and a sentence in a detention center. It is also illegal for anyone under 21 to buy or possess alcohol. An underage person who is caught driving while intoxicated will lose his or her license. Adults who sell alcohol to anyone under 21 are also breaking the law.

Involvement with alcohol or other drugs often leads teens to commit other crimes. A person is more likely to become violent while under the influence of alcohol or other drugs. Teens who use substances are also at risk for becoming victims of crime. Because people are often unable to make responsible decisions when they are under the influence of alcohol or drugs, they risk injury or death.

Stores that sell alcohol to underage customers face stiff fines.

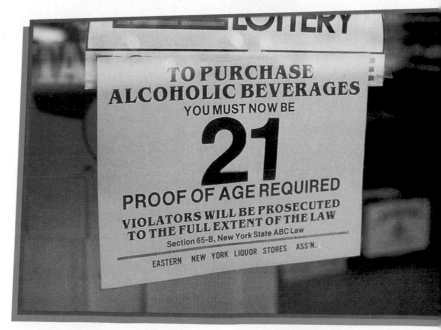

Getting Help

People who are addicted to alcohol, drugs, or other substances may try to hide the problem or deny that one exists. You can get help for yourself, a friend, or a family member who has an alcohol or drug problem. First, try going to trusted adults: parents, teachers, religious leaders, or counselors. You may feel uncomfortable talking about such a big problem with someone close to you. If so, you can turn to organizations that offer counseling and treatment. Sources of help include support groups, alcohol or drug treatment centers, and toll-free drug hot line counselors.

Reasons to Avoid Alcohol and Drugs

There are no healthful reasons to try alcohol or drugs. However, there are many good reasons to avoid them. Remind yourself:

- I don't show respect for myself if I use alcohol or drugs.
- My future means too much to me to ruin it.
- I'd rather be in control of what I do.
- Alcohol and drugs can harm my health.
- Using alcohol or drugs means breaking the law.
- My true friends don't try to convince me to use drugs.
- Alcohol and drugs can take away my energy.

Alternatives to Substance Use

Many teens turn to substance use because they are already having other problems. Dealing with the issues that are causing the problems—instead of experimenting with alcohol and drugs—is one way to avoid substance use. Don't give in to feelings of low self-esteem. Instead, find a healthy way to spend time. Learn to do something you've always wanted to try. Join an activity at school, or volunteer—hospitals, homeless shelters, child-care centers, and soup kitchens can use your time and enthusiasm. Identify and participate in any alcohol- and drug-free events taking place in your community. Remember that your healthy, successful future depends on your choice to avoid using alcohol, drugs, and other harmful substances.

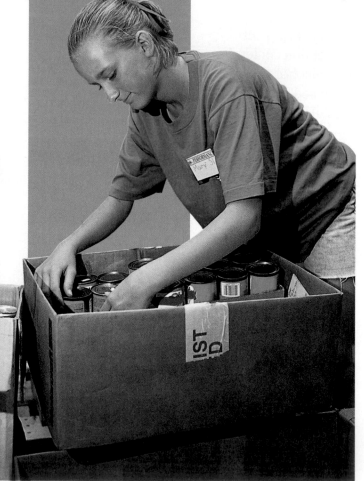

Teens who have a sense of purpose can more easily avoid alcohol and drugs. Volunteering is a great way to use your time and talents to care for people in need.

Refusing to Use Alcohol and Drugs

Many teens name peer pressure as their main reason for using alcohol or drugs. One way to deal with peer pressure is to avoid social situations where substance use might take place. When you can't avoid these situations, it's easier to say no if you're prepared. You need to be **assertive**, or *willing to stand up for yourself in a firm but positive way.* You also need effective refusal skills.

HEALTH SKILLS ACTIVITY

REFUSAL SKILLS

Refusing to Use Drugs

Lately, Caitlyn's friend Beth has become distant. Sometimes she's barely able to follow a conversation.

One night while Caitlyn and Beth are hanging out at the mall, one of Beth's new friends comes over and presses something into her hand. Beth shows it to Caitlyn: pills. She tells Caitlyn how good they make her feel and tries to press a pill into her hand.

Caitlyn knows that she doesn't want to use drugs. However, she wants to stay friends with Beth. What should Caitlyn do?

WHAT WOULD YOU DO?

Role-play how Beth and Caitlyn interact at the moment when Beth tries to put a pill into Caitlyn's hand. How might Caitlyn use S.T.O.P. in this situation? Predict how Beth might react.

SAY NO IN A FIRM VOICE.
TELL WHY NOT.
OFFER ANOTHER IDEA.
PROMPTLY LEAVE.

Lesson 5 Review

Using complete sentences, answer the following questions on a sheet of paper.

Reviewing Terms and Facts

1. **List** Name five mental/emotional effects of alcohol and drug use.
2. **Identify** List three problems teens who use alcohol or drugs may have in school.
3. **Vocabulary** Define the term *assertive*.
4. **List** Identify some activities that are healthy alternatives to substance use.

Thinking Critically

5. **Apply** What is the most important reason for you to stay substance free?

6. **Hypothesize** How might you be affected if one of your close friends developed a substance use problem?

Applying Health Skills

7. **Accessing Information** Do some research to identify any alcohol- and drug-free events taking place in your community. Make a list of these events and share them with the class. Choose an upcoming event to participate in. Encourage your peers to attend as well.

Quiz

1. All teens tend to be very moody.
   a. True   b. False

2. Someone may be depressed if
   a. everything gets on that person's nerves.
   b. he or she keeps having headaches or other health problems that a doctor can't determine a cause for.
   c. that person's grades are dropping—and he or she doesn't care.
   d. All of the above

3. Depression often goes hand in hand with which of the following?
   a. An eating disorder
   b. Obsessive-compulsive disorder
   c. Learning disabilities
   d. All of the above

4. Which of the following can help someone recover from depression?
   a. Winning the lottery
   b. Antidepressant drugs and psychiatric treatment
   c. Getting straight As
   d. All of the above

5. A person who is seriously depressed is at a much higher risk of attempting suicide.
   a. True   b. False

6. If someone is strong enough, he or she can tackle a bout of depression alone.
   a. True   b. False

Answers: 1.b.; 2.d.; 3.d.; 4.b.; 5.a.; 6.b.

Check out the explanations on the next page!

What Is Depression?

Test your knowledge on the difference between feeling blue and being depressed.

Symptoms of Depression

Depression is a serious medical condition—a person's life could depend on getting treatment. According to the National Institute of Mental Health, if someone experiences five or more of the following symptoms for more than two weeks, he or she may be clinically depressed.

If this applies to you or someone you know, talk to a parent, teacher, or counselor about the problem.

- Feeling sad or crying a lot
- Feeling guilty for no reason, feeling worthless, loss of confidence
- Feeling hopeless
- Loss of interest in school, friends, or activities
- Difficulty concentrating or making decisions
- Feeling irritable, overreacting
- Sleeping a lot more or having trouble falling asleep at night
- Loss of appetite or overeating
- Feeling restless or tired most of the time
- Having thoughts about death, dying, or suicide

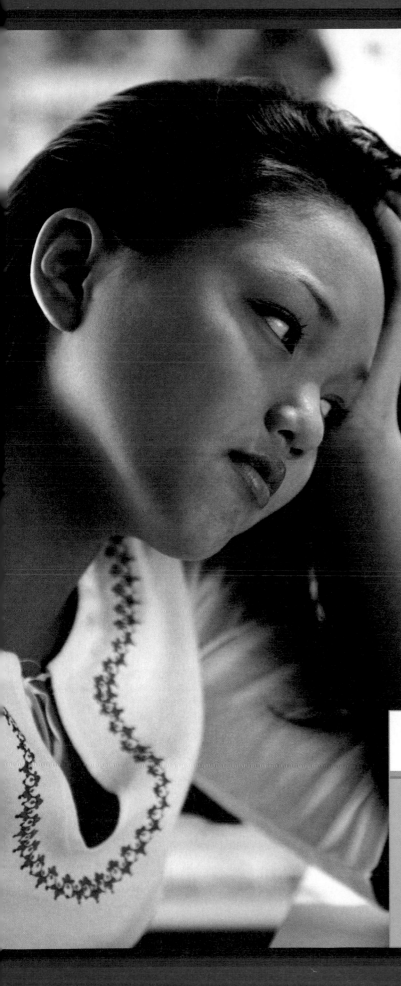

Explanations

1. While **most adolescents feel sad every now and then,** they tend to feel better quickly. However, the medical condition known as depression is disabling, lasting, and requires professional treatment.

2. **Irritability, unexplained physical ailments, and slipping grades are key signs of depression.** A person may also lose interest in friends and activities.

3. **Often, depressed teens will have other mental health issues,** says James Chandler, M.D., a psychiatrist in Yarmouth, Nova Scotia, Canada. Sometimes the more obvious emotional distress gets all the attention, but both issues need to be treated.

4. If a person is clinically depressed, no news—no matter how good—will make him or her feel better. **What works: counseling and, sometimes, antidepressants.** These prescription drugs should be accompanied by psychotherapy. Dr. David Fassler, chair of the American Psychiatric Association's Council on Children, Adolescents and Their Families, warns that "medication alone is rarely appropriate."

5. Statistics show that **teens who have a mental illness and those who have previously tried to kill themselves are among the most likely to commit suicide.**

6. Like diabetes or asthma, **depression is an illness that calls for medical treatment.** "There's a misperception that you can just get over this," says Dr. Fassler. "The tragedy is that [most depressed] teens aren't getting help." ◾

TIME TO THINK...

About Depression
Use reliable online resources or your school's media center to learn more about depression. Find statistics on how widespread the disorder is. Research past and present views of and treatments for depression. Summarize your findings in a brief report.

REFUSE TO USE ALCOHOL AND DRUGS

Model

Andie and her friend Donna are watching television at Donna's house when Donna's cousin Nick shows up. He lights up a joint and holds it out to Andie. She shakes her head no. He tells her that she should try it. "Smoking pot is no big deal," he says. "Everybody does it." Andie is surprised and a little afraid. She thinks quickly and remembers a conversation she had with her older brother about what to do if anyone ever offered her drugs. She uses S.T.O.P.

> No way. I don't do drugs.

> A friend of mine got into serious trouble with drugs. I don't want that to happen to me.

> Let's go over to Jim's and see what he's doing.

> Are you sure you don't want to go to Jim's? Okay, well, it's getting late. I'll see you tomorrow.

Say no in a firm voice.

Tell why not.

Offer another idea.

Promptly leave.

Practice

It takes courage to be able to resist negative peer pressure. It also takes a strategy. Read the following scenario about a teen who is offered alcohol.

Ron meets his friend Dennis to play basketball at the park. Before they start, Dennis reaches into his gym bag and takes out two beers. He offers one to Ron with a smile, saying, "It's going to be hot today—better get some fluids in you." Ron doesn't drink alcohol because he knows that it's illegal and that it can have dangerous effects on the body.

In small groups, discuss how Ron could refuse alcohol. Have members of your group take turns role-playing Ron's refusal for the class.

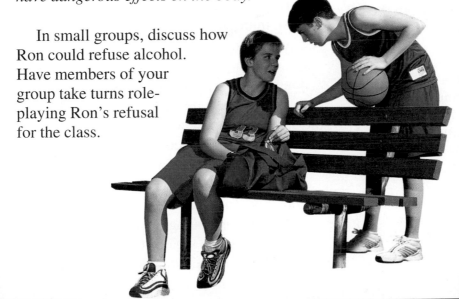

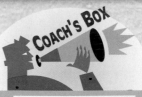

Refusal Skills

S.T.O.P. is an easy way to remember how to use refusal skills.

S Say no in a firm voice.

T Tell why not.

O Offer another idea.

P Promptly leave.

Self-✓Check

- Does the teen in my story use S.T.O.P. successfully?
- Does my story include at least one pressure statement and one response from my list?
- Does the teen in my story mention his or her personal reason(s) for staying alcohol and drug free?
- Is my story realistic?

Apply/Assess

Think of statements that people use to pressure others to try alcohol or drugs. Create a two-column chart. In the left column write down several of these pressure statements. In the right column write a possible response to each statement. Then use your list to create a short story. The story should show how a teen stands up to peer pressure by using S.T.O.P. and the response items on your list. Don't forget to include your character's personal reasons for staying alcohol and drug free. Swap short stories with a classmate. How did your classmate use S.T.O.P. in his or her story?

After You Read

Use your completed Foldable to review the information on the safe use of medicines.

FOLDABLES™
Study Organizer

Reviewing Vocabulary and Concepts

On a sheet of paper, write the numbers 1–6. After each number, write the term from the list that best completes each sentence.

> - alcohol
> - alcoholism
> - cirrhosis
> - intoxicated
> - over-the-counter medicine
> - prescription medicine

Lesson 1

1. A cold remedy that you buy at a supermarket is an example of a(n) _____.

2. Medicine that you can get only with a doctor's written order is a(n) _____.

Lesson 2

3. People who start drinking in their early teen years may become dependent on _____.

4. Long-term drinking may cause _____, a disease that destroys liver tissue.

5. A(n) _____ driver is dangerous to other drivers, pedestrians, passengers, and himself or herself.

6. _____ is an illness characterized by a physical and psychological need for alcohol.

On a sheet of paper, write the numbers 7–10. Write *True* or *False* for each statement below. If the statement is false, change the underlined word or phrase to make it true.

Lesson 3

7. People may take <u>depressants</u> to feel more energetic and powerful.

8. Glue, gasoline, and spray paint are examples of <u>narcotics</u>.

Lesson 4

9. The <u>neuron</u> is the largest organ of the central nervous system.

10. An injury to the <u>spinal cord</u> can cause paralysis.

On a sheet of paper, write the numbers 11–13. After each number, write the letter of the answer that best completes each statement.

11. Teens who use alcohol, drugs, or other substances risk all of the following consequences, *except*
  a. injury and death.
  b. lying or stealing to support the habit.
  c. getting into serious trouble with the law.
  d. improved relationships with family and friends.

12. You can get help for yourself, a friend, or a family member who has an alcohol or drug problem from
  a. a support group.
  b. an alcohol or drug treatment center.
  c. a drug hot line counselor.
  d. all of the above.

13. If you stand up for yourself in a firm but positive way, you are being
  a. addicted.
  b. intoxicated.
  c. assertive.
  d. drunk.

Thinking Critically

Using complete sentences, answer the following questions on a sheet of paper.

14. **Explain** Why is alcohol and drug use considered a preventable cause of nervous system disorders?
15. **Hypothesize** Why might someone ignore the risks of alcohol and drug use?
16. **Apply** How could a teen use positive peer pressure to counteract the negative effects of living with a family member who is abusing alcohol or drugs?
17. **Explain** How can avoiding alcohol and other drugs support a teen's decision to abstain from sexual activity?

Career Corner

Neurologist A person who has a nervous system disorder may need treatment from a neurologist. A neurologist is a medical doctor who specializes in diseases and disorders of the brain and nervous system. These professionals complete a four-year college degree, four years of medical school, and one to seven years of residency training. Learn more about this and other health careers by clicking on Career Corner at health.glencoe.com.

Standardized Test Practice

Math

Read the paragraph below and then answer the questions.

One of the main causes of accidents on the road is drinking alcohol and driving. According to the National Commission Against Drunk Driving, the three age groups that are most likely to drive after drinking include young adults and underage drinkers. Underage drinkers are especially dangerous on the road because they are not experienced drivers. They are more likely to be involved in alcohol-related crashes than any other age group.

Even one drink can impair judgment, coordination, and reflexes. Drinking alcohol and then getting behind the wheel is a potentially lethal combination.

1. An average of eight young people die each day in alcohol-related crashes. What does the number "eight" in this statement represent?
   - (A) median
   - (B) mode
   - (C) mean
   - (D) first quartile

2. Two out of every five people will, at some time, be involved in an alcohol-related accident. What percent of the population does this number represent?
   - (A) 4%
   - (B) 10%
   - (C) 25%
   - (D) 40%

3. Survey your classmates about whether they think drinking and driving is a serious problem in the community. What percent of the class thinks that this is the case?

CHAPTER 12

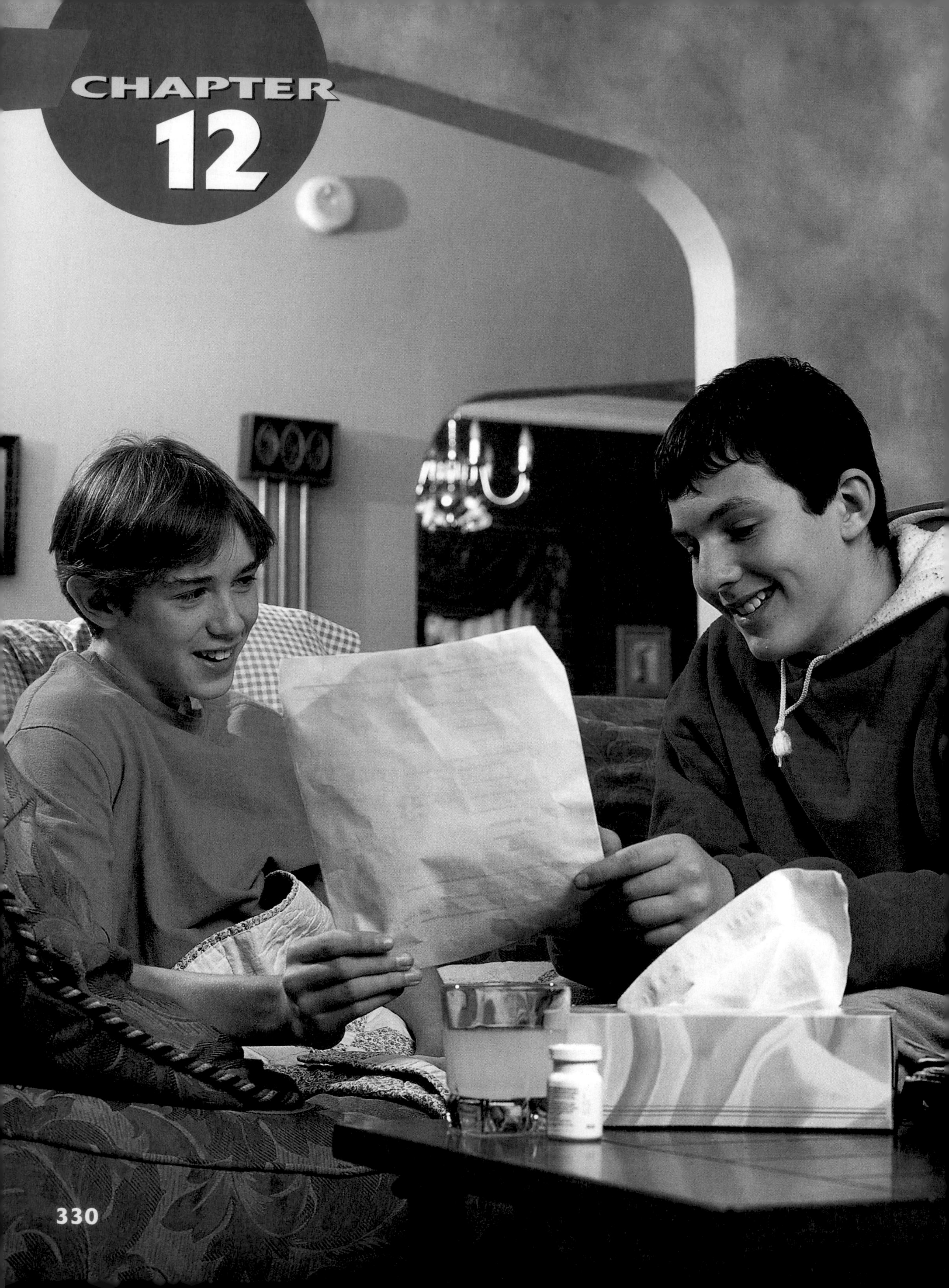

Understanding Communicable Diseases

HEALTH *Online*

Do you make healthful choices when it comes to avoiding and preventing the spread of communicable diseases? Find out by taking the Chapter 12 Health Inventory at health.glencoe.com.

FOLDABLES™
Study Organizer

Before You Read

Make this Foldable to help you record main ideas about the causes of communicable diseases. Begin with a plain sheet of 8½" × 11" paper.

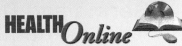

Step 1

Fold the sheet of paper along the long axis, leaving a ½" tab along the side.

Step 2

Turn the paper. Fold in half, then fold in half again.

Step 3

Unfold and cut the top layer along the three fold lines. This makes four tabs.

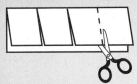

Step 4

Label the tabs as shown.

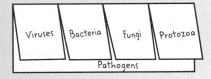

As You Read

Under the appropriate tab, summarize what you learn about each type of pathogen.

Quick Write

What do you think it means to "catch" a cold? Jot down one or two sentences to explain your answer.

LEARN ABOUT...

- types of germs that can cause disease.
- what an infection is.
- how germs are spread.

VOCABULARY

- disease
- communicable disease
- germs
- pathogens
- infection
- viruses
- bacteria
- fungi
- protozoa

Causes of Communicable Diseases

Germs and Disease

If you have ever had a cold or the flu, then you have had a disease. A **disease** is *any condition that interferes with the proper functioning of the body or mind.* Diseases are either communicable or noncommunicable. A **communicable** (kuh·MYOO·ni·kuh·buhl) **disease** is *a disease that can be spread to a person from another person, an animal, or an object.* A cold is a communicable disease.

All communicable diseases are caused by **germs**, *organisms that are so small that they can be seen only through a microscope.* The environment is filled with many different types of germs, most of which are harmless and some of which are helpful. *The germs*

FIGURE 12.1

PATHOGENS AND THE DISEASES THEY CAUSE

Pathogens	Diseases
Viruses	AIDS, chicken pox, colds, hepatitis, herpes, influenza, measles, mononucleosis, mumps, polio, rabies, smallpox, viral pneumonia
Bacteria	bacterial pneumonia, diphtheria, most foodborne illnesses, gonorrhea, Lyme disease, pinkeye, strep throat, tuberculosis
Fungi	athlete's foot ringworm
Protozoa	amebic dysentery malaria

that are responsible for causing disease are known as **pathogens**. An **infection** is *a condition that occurs when pathogens enter the body, multiply, and damage body cells*. If the body is not able to fight off the infection, a disease develops.

Types of Pathogens

All pathogens are not alike. Types of pathogens include viruses, bacteria, fungi, and protozoa. **Figure 12.1** on the previous page shows some of the diseases caused by these four types of pathogens.

Viruses (VY·ruh·suhz), *the smallest and simplest disease-causing organisms,* cause a wide range of health problems. Fortunately, scientists have developed ways to prevent many of the diseases caused by viruses. Bacteria are another common kind of pathogen. **Bacteria** are *tiny one-celled organisms that live nearly everywhere.* Many bacteria are harmless, and some are actually helpful. For example, bacteria in your intestines aid digestion. However, certain bacteria are harmful and can cause disease. **Fungi** (FUHN·jy) are *primitive life-forms, such as molds or yeasts, that cannot make their own food.* Most fungi are harmless, but some can cause health problems. **Protozoa** (proh·tuh·ZOH·uh) are *one-celled organisms that have a more complex structure than bacteria.* While many are harmless, some types are harmful and can cause serious diseases. These diseases are less common in the United States than in many other parts of the world.

How Pathogens Are Spread

Knowing how pathogens can be spread can help you protect yourself from them. This will reduce your risk of contracting communicable diseases. Pathogens can be spread in several ways:

- **Direct contact with others.** You can get pathogens on your skin through direct contact with another person. For example, suppose someone who has a cold coughs into his or her hand. If you then shake hands with that person, the cold pathogens will be transferred to your hand. If you touch your eyes or nose, the pathogens can enter your body.
- **Indirect contact.** When people sneeze, they expel pathogens into the air. Other people in the area then breathe in these pathogens. This is one way in which indirect contact leads to the spread of diseases such as colds, flu, and tuberculosis. How often have you taken a sip out of a friend's glass? That is another way you can pick up pathogens: by sharing drinking glasses, food, eating utensils, and other personal

Reading Check
Understand word parts. Use a dictionary to identify the meanings of each part of the word *communicable*.

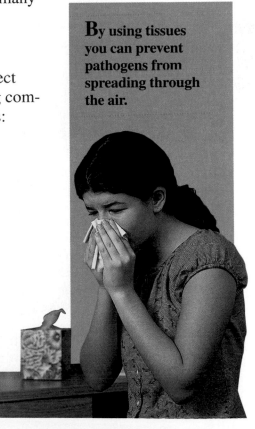

By using tissues you can prevent pathogens from spreading through the air.

items. Pathogens may also be spread when you touch a surface—a doorknob or a telephone receiver, for example—that is contaminated with another person's germs.

- **Contact with animals or insects.** Animal and insect bites can also spread pathogens. For example, the bite of a rabid animal spreads rabies. The bite of a deer tick may transmit Lyme disease to humans and animals.
- **Contaminated food and water.** A mountain stream or rare burger can look pretty inviting. However, pathogens can be spread through contaminated water or raw or undercooked food. Illnesses that result from eating unsafe food are known as foodborne illnesses.

Hands-On Health

OBSERVING BACTERIA

You cannot see an individual bacterium (singular of *bacteria*) without a microscope. However, given the right nutrients, bacteria will increase in number until they form a group or colony that can be seen with the unaided eye.

WHAT YOU WILL NEED
- three petri dishes filled with agar
- sterile swabs
- labels
- disinfectant soap

WHAT YOU WILL DO
1. Choose two places to collect samples of bacteria, such as your unwashed hands, doorknobs, floors, or furniture.
2. Wipe the object with a sterile swab and touch the swab to the agar.
3. Cover the dish immediately. On a label, write down exactly where you collected the sample. Attach the label to the dish.
4. Wash and dry your hands.
5. Repeat the procedure with the second sample.
6. For the third sample, wash your hands carefully with disinfectant soap and dry them on a paper towel. Then press your fingers against the agar in the third dish.

7. Cover the third dish and label it "Clean Hands."
8. Keep dishes in a warm, dark place for five days. For safety reasons, do not remove the lids.

IN CONCLUSION
1. Which container shows the greatest growth of bacteria? Which shows the least?
2. What conclusions can you draw from your observations?

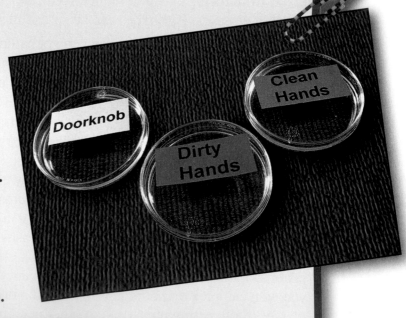

For example, *E. coli* bacteria, found in raw or undercooked ground meat, can cause severe illness and even death.

- **Contact with someone else's blood.** Certain viruses, such as HIV, can be transmitted through contact with an infected person's blood. This contact can occur through sharing needles that are used to inject drugs. Donated blood is screened carefully to prevent such infections from being transmitted.
- **Sexual contact.** Certain diseases are transmitted through sexual contact. You will learn more about these diseases in Lesson 4.

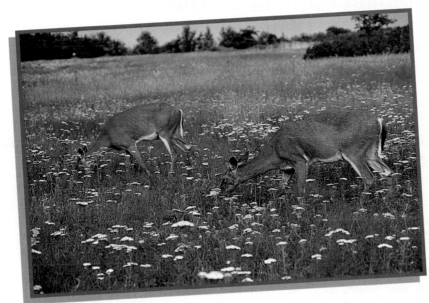

To prevent Lyme disease, wear long-sleeved shirts, light-colored clothing, and high boots when hiking through deer habitats. Tucking your pants into your boots or socks and using tick repellent will also help.

Lesson 1 Review

Using complete sentences, answer the following questions on a sheet of paper.

Reviewing Terms and Facts

1. **Vocabulary** Define the terms *disease* and *communicable disease.*
2. **Describe** What is a *pathogen?* Identify four types of pathogens, and list their characteristics.
3. **Identify** List two diseases caused by each of the four kinds of pathogens.
4. **Recall** What are six ways in which pathogens are spread?

Thinking Critically

5. **Explain** Suppose that you were hiking with a friend who wanted to drink water from a stream. What would you tell your friend?
6. **Evaluate** Is it more difficult to protect yourself from pathogens that are spread through direct contact or indirect contact? Explain your answer.

Applying Health Skills

7. **Advocacy** Use library resources and the Internet to learn more about Lyme disease. Create a pamphlet to educate others about how they can protect themselves from Lyme disease.

Lesson 2

The Immune System

Quick Write

List some of the signs that let you know when you have come down with an illness.

LEARN ABOUT...

- the function of the immune system.
- how antibodies protect the body from pathogens.
- how you can develop immunity to a disease.

VOCABULARY

- immune system
- inflammation
- lymphatic system
- lymphocytes
- antigens
- antibodies
- immunity
- vaccine

Keeping Pathogens Out

Each day you are exposed to countless pathogens. Fortunately, your body can repel, trap, or destroy most of these pathogens before they can do any damage. The five major barriers against such invaders are explained in **Figure 12.2**.

Sometimes, however, pathogens break through these barriers. That's when your immune system springs into action. The **immune** (i·MYOON) **system** is *a combination of body defenses made up of cells, tissues, and organs that fight off pathogens.*

FIGURE 12.2

THE FIVE MAJOR BARRIERS

Pathogens have to get through your body's defenses before they can begin to do harm. ***What defense does your body use when a foreign object gets into your eye?***

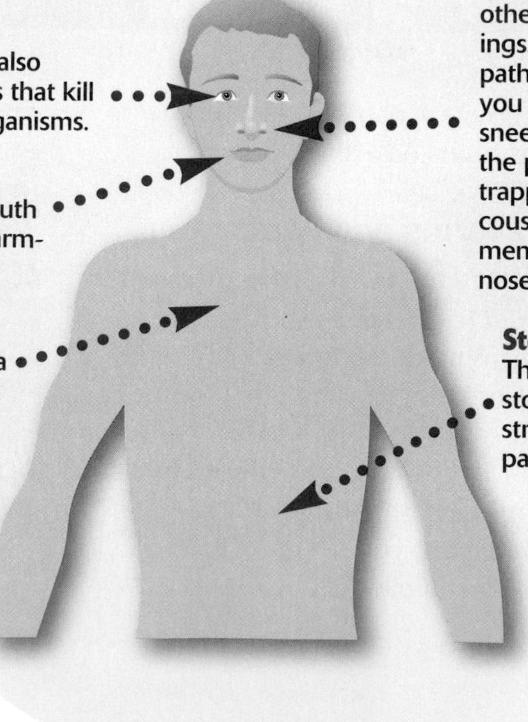

Tears
Tears wash away pathogens. They also contain chemicals that kill some harmful organisms.

Saliva
Saliva in your mouth destroys many harmful organisms.

Skin
Your skin acts as a protective barrier. Pathogens may get through this barrier when you have a cut, burn, or scrape.

Mucous Membranes
These tissues line your mouth, nose, throat, eyes, and other body openings. They trap pathogens. When you cough or sneeze, you expel the pathogens trapped by the mucous (MYOO·kuhs) membranes in your nose and throat.

Stomach Acid
The acid in your stomach destroys many pathogens.

The Immune System's Nonspecific Response

If pathogens enter the body, the immune system launches an attack. The immune system's nonspecific response is always the same, no matter what type of foreign substance invades your body.

The inflammatory response is a nonspecific response that occurs if a foreign invader gets past the five major barriers. This response occurs in the blood and tissues.

First the blood supply to the affected area increases, and circulation in that area slows down. This raises the blood pressure in the region, causing fluid to leak from the blood vessels. As a result, surrounding tissues swell. Special white blood cells called phagocytes (FA·guh·syts) attack the invading pathogens. The phagocytes surround the invaders, take them apart, and "eat" them.

You can see the inflammatory response if you have a cut, bee sting, or splinter. There will be **inflammation**, which is *the body's response to injury or disease, resulting in a condition of swelling, pain, heat, and redness.*

The inflammatory response has other components as well. The phagocytes release special proteins to help defend the body. One of these proteins, interferon (in·ter·FIR·ahn), stops viruses from reproducing and helps the cells that fight infection. If the infection has spread throughout the body, a fever becomes part of the inflammatory response. Fever signals the body to produce more white blood cells, and also makes it difficult for some pathogens to reproduce. **Figure 12.3** shows the inflammatory response in action.

Reading Check

Identify cause and effect. Describe the cause or effect for each of the following: *fever, inflammation, bee sting, body tissue swells.*

FIGURE 12.3

INFLAMMATION

During the inflammatory response, more blood flows to the infected area, and phagocytes rush in to destroy the invading pathogens.

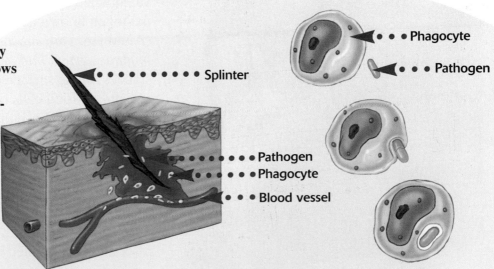

Splinter

Phagocyte

Pathogen

Pathogen

Phagocyte

Blood vessel

The Immune System's Specific Response

Sometimes pathogens are able to survive the inflammatory response. When this happens, the body counters with a specific response. This response is tailored to a particular pathogen and the poisons that it produces. Often the specific response not only defends the body against an invading pathogen but also allows the immune system to "remember" that particular type of pathogen. As a result, the pathogen may be destroyed more swiftly if the body encounters it again.

The Lymphatic System

The body calls upon the lymphatic system to fight against specific pathogens. The **lymphatic** (lim·FA·tik) **system** is *a secondary circulatory system that helps the body fight pathogens and maintain its fluid balance.* The lymphatic system circulates a watery fluid known as lymph (LIMF). *Special white blood cells in the lymph are called* **lymphocytes** (LIM·fuh·syts). There are three types of lymphocytes: B cells, T cells, and NK cells. All are important in fighting off pathogens and disease. The lymph also contains phagocytes called macrophages (MA·kruh·fay·juhz) that digest and process invading pathogens and then help the lymphocytes identify them.

The first two types of lymphocytes are named for the places in the body in which they are formed. B cells are formed in bone marrow, and T cells develop in the thymus gland. The third type of lymphocyte is the natural killer cell, or NK cell. NK cells attack cancerous growths.

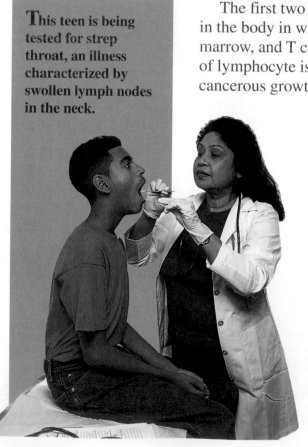

This teen is being tested for strep throat, an illness characterized by swollen lymph nodes in the neck.

Antibodies

All three types of lymphocytes are activated when the body recognizes a part of a pathogen known as an antigen. **Antigens** (AN·ti·jenz) are *substances that send the immune system into action.* For example, substances on the surface of a bacterium can be antigens. Blood cells of a blood type different from your own have different antigens on their surfaces. Your body reacts to antigens by producing **antibodies**, *proteins that attach to antigens, keeping them from harming the body.* B cells produce specific antibodies to fight a particular type of antigen. A complete explanation of the immune system's specific response is illustrated in **Figure 12.4.**

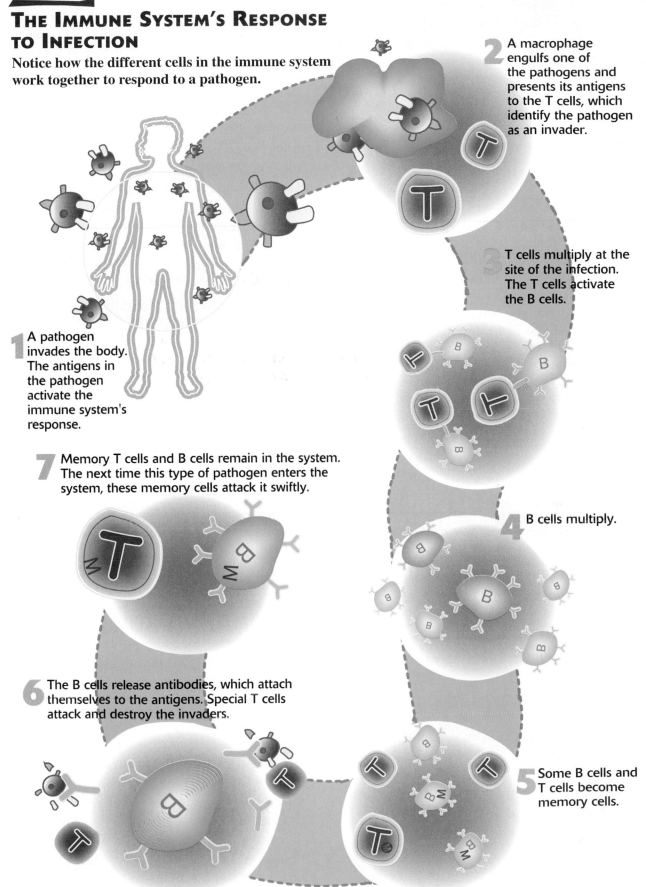

FIGURE 12.4

THE IMMUNE SYSTEM'S RESPONSE TO INFECTION

Notice how the different cells in the immune system work together to respond to a pathogen.

2 A macrophage engulfs one of the pathogens and presents its antigens to the T cells, which identify the pathogen as an invader.

3 T cells multiply at the site of the infection. The T cells activate the B cells.

1 A pathogen invades the body. The antigens in the pathogen activate the immune system's response.

7 Memory T cells and B cells remain in the system. The next time this type of pathogen enters the system, these memory cells attack it swiftly.

4 B cells multiply.

6 The B cells release antibodies, which attach themselves to the antigens. Special T cells attack and destroy the invaders.

5 Some B cells and T cells become memory cells.

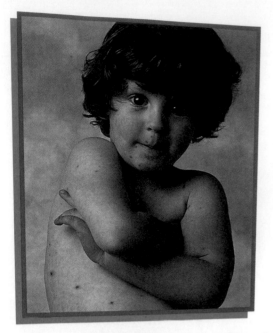

Immunity

Your body's ability to resist the pathogens that cause a particular disease is called **immunity**. You were born with some immunities that were passed on to you from your mother. These immunities lasted for a few months, after which you began to produce antibodies on your own.

Another way your body builds immunity is by being exposed to pathogens and by having certain diseases. When your body encounters an antigen, it produces memory B cells and T cells, as shown in **Figure 12.4** on page 339. Often these memory cells stay in your blood. If the same type of pathogen returns, your immune system remembers it and fights the invader so that it does not make you ill a second time.

If you've already had chicken pox or received the chicken pox vaccine, your immune system has memory cells for that virus, and you won't get chicken pox again.

You don't have to get a disease to acquire immunity to it. You can receive an immunization, or vaccine. A **vaccine** (vak·SEEN) is *a preparation of dead or weakened pathogens that is injected into the body to cause the immune system to produce antibodies.* This process is called immunization because the antibodies your body produces in response to the vaccine will build immunity. Since the pathogens used in vaccines are dead or weakened, vaccination won't cause you to develop the disease you're vaccinated against. Vaccines have been developed to prevent many diseases, including polio, measles, and mumps.

Lesson Review

Using complete sentences, answer the following questions on a sheet of paper.

Reviewing Terms and Facts

1. **Vocabulary** Define the term *immune system.*
2. **Identify** What are the body's five major barriers against pathogens?
3. **Describe** What is *inflammation*?
4. **Distinguish** Explain the difference between antigens and antibodies.
5. **Recall** Explain the role of immunizations in disease prevention.

Thinking Critically

6. **Evaluate** What changes could you make in your lifestyle to strengthen and protect your immune system?
7. **Conclude** Why do you think diseases that damage the immune system are so dangerous to the body?

Applying Health Skills

8. **Accessing Information** Use Internet and library resources to research the development of vaccines for smallpox and influenza. Find out when each vaccine was developed, by whom, and how much time it took. Write a brief report on your findings, and share it with your class.

Communicable Diseases

Facts About the Common Cold

Your nose is stuffy and runny, your throat is sore, you're tired, and your body aches. You probably have a cold, one of the most frequently occurring communicable diseases. One reason colds are so common is that cold pathogens are spread in several ways, by both direct and indirect contact.

Hundreds of different viruses can cause colds. Each cold you have during the year is probably caused by a different virus. This is why no one has been able to develop a cold vaccine. A vaccine that would give you immunity to one cold virus would not protect you against the others. You would need a different vaccine for each one!

Quick Write

List some risk factors that make it more likely for people to catch a cold. Which of these risk factors can you control?

LEARN ABOUT...

- the differences between a cold and the flu.
- some common communicable diseases.
- which communicable diseases can be prevented by vaccination.

VOCABULARY

- influenza
- contagious period
- mononucleosis
- hepatitis
- tuberculosis (TB)
- pneumonia
- strep throat

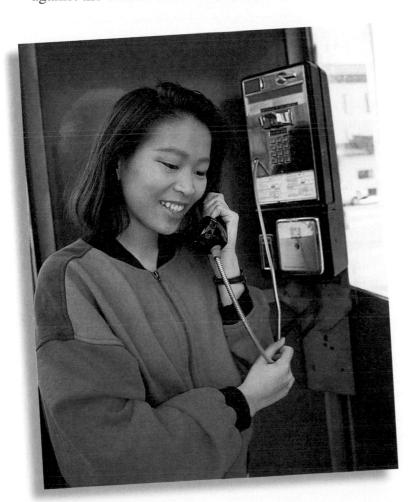

You can catch a cold by touching objects that someone with a cold has touched.

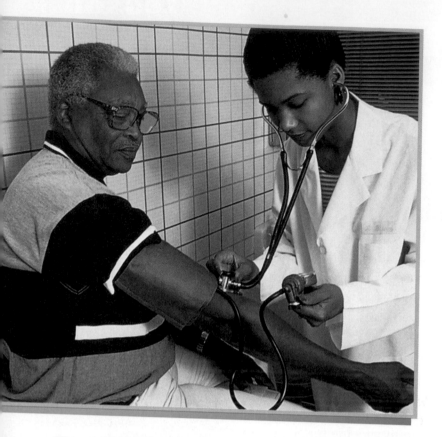

Facts About the Flu

Sometimes you might not know whether you have a cold or the flu because some of the symptoms of these two diseases are the same. However, different viruses cause colds and the flu, or influenza. **Influenza** (in·floo·EN·zuh) is *a communicable disease characterized by fever, chills, fatigue, headache, muscle aches, and respiratory symptoms.*

The flu begins more suddenly than a cold, and it lasts longer. As with a cold, you can catch the flu through direct and indirect contact. The peak months of flu season are December through early March. Each year different strains of flu viruses are responsible for the disease.

Because flu symptoms can be more severe in older adults, it is recommended that people over the age of 65 get yearly flu shots as part of a routine medical checkup. People with heart or lung diseases or weakened immune systems should also receive yearly flu vaccines.

Chicken Pox, Measles, and Mumps

The **contagious period** is *the length of time that a particular disease can be spread from person to person.* Depending on the disease, this period may be unknown or may vary. Chicken pox, measles, and mumps, however, are diseases with well-defined contagious periods.

- **Chicken pox** involves an itchy rash, fever, headache, and body aches. The rash begins as small red bumps that develop into blisters. Chicken pox can be passed to others from two days before the rash appears until about six days after. There is now a chicken pox vaccine.
- **Measles** is characterized by a rash accompanied by fever, runny nose, and coughing. People with measles can infect others from several days before the rash appears until about five days after. Measles has become less common in the United States due to a measles vaccine that is routinely given to children.
- **Mumps** causes a fever, headache, and swollen salivary glands. It is most easily passed to others around the time when the symptoms appear, but it may be passed on from as long as seven days before the symptoms appear until nine days after. Like measles, mumps is now uncommon because a vaccine has been developed.

Other Communicable Diseases

There are several other common communicable diseases. They vary in severity and in the way they are spread.

Mononucleosis

Commonly known as "mono," **mononucleosis** (MAH·noh·noo·klee·OH·sis) is *a disease characterized by swelling of the lymph nodes in the neck and throat.* Other symptoms may include fatigue, loss of appetite, fever, headache, and sore throat. The disease is caused by a virus and is most common in teens and young adults.

Mononucleosis can be spread through kissing and by sharing drinking glasses or eating utensils. Treatment for mononucleosis includes rest and pain relievers. Most symptoms will go away in three to six weeks.

Hepatitis

Hepatitis (he·puh·TY·tis) is *an inflammation of the liver characterized by yellowing of the skin and the whites of the eyes.* Other symptoms may include weakness, nausea, fever, headache, sore throat, and loss of appetite. The three most common types of hepatitis are hepatitis A, B, and C; each is caused by a different virus.

You can contract hepatitis A from contaminated food or water. People who travel to or live in regions with poor sanitation are particularly at risk for hepatitis A. Hepatitis B and C, which can permanently damage the liver, are usually spread through contact with the blood or other body fluids of an infected person. This can occur when drug users share needles. Hepatitis, particularly hepatitis B, can also be spread through sexual contact.

Hepatitis is treated with rest and a healthful diet. Most people recover completely, but those infected with hepatitis B can remain contagious for the rest of their lives. Vaccines are available for hepatitis A and B. Hepatitis C can be treated with medication.

Tuberculosis

After many years of decline, cases of tuberculosis are increasing in many parts of the world, including the United States. **Tuberculosis** (too·ber·kyuh·LOH·sis), or TB, is *a bacterial disease that usually affects the lungs.* Symptoms may include cough, fatigue, night sweats, fever, and weight loss. TB is spread when infected people cough or sneeze droplets into the air. It can be treated with antibiotics. A TB vaccine is also available.

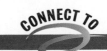

CONNECT TO
Social Studies

TAKING PRECAUTIONS
People throughout the world take many different precautions to prevent the spread of pathogens. In Japan, for example, people who have colds or the flu may wear a mask to keep germs from spreading. *Ask your parents and older relatives to describe some common ways to prevent illness when they were growing up. Use this information in a paragraph describing health behaviors or health knowledge unique to different generations, populations, or cultures.*

Pneumonia

Pneumonia (nu·MOHN·yuh) is *a serious inflammation or infection of the lungs.* Symptoms of pneumonia may include fever, cough, weakness, chills, and difficulty breathing. Pneumonia may be caused by viruses or bacteria. People may catch pneumonia by inhaling airborne pathogens or by having direct contact with an infected person.

Treatment of the disease varies, depending on the type of pneumonia and how serious the case is. Bacterial pneumonia can be treated with antibiotics. Regardless of the type of pneumonia, rest and plenty of fluids are recommended.

Strep Throat

Strep throat is *a sore throat caused by streptococcal bacteria.* Symptoms include a red and painful throat, fever, and swollen and tender lymph nodes in the neck. Headache, nausea, and vomiting may also occur. Strep throat is usually spread through direct contact or when infected people breathe or cough droplets into the air. To determine whether a person has strep throat, doctors perform a test known as a throat culture.

Strep throat can be treated with antibiotics. See a doctor if you think that you have strep throat or if you suddenly develop a sore throat accompanied by a fever. Left untreated, strep throat can lead to serious complications such as rheumatic fever, a condition that can damage the heart.

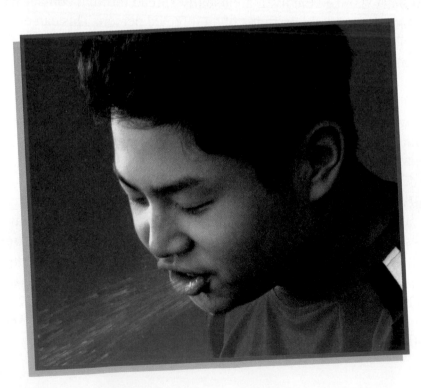

Respiratory diseases such as TB and pneumonia can be transmitted by airborne pathogens.

Vaccination Schedules

Some communicable diseases used to be much more common than they are now. The immunization of infants and children is making such diseases increasingly rare. **Figure 12.5** shows a typical vaccination schedule. Vaccinations are often given at wellness exams.

FIGURE 12.5

VACCINATION SCHEDULE

Vaccine: Diseases It Protects Against	Typical Vaccination Schedule
Hep B: hepatitis B	Series of three injections: birth–2 months, 1–4 months, and 6–18 months
DTaP: diphtheria, tetanus (lockjaw), and pertussis (whooping cough)	Series of five injections: 2 months, 4 months, 6 months, 15–18 months, and 4–6 years (before starting school); Td (tetanus and diphtheria toxoid) booster given at 11–12 years and every 10 years thereafter
Hib: *Haemophilus influenzae* type b bacteria	Series of three injections: 2 months, 4 months, and 6 months; booster dose given at 12–15 months
IPV: polio	Four doses: 2 months, 4 months, 6–18 months, and 4–6 years
PCV: pneumococcal infections (such as bacterial meningitis)	Series of four injections: 2 months, 4 months, 6 months, and 12–15 months
MMR: measles, mumps, and rubella (German measles)	Two doses: 12–15 months and 4–6 years; schedule should be completed by age 11–12
Varicella: chicken pox	One dose: 12–18 months
Hep A: hepatitis A	Two doses, given at least 6 months apart: 2–18 years; used only in high-risk areas or for high-risk groups

Source: Table based on immunization schedule recommended by the Centers for Disease Control and Prevention, the American Academy of Pediatrics, and the American Academy of Family Physicians

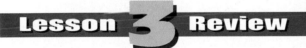

Lesson 3 Review

Using complete sentences, answer the following questions on a sheet of paper.

Reviewing Terms and Facts

1. **Vocabulary** Define the term *influenza.* Then explain the difference between a cold and influenza.
2. **Identify** Define the term *contagious period.* What diseases have well-defined contagious periods?
3. **Describe** What is *mononucleosis?* How is it spread?
4. **Explain** What are the symptoms of strep throat? How is it treated?

Thinking Critically

5. **Hypothesize** Why would it be important to know a disease's contagious period?
6. **Analyze** Schools often require that children have certain vaccinations before they are allowed to attend. Why do you think this is so?

Applying Health Skills

7. **Practicing Healthful Behaviors** Talk with your parents or guardians to determine when illness can be treated at home and when and how to seek medical care. Summarize your discussion in a brief paragraph.

Lesson 4

Sexually Transmitted Diseases and HIV/AIDS

Quick Write

Where could you go to get reliable information about sexually transmitted diseases? Write down one or two sources.

Learn About...

- common STDs.
- how people may become infected with HIV and develop AIDS.
- what is being done to fight AIDS.
- how to protect yourself from STDs.

Vocabulary

- sexually transmitted diseases (STDs)
- chlamydia
- genital warts
- genital herpes
- gonorrhea
- syphilis
- HIV (human immunodeficiency virus)
- AIDS (acquired immunodeficiency syndrome)

What Are Sexually Transmitted Diseases?

Sexually transmitted diseases (STDs), also known as sexually transmitted infections (STIs), are *infections that are spread from person to person through sexual contact.* Knowing the causes of STDs and their symptoms can help keep you safe from these serious infections. See **Figure 12.6** for some important facts about STDs.

FIGURE 12.6

The Facts About STDs

When you know the facts about STDs, you have the power to avoid them.

Someone who has an STD may not have visible symptoms or may have symptoms that come and go. However, such a person may be contagious even when there are no symptoms.

STDs can make a person sterile or infertile.

Not all STDs are curable, and some are even fatal.

A person who suspects that he or she is infected with an STD *must* see a doctor.

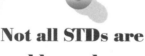

STDs can be prevented by avoiding sexual activity and by not injecting drugs.

Vaccines are not available for most STDs.

Common STDs

Some common STDs are described below.

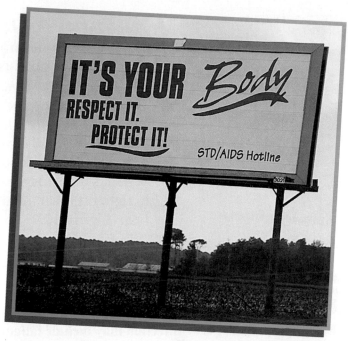

- **Chlamydia** (kluh·MI·dee·uh) is *a bacterial STD that may affect the reproductive organs, urethra, and anus.* Symptoms, which are not present in many cases, may include a genital discharge and a burning sensation during urination. If left untreated, chlamydia can cause pelvic pain, infertility, and other infections. Chlamydia can be treated with antibiotics.
- **Genital** (JEN·i·tuhl) **warts** are *growths or bumps in the genital area caused by certain types of the human papillomavirus (HPV).* HPV infection is the most common STD in the United States. Many people will not develop warts until long after they have been exposed, so they may not know that they are passing the virus to others. The infection cannot be cured, although the warts can be treated. This STD has been linked to cervical cancer.
- **Genital herpes** (JEN·i·tuhl HER·peez*)* is *a viral STD that produces painful blisters in the genital area.* The herpes virus may remain inactive in a person's body, causing no symptoms. Some people, though, have periodic outbreaks of painful blisters or sores. Genital herpes can be transmitted to others whether or not symptoms are present. There is no cure for genital herpes, but medications can relieve symptoms.
- **Gonorrhea** (gah·nuh·REE·uh*)* is *a bacterial STD that affects the mucous membranes of the body, particularly in the genital area.* As with some other STDs, a person may be unaware that he or she is infected. Symptoms of gonorrhea may include a thick, yellow discharge from the genitals and burning during urination. If left untreated, this infection can cause sterility in men and infertility in women. Gonorrhea is treated with antibiotics.
- **Syphilis** (SI·fuh·luhs*)* is *a bacterial STD that can affect many parts of the body.* Symptoms vary as the disease progresses. Early symptoms may include only a painless sore at the site where the infection entered the body and swollen lymph glands in the genital area. If left untreated, syphilis may cause brain damage, heart disease, and eventual death. If treated early, syphilis can be cured by antibiotics.
- **Hepatitis B**, a liver disease that can be transmitted through sexual contact, is the only STD for which a vaccine is available.

It is estimated that more than 15 million cases of STDs occur each year in the United States. *What do you think can be done to help stop this epidemic (disease that affects a large population)?*

HIV and AIDS

HIV (human immunodeficiency virus) is *the virus that causes AIDS.* **AIDS (acquired immunodeficiency syndrome)** is *a deadly disease that interferes with the body's ability to fight infection.* A person who is infected with HIV may not show any signs of illness for a long time. In fact, an average of ten years may pass before AIDS develops. Nevertheless, during this time the virus seriously damages the infected person's immune system. When the system's defenses are critically weakened, the body becomes unable to fight off other infections and diseases, which eventually prove fatal. **Figure 12.7** shows how HIV attacks the body.

FIGURE 12.7

HOW HIV ATTACKS THE BODY

Early symptoms of HIV infection may include fatigue, rash, fever, swollen lymph nodes, and diarrhea.

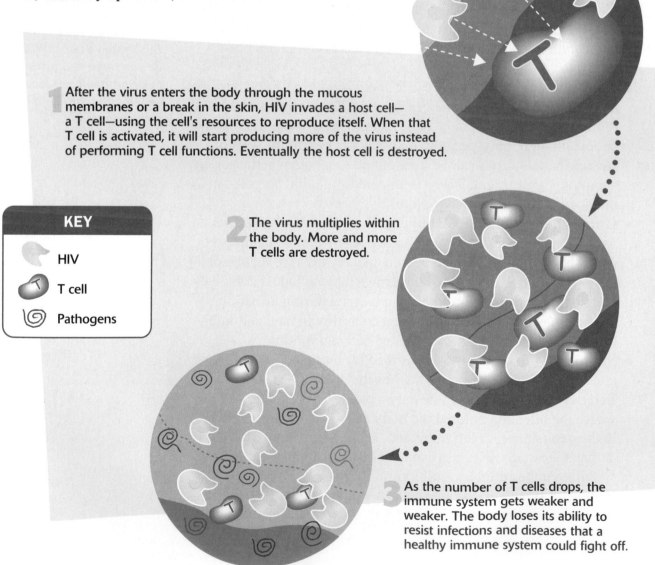

1 After the virus enters the body through the mucous membranes or a break in the skin, HIV invades a host cell— a T cell—using the cell's resources to reproduce itself. When that T cell is activated, it will start producing more of the virus instead of performing T cell functions. Eventually the host cell is destroyed.

KEY

- HIV
- T cell
- Pathogens

2 The virus multiplies within the body. More and more T cells are destroyed.

3 As the number of T cells drops, the immune system gets weaker and weaker. The body loses its ability to resist infections and diseases that a healthy immune system could fight off.

The Spread of HIV

HIV is almost always spread in one of the following ways:

- **Having any form of sexual intercourse with an infected person.** This is the most common way of becoming infected with HIV. HIV circulates in the bloodstream and in other body fluids, such as semen and vaginal fluid. Therefore, an infected person can pass on the virus even if he or she has no symptoms. People who have sex with multiple partners are at highest risk. *Avoiding sexual intercourse is the only sure way to protect yourself against this method of transmission.*

- **Using a contaminated needle.** A drop of blood left on a needle can transmit the virus. To protect yourself, avoid injecting drugs, and be sure that any procedure involving needles or blood is performed by a health care professional.

- **Other modes of transmission.** In rare cases, HIV is transmitted through transfusions of blood received from an infected person. Most people infected with HIV in this way were infected before 1985. Since then, all donated blood in the United States has been routinely tested for HIV. The infection may also be transmitted from mother to child, before birth, during birth, or through breast-feeding. A treatment is available that reduces the chances of an infected mother transmitting HIV to her unborn child.

FIGURE 12.8

HOW HIV IS *NOT* SPREAD

You *cannot* get HIV in any of the ways shown here. *Why might people think that HIV can be transmitted in these ways?*

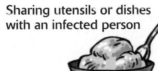
Sharing utensils or dishes with an infected person

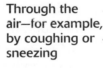
Through the air—for example, by coughing or sneezing

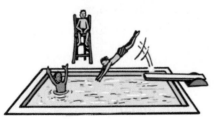
Swimming in the same pool as an infected person

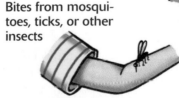
Bites from mosquitoes, ticks, or other insects

Using the same telephone, shower, bathtub, or toilet as an infected person

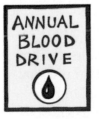
Donating blood

Nonsexual contact with an HIV-infected person, such as shaking hands or hugging

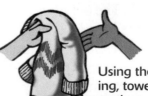
Using the same clothing, towel, sports equipment, comb, or furniture as an infected person

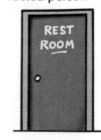

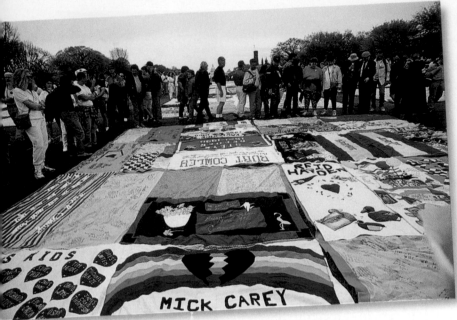

Battling AIDS

With more and more people around the world becoming infected with HIV, a critical situation has developed. Scientists, health care professionals, educators, and many others have joined the fight against AIDS.

Combinations of powerful drugs can dramatically reduce HIV levels in the blood and prolong the life expectancy of many HIV-infected people. Other drugs can help control infections in people with AIDS. However, many of these drugs have serious side effects, and they do not work for everyone. These drugs are also very expensive.

The AIDS Memorial Quilt has more than 44,000 panels commemorating the lives of those lost to AIDS. *How is the quilt an educational tool?*

Scientists are also working to develop an HIV vaccine. However, because the virus occurs in many forms, a vaccine that works against one form of HIV may not work against another. Most researchers believe that the development of an effective vaccine for HIV is still many years away.

With neither a cure for AIDS nor an effective HIV vaccine currently available, educating people about preventing the spread of HIV is crucial. Health care professionals; educators; and workers in federal, state, and local governments are making an all-out effort to teach the public how HIV is spread and how its transmission can be prevented.

Abstinence Before Marriage

The media often portray sexual activity as exciting and important in a relationship. What the media don't reveal are the high costs of sexual activity before marriage. The physical consequences can include STDs and unplanned pregnancy. Less obvious are the social problems and emotional trauma associated with adolescent sexual activity.

The only 100 percent effective method of protecting yourself from the harmful consequences of sexual activity is abstinence from sexual activity before marriage. You protect yourself against unplanned pregnancy and STDs, including HIV infection. You get to know someone in a way that goes beyond physical attraction. You show respect for the wishes of your family. You can remain committed to your long-term goals, such as education, career, and family.

It is normal to feel physically attracted to another person and have sexual feelings. If you have questions about these feelings, discuss them openly and honestly with your parents or guardians. You can acknowledge your feelings responsibly by showing affection in ways that don't risk your health or compromise values. Appropriate ways for teens to show affection include holding hands and complimenting someone. By practicing abstinence from sexual activity before marriage you can be sure that your relationships are built on shared interests and mutual trust rather than on sexual attraction. Practicing abstinence now means that you are more likely to enjoy a mutually faithful sexual relationship with your future mate.

Affection for another person can be expressed in ways that don't compromise either person's health or values. *How might a mutual decision to practice abstinence improve a relationship?*

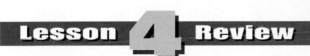

Lesson 4 Review

Using complete sentences, answer the following questions on a sheet of paper.

Reviewing Terms and Facts

1. **Vocabulary** Define the term *sexually transmitted diseases*.
2. **Compare** How are genital warts different from genital herpes?
3. **Identify** What are the symptoms of gonorrhea? How is it treated?
4. **Distinguish** What is the difference between HIV and AIDS?
5. **List** Summarize the facts related to HIV infection and STDs.

Thinking Critically

6. **Analyze** What factors do you think make STDs especially dangerous?
7. **Explain** Why do you think people often postpone seeing a doctor if they think that they might have an STD?

Applying Health Skills

8. **Advocacy** Create a pamphlet for teens that analyzes the importance of abstinence from sexual activity as the preferred choice of behavior in relationship to all sexual activity for unmarried persons of school age.

Lesson 5

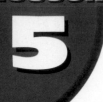

Preventing the Spread of Disease

Quick Write

Make a list of things you do on a regular basis to stay healthy.

LEARN ABOUT...

- how to protect yourself from pathogens.
- how to avoid spreading pathogens to others when you are sick.
- habits that can help you stay healthy.

VOCABULARY

- hygiene

Stop Pathogens from Spreading

Although you can't see the pathogens that surround you, you can defend yourself against them. Good personal **hygiene**, or *cleanliness,* and other healthful habits, such as getting enough physical activity and rest, can help you stay well. Making sure that your environment is kept clean is another important part of preventing the spread of pathogens.

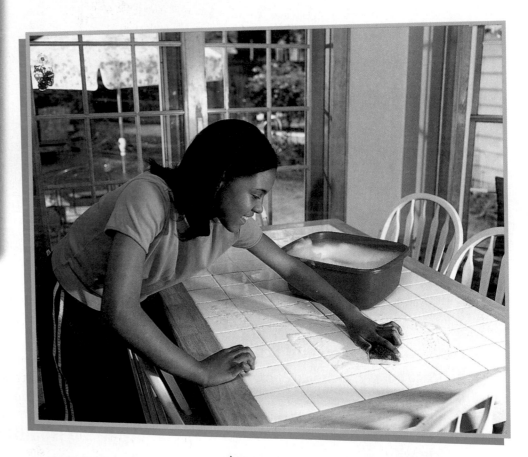

A clean environment is one of the most important factors in preventing disease. *What can you do to keep your kitchen clean?*

Protect Yourself

Common sense will help you to stay healthy. Be smart—avoid taking risks with your health. Here are some guidelines to follow.

- Avoid close contact with people who are ill, especially during the contagious period of a disease.
- Do not share eating utensils, dishes, glasses, bottles, or cans.
- Wash your hands often, especially when you have been around someone with a contagious disease. Be sure to wash your hands before handling food and after using the bathroom, playing with a pet, handling garbage, or touching any other obvious source of germs. See **Figure 12.9** for some handwashing tips. Good personal hygiene prevents the spread of disease.
- Keep your hands away from your mouth, nose, and eyes.
- Take proper precautions against known factors that may cause disease, such as ticks.
- Follow safe practices in handling, preparing, and storing food to avoid foodborne illnesses.
- Simple actions—such as wiping counters and tables with warm, soapy water and disposing of garbage properly—help keep pathogens from spreading.

☑
Reading Check
Build vocabulary. Find synonyms for each of the following words in the text or in a thesaurus: *hygiene, simple, sick.*

FIGURE 12.9

HANDWASHING

Frequent handwashing will help keep pathogens from entering your body. *Why is it important to wash your hands before eating?*

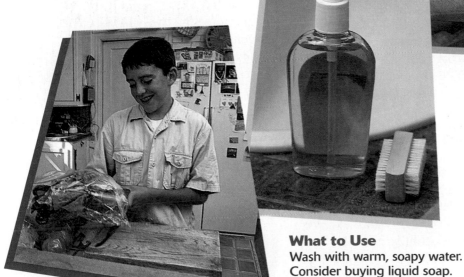

When to Wash
Always wash your hands before handling or eating food.

What to Use
Wash with warm, soapy water. Consider buying liquid soap. Use a brush to scrub under nails. Be sure to carry moist towelettes or a small bottle of waterless hand sanitizer if you go to a place where you won't have access to soap and water.

How to Wash
First wet your hands under warm running water and apply soap. Then rub your hands together vigorously, and scrub all surfaces for at least 15 seconds. Finally, rinse well and dry your hands, using a clean or disposable towel. If you are using a public rest room, turn the faucet off with a paper towel. Also use a paper towel when you turn the doorknob to avoid touching germs after washing your hands.

Protect Others

As a responsible person, you should do whatever you can to avoid spreading pathogens to other people. Here are some ways to protect others.

- If you are ill, stay home from school during the contagious period of the disease, and avoid close contact with other people. Wash your hands frequently.
- Cover your mouth and nose when you cough or sneeze, and turn your head away from others. Use tissues and dispose of them properly. If you don't have a tissue handy, turn your head and cough or sneeze into the crook of your elbow. That way you will be less likely to transfer pathogens to everything you touch. Wash your hands immediately afterward or as soon as possible.
- Get medical treatment if you need it. Delaying a visit to the doctor may allow your condition to worsen while increasing the chances that you'll spread pathogens to others.
- When you take a prescribed medication, follow the directions and your physician's orders carefully. Take the entire cycle of prescribed medication. Don't stop taking it just because you feel better.
- Encourage other people to follow wise health practices.

HEALTH SKILLS ACTIVITY

PRACTICING HEALTHFUL BEHAVIORS

Protecting Your Immune System

You can play an active role in maintaining and boosting the function of your immune system. A strong immune system means that your body will be better able to fight off infection. Follow these tips to help keep your immune system in peak condition.

- Participate in regular physical activity.
- Eat plenty of vitamin-rich fruits, vegetables, and whole grains. Make sure that you get the recommended servings of calcium-rich foods. Go easy on high-fat and sugary snacks. Eating healthfully is a key factor in fighting off disease.
- Learn to manage stress. Reducing stress in your life can help your immune system respond more effectively to invading pathogens.
- Get enough sleep. This strengthens the body's defenses and reduces your chances of becoming ill.

WITH A GROUP
Use library resources to find articles that explain how vitamins and minerals affect the immune system. Create a chart that describes at least five vitamins and minerals that strengthen the immune system and the food sources that provide them.

Develop a Healthy Lifestyle

If you were to evaluate your lifestyle, you might think that it was pretty healthy. You eat a balanced diet, participate in regular physical activity, get enough rest, bathe or shower daily, and avoid harmful behavior such as using tobacco, alcohol, and other drugs. These healthful habits are important weapons in the fight against pathogens. However, you can do even more to help your body stay healthy.

- When you are sick, avoid strenuous activity. Allow your body to use its energy to fight the infection.
- Be sure that you are immunized against diseases for which a vaccine exists. If you're not sure which immunizations you need, ask your doctor or your school nurse.
- Learn to manage stress. Stress makes you vulnerable to illness if you do not find ways to avoid it or deal with it effectively.
- Get regular health screenings. Cooperate with your health care provider—follow recommended instructions to recover from illness.

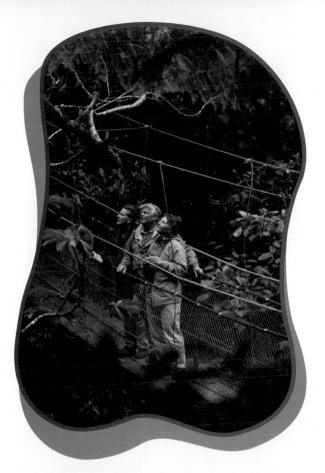

You may have to take extra precautions to prevent illness when you travel to a foreign country. *Aside from being vaccinated beforehand, what measures might you have to take in a foreign country to stay healthy?*

Lesson 5 Review

Using complete sentences, answer the following questions on a sheet of paper.

Reviewing Terms and Facts

1. **Vocabulary** Define *hygiene*.
2. **Identify** List five ways to protect yourself against communicable diseases.
3. **Explain** Describe the procedures of thorough handwashing.
4. **Recall** Name three ways to avoid spreading pathogens to others.

Thinking Critically

5. **Analyze** Why do you think it is important to wash your hands after playing with a pet?

6. **Decide** A friend tells you that she's planning to go to school even though she has the flu. What would you tell her?

Applying Health Skills

7. **Communication Skills** Taking an active role in the treatment of a communicable disease involves communicating effectively. Write a dialogue in which a teen uses effective communication skills to talk to parents or a health care provider about his or her illness. Read your dialogue to the class.

One Bad Bug

Will the flu bug bite you?

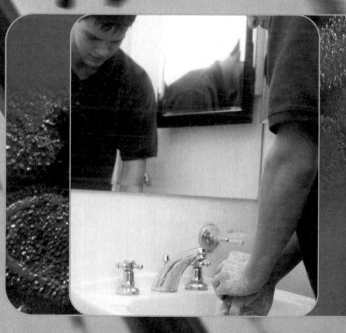

There's nothing gradual about the flu: It slams you like a hammer. One minute you're feeling fine. Next thing you know, you're shivering, you're burning up, then shivering again. In minutes, your legs turn to jelly and your whole body aches.

Flu season lasts from November through April. Each year, the bug infects about one in 10 Americans. A look at those empty desks at school tells you that kids are the most frequent victims.

Tiny Viruses, Big Miseries

Like the common cold, influenza is caused by a microscopic virus. Several million flu bugs could fit on the period at the end of this sentence. The virus spreads from person to person on the tiny droplets produced by a sneeze or a cough.

FLU-FIGHTING TIPS

1. **Always cover your nose and mouth with a tissue when you cough or sneeze. Encourage others to do the same.**
2. **Wash your hands often, especially before eating.**
3. **Avoid rubbing your eyes or nose.**
4. **Don't share food, dishes, or eating utensils with anyone. Even people who appear healthy can spread the flu virus.**

Once inside the body, flu viruses settle into the delicate cells that line the lungs, nose, and throat. There the sneaky invaders use your cells' own machinery to create billions of copies of themselves. These viruses quickly spread into more cells. Most flu symptoms—fever, runny nose, body aches—are caused not by the virus itself but by your body's attempt to get rid of it.

A healthy person can fight off the flu in three to five days, though a cough and fatigue can last about two more weeks. Often an attack of the flu is followed by another illness. That's what happened to middle-school student Phillip Winston of New City, New York. After a week of headaches, dizziness, and fevers as high as 104°F, he finally beat the flu. "Then I got an ear infection, and I'm still taking medicine for it," he says.

Doctors believe that the damage done by the flu virus makes it easier for other germs to attack, including the bacteria that cause ear infections and pneumonia. The one-two punch of flu followed by pneumonia is the sixth leading cause of death in the United States. Nine out of 10 of these deaths occur in older adults.

The lesson for people of any age: If you aren't getting better after four or five days of the flu, or if you get better and then get worse, see a doctor.

Medical Weapons

Doctors recommend that older adults, or people of any age with heart or lung problems such as asthma, get an annual flu shot. Because flu viruses change all the time, a new vaccine must be prepared each year to protect against the latest versions. A medical team at the Centers for Disease Control and Prevention (CDC) in Atlanta, Georgia, and others in Britain, Japan, and Australia are always studying the current crop of flu viruses to develop next year's shot.

Should healthy kids get the vaccine? "That's something to talk over with a doctor," says Dr. Carolyn Bridges, a flu expert at the CDC. The main side effect, she notes, "is a sore arm." If that sounds bad, stay tuned. Researchers are developing a new kind of vaccine that enters the body through the nose. ◢

TIME TO THINK...

About the Flu

Millions of people worldwide died during an outbreak of the Spanish flu in 1918. Using reliable online and print resources, research this global disaster, and write a report on your findings. Describe how this outbreak was different from most other flu outbreaks and explain whether you think an epidemic this bad could happen again.

MEDIA MESSAGES ABOUT SEX

Model

Read about Susanna and the influences that affect her choice about sexual activity.

Susanna has been learning about STDs in her health class. For a homework assignment, she analyzed television's portrayal of the relationship between sex and STDs. As she watched television over a one-week period, she realized that although a lot of shows had characters who engaged in sexual activity, the possibility of catching an STD was rarely mentioned. This made Susanna think about how the media might influence her if she weren't aware of the facts about STDs. Most shows give the impression that sex doesn't have any consequences. Susanna knows that shows usually don't claim to be exactly like real life. However, she also knows that lots of teens want to be like television characters.

Fortunately, Susanna is more strongly influenced by her parents. They have talked to her about abstinence from sexual activity and the dangers of STDs. These and other influences have convinced her that her best choice is to abstain from sexual activity.

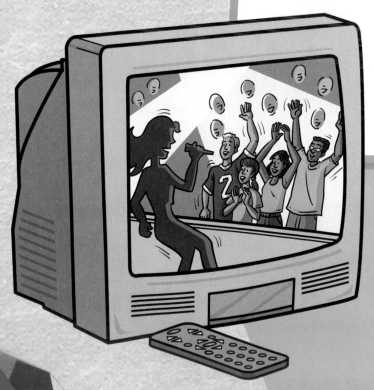

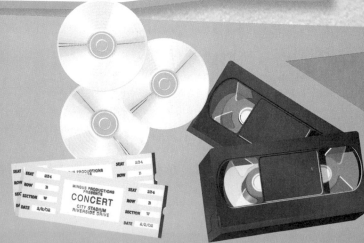

Practice

Joseph and his friend Steve like to hang out and listen to music or watch music videos. Joseph is concerned, however, because song lyrics are often about sex, and videos frequently portray sex without any consequences. Read the conversation between these friends and answer the questions that follow.

STEVE: *Cool! I love this video! The words to this song are really good.*

JOSEPH: *I like this song, too. I don't know, though. I don't think I'd want my younger sister to see this video.*

STEVE: *What do you mean?*

JOSEPH: *Well, my sister and her friends really like this singer—they even dress like her. But this song and the video make it seem like you can have sex without risks. What if the other person has HIV or AIDS?*

STEVE: *I guess I see what you mean.*

1. What message does Joseph think that the video and song send about STDs?
2. How does Joseph think that the singer, her song, and her video might influence teens?

Apply/Assess

Many magazines are marketed to teens. Along with articles and information, these magazines are full of advertisements. Often these advertisements use sexy images to sell their products.

Look at a teen magazine and make a list of how many advertisements use sexual images. Write a brief report explaining what sort of overall message the magazine sends about sex and its possible consequences and how much influence you think the magazine has on your thoughts and actions.

COACH'S BOX

Analyzing Influences

Both internal and external influences affect your choices. These influences may include:

Internal
- Interests
- Likes/dislikes
- Fears
- Curiosity

External
- Family
- Friends
- Media
- Culture

Self-√Check

- Did I explain the overall message the magazine conveys about sex?
- Did I explain the influence of the magazine on my thoughts and actions?

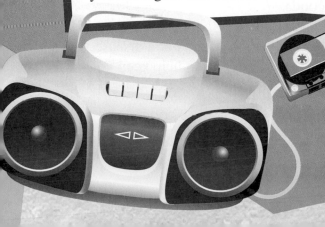

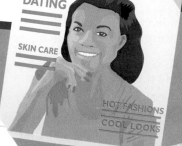

Today's Teen

DATING

SKIN CARE

HOT FASHIONS
COOL LOOKS

After You Read

Use your completed Foldable to review the information on the four types of pathogens.

FOLDABLES™
Study Organizer

Reviewing Vocabulary and Concepts

On a sheet of paper, write the numbers 1–7. After each number, write the term from the list that best completes each sentence.

- immunity
- Lyme disease
- infection
- lymphatic system
- vaccine
- lymphocytes
- germs

Lesson 1

1. _____ are organisms that are so small that they can be seen only through a microscope.
2. A(n) _____ occurs when pathogens get inside the body, multiply, and damage body cells.
3. Bites from deer ticks can cause _____.

Lesson 2

4. The _____ is a secondary circulatory system that helps the body fight pathogens and maintain its fluid balance.
5. Special white blood cells in the lymph are called _____.
6. You can develop _____, or the ability to resist the pathogens that cause a particular disease.
7. A(n) _____ is a preparation of dead or weakened pathogens that causes the immune system to produce antibodies.

Lesson 3

On a sheet of paper, write the numbers 8–10. After each number, write the letter of the answer that best completes each statement.

8. Yellowing of the skin and the whites of the eyes is a sign of
   a. influenza.
   b. mononucleosis.
   c. hepatitis.
   d. strep throat.
9. Which disease is *not* caused by a virus?
   a. tuberculosis
   b. mononucleosis
   c. hepatitis
   d. influenza
10. Pneumonia is usually caused by
    a. fungi.
    b. protozoa.
    c. parasites.
    d. viruses or bacteria.

On a sheet of paper, write the numbers 11–16. Write *True* or *False* for each statement below. If the statement is false, change the underlined word or phrase to make it true.

Lesson 4

11. <u>Chlamydia</u> is an STD that may affect the reproductive organs, urethra, and anus.
12. If left untreated, <u>gonorrhea</u> may lead to heart disease, brain damage, and death.
13. <u>Abstinence</u> is the one guaranteed way to avoid STDs.

Lesson 5

14. You should wash your hands for at least <u>five</u> seconds.
15. It is important to avoid contact with others during the <u>contagious period</u> of a disease.
16. Good personal <u>hygiene</u> can help keep you from getting sick.

Thinking Critically

Using complete sentences, answer the following questions on a sheet of paper.

17. Analyze How can understanding the ways in which pathogens are spread help people stay healthy?

18. Describe Explain how lymph, the lymph nodes, and lymphocytes work within the lymphatic system to fight against specific pathogens.

19. Analyze The following diseases are caused by pathogens: a cold, the flu, mononucleosis, and TB. What are the risks for contracting each disease?

Career Corner

School Nurse Would you like to help young people feel better when they're sick? If so, you might consider a career as a school nurse. School nurses care for sick or injured students, help in emergencies, and perform health screenings. These professionals also teach behaviors that reduce the spread of germs. To become a nurse, you need a four- to five-year nursing degree. Volunteering at a local hospital is one way to see if you would enjoy this work. Learn about nursing and other health careers by clicking on Career Corner at health.glencoe.com.

Standardized Test Practice

Reading & Writing

Read the paragraphs below and then answer the questions.

Black Death, also known as the plague, swept through Europe, North Africa, and parts of Asia in the fourteenth century. It was the worse epidemic in history.

Black Death first struck Europe in 1347, when a fleet of trading ships landed in Sicily, Italy. When their journey began, the traders on these ships had no way of knowing that the black rats on board were the hosts for plague-bearing fleas. By the time these traders reached Sicily, the crew was dead or dying and the rats slipped unnoticed to the shores of Europe. The plague struck the port cities and then followed trade routes, raging through Italy, France, Britain, over the Alps into Switzerland and then east. Everywhere it went, people fell sick and died.

Since people at that time knew little about disease transmission, no one figured out what was causing the epidemic. Many believed that it was divine punishment on a sinful world.

1. In the second paragraph, the phrase "were the hosts" means that

   A the rats were carrying the fleas.

   B the rats were guests of the fleas.

   C the rats already had the plague.

   D the traders were infected.

2. What is the second paragraph about?

   A how people reacted to the plague

   B the symptoms of the plague

   C how people discovered the cause of the plague

   D how the plague spread throughout Europe

3. Write a paragraph describing why you think people believed the plague was a punishment.

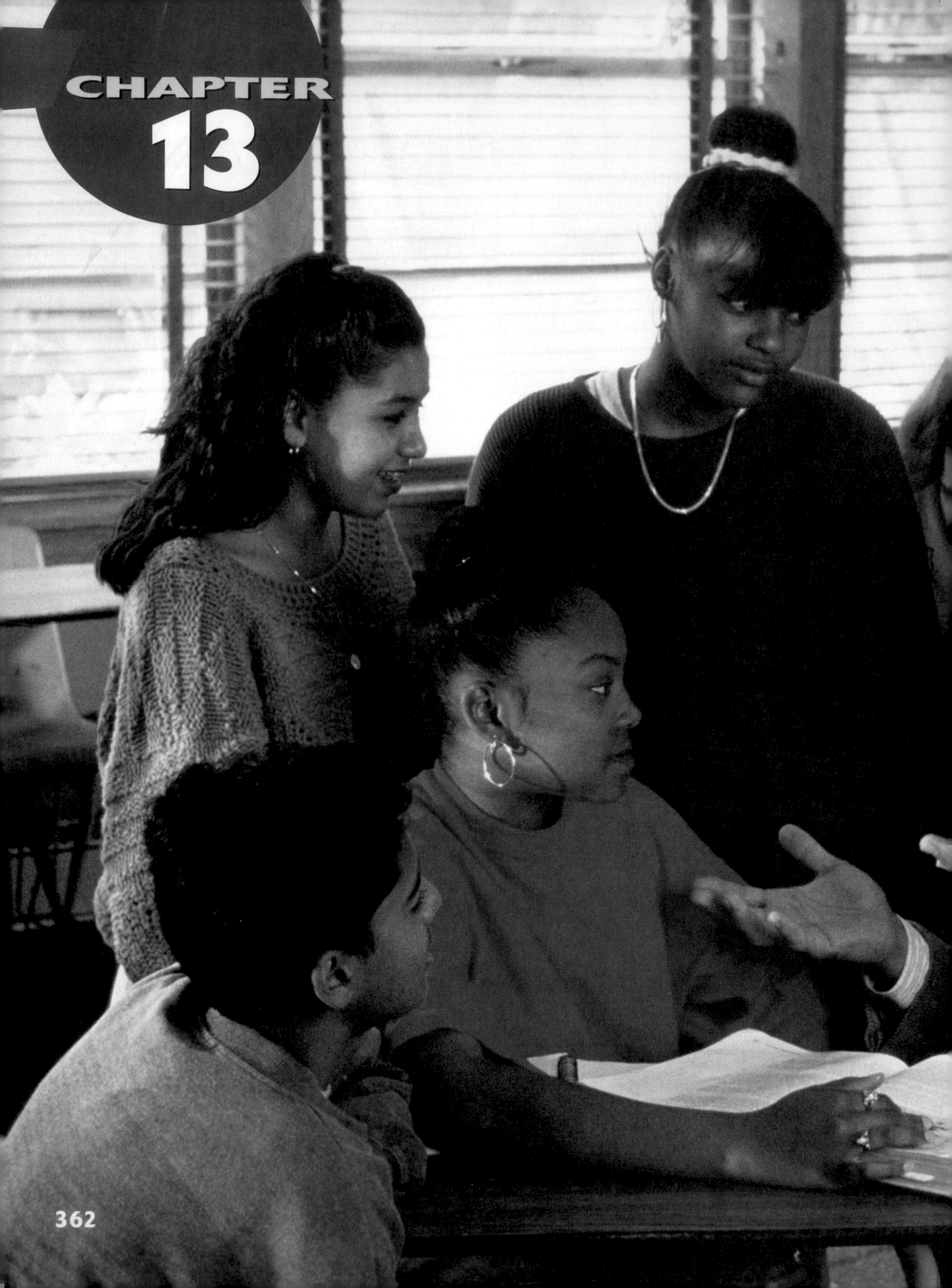
CHAPTER
13

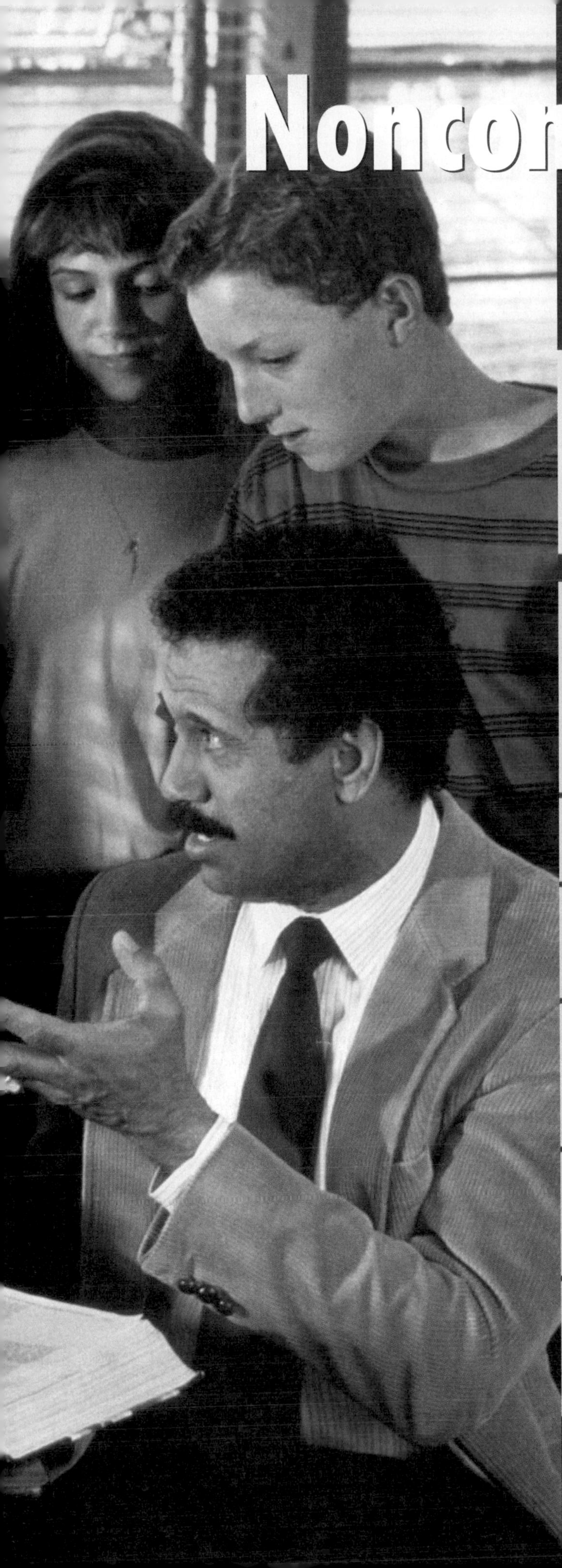

Noncommunicable Diseases

HEALTH *Online*

Do your habits protect your lifelong health? Use the Chapter 13 Health Inventory at health.glencoe.com to rate your behaviors and choices.

FOLDABLES™ Study Organizer

Before You Read

Make this Foldable to help you organize the information on allergies and asthma in Lesson 1. Begin with a plain sheet of 11″ × 17″ paper.

Step 1

Fold a sheet of paper in half along the short axis, then fold in half again. This forms four columns.

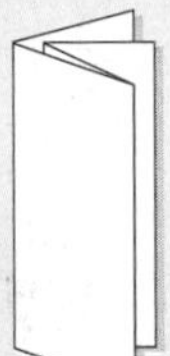

Step 2

Open the paper and refold it into thirds along the long axis. This forms three rows.

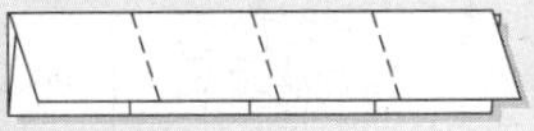

Step 3

Unfold and draw lines along the folds.

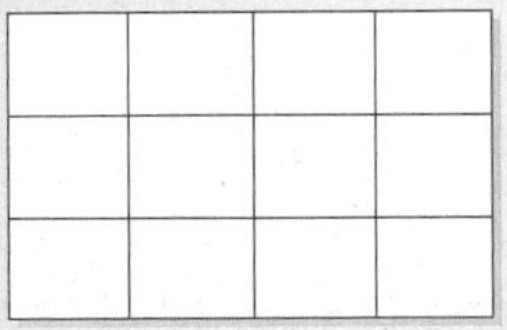

Step 4

Label the chart as shown.

Noncommun-icable Diseases	Causes	Effects	Treatment
Allergies			
Asthma			

As You Read

Write down information on the causes, effects, and treatments of allergies and asthma in the appropriate section of the chart.

Understanding Allergies and Asthma

Quick Write

You have probably seen TV commercials for allergy medications. What types of allergies do these medications treat?

LEARN ABOUT...

- types of noncommunicable diseases.
- what allergies are and how they're treated.
- what asthma is and how it's treated.

VOCABULARY

- noncommunicable disease
- chronic
- allergy
- allergen
- pollen
- histamine
- antihistamine
- asthma
- bronchodilator

Noncommunicable Disease

A **noncommunicable disease** is *a disease that cannot be spread from person to person.* Common examples are asthma, cancer, and heart disease. Most noncommunicable diseases are caused by changes within the body. Take a look at **Figure 13.1** to learn more about different types of noncommunicable diseases.

FIGURE 13.1

TYPES OF NONCOMMUNICABLE DISEASES

Noncommunicable diseases can be organized into several different categories, based on their causes. However, most noncommunicable diseases have multiple causes. Compare this figure to Figure 12.1 on page 332. Describe the differences in risk factors between communicable and noncommunicable diseases.

Type	Causes/Risk Factors	Examples
Present at birth	Diseases that are caused by hereditary factors or that result from problems during a baby's development or birth	• Cystic fibrosis • Sickle-cell anemia • Cerebral palsy
Behavior choices	Diseases to which unhealthful behavior choices often contribute (i.e., eating high-fat foods; being physically inactive; using tobacco, alcohol, or other drugs; failing to manage stress properly)	• Many types of heart disease • Most cases of lung cancer • Cirrhosis of the liver
Environmental factors	Diseases that are caused by exposure to specific substances in the environment or to environmental hazards, such as pollution, toxic wastes, and secondhand smoke	• Some types of allergies • Lung cancer caused by breathing in asbestos particles • Respiratory diseases caused by breathing in certain substances in polluted air
Unknown causes	Diseases whose causes are unknown	• Alzheimer's disease • Rheumatoid arthritis • Chronic fatigue syndrome

Many noncommunicable diseases are **chronic** (KRAH·nik), or *present continuously or on and off over a long period of time.* Allergies and asthma are two examples.

Allergies

In the United States, more than 50 million people have allergies. An **allergy** is *an extreme sensitivity to a substance.* As you know, the immune system fights and destroys pathogens. In a person who has allergies, however, the immune system is overly sensitive to certain substances that are normally harmless. The immune system's response to these substances triggers an allergic reaction. *The substances that cause an allergic reaction* are called **allergens** (AL·er·juhnz). One of the most common allergens is **pollen**, *a powdery substance released by the flowers of certain plants.* Trees, grasses, and weeds all release pollen into the air. **Figure 13.2** shows some common allergens in the environment.

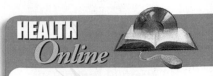

Topic: Allergies and asthma

For links to more information on allergies and asthma, go to **health.glencoe.com.**

Activity: Using the information provided at these links, create a fact sheet on allergies and asthma.

FIGURE 13.2

COMMON ALLERGENS

Allergens can be found both indoors and outdoors and in any season. *Which of these allergens might be difficult to avoid? Why?*

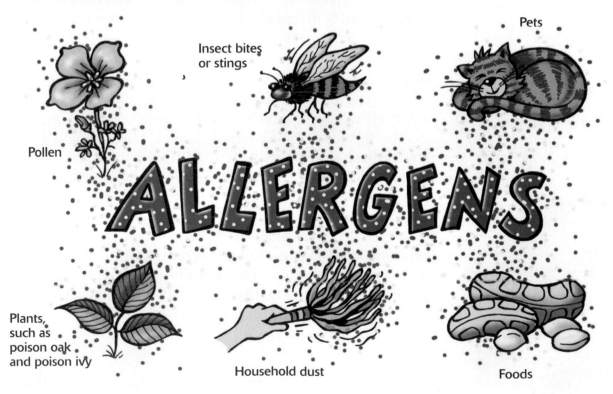

Insect bites or stings

Pets

Pollen

Plants, such as poison oak and poison ivy

Household dust

Foods

Reading Check
Understand text organi-
zation. Look at the lists
on these two pages. What
are their similarities and
differences?

Allergic Reactions

When a person who has an allergy breathes in, touches, or swallows an allergen, the allergen locks onto the body's lymphocytes. These cells then release **histamines** (HIS·tuh·meenz), *the chemicals in the body that cause the symptoms of an allergic reaction.* Allergic reactions may involve the following parts of the body:

- **Eyes.** Allergies can make the eyes red, watery, and itchy.
- **Nose.** Common allergy symptoms include a runny nose and sneezing.
- **Throat.** Some food allergies can make swallowing difficult. In extreme reactions the throat can swell and close up.
- **Skin.** An allergic reaction can cause the skin to break out in a rash. It can also cause hives, which are raised, itchy areas.
- **Respiratory system.** Allergies can cause coughing and difficulty breathing.
- **Digestive system.** An allergic reaction to food may cause stomach pain, cramps, and diarrhea.

Treating Allergies

How do you know what substances, if any, you're allergic to? Sometimes the answer is obvious. For example, if you touch poison oak or ivy, you may develop a rash. Sometimes the source of an allergic reaction isn't so obvious. In these cases a doctor can perform tests to try to find out the cause. Once the specific allergen is known, the person who has the allergy can use one of the following methods to cope with it.

- **Avoid the allergen.** If you're allergic to a certain food, you can prevent a reaction by not eating it. Sometimes, however, you may have to check labels carefully to determine whether a product contains that food. Some allergens, such as dust and pollen, are more difficult to avoid.
- **Take medication.** If you can't avoid the allergen, antihistamines may relieve symptoms. **Antihistamines** are *medications that relieve the symptoms of allergic reactions by suppressing the production of histamines.*
- **Get injections.** A person who has severe allergies can undergo a long-term series of injections. Each injection contains a tiny amount of the allergen to help a person overcome his or her sensitivity to it.

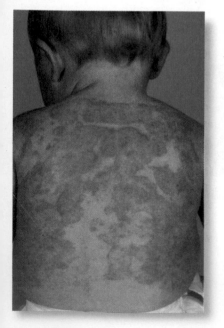

Hives are raised, itchy patches on the skin caused by an allergic reaction to anything from food to plants. *Do you have any allergies?*

Asthma

Asthma (AZ·muh) is *a chronic respiratory disease that causes air passages to become narrow or blocked, making breathing difficult.* The number of people with asthma, especially children, has risen in the last 20 years. Nearly 5 million Americans under the age of 18 have asthma.

Many of the same substances that cause allergies also cause asthma. These substances and certain conditions or situations are called asthma triggers. Common triggers include

- certain allergens, such as pollen, dust, pets, and mold.
- strenuous physical activity, especially in cold weather.
- infections of the respiratory system, such as colds and flu.
- irritants such as cigarette smoke and air pollution and fumes from paint, gasoline, and other toxic substances.
- situations in which the person's breathing rate increases, such as stressful events and vigorous laughing or crying.
- weather and climate changes and cold air.

A Typical Asthma Attack

The symptoms of an asthma attack may include wheezing, shortness of breath, a feeling of gagging or choking, and tightness in the chest. **Figure 13.3** shows how an asthma attack affects the airways to the lungs.

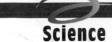
CONNECT TO
Science

REDUCING DUST MITES
Dust mites—microscopic bugs that live in bedding, carpeting, furniture, and drapes—are a common allergy and asthma trigger. Research ways to reduce household dust mites. Discuss these measures with your parents or guardians.

FIGURE 13.3

EFFECTS OF AN ASTHMA ATTACK

The changes caused by an asthma attack make the airways narrow so that breathing becomes more difficult. *What are some of the symptoms of an asthma attack?*

Normal airway

Swollen airway and contracted muscle

Narrowed airway

Mucus

During normal breathing, the lungs' airways are wide open. Air passes freely in and out through these tubes.

During an asthma attack, the lining of the airways becomes swollen, and the muscles around the tubes tighten. Extra mucus is produced, further clogging the airways.

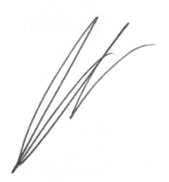

Managing Asthma

With the help of parents or guardians and a doctor or other health care provider, a person with asthma can develop a plan that will keep the condition under control. The following strategies can help people with asthma feel better and avoid asthma attacks:

- **Monitor the condition.** Because asthma is a chronic disease, people who have it need to be aware of their condition. Many doctors suggest using an instrument called a peak flow meter to monitor lung capacity regularly. By blowing into this device when the asthma is under control, the person can determine her

Hands-On Health

DETERMINING LUNG CAPACITY

In this activity you will work with a partner to measure the air capacity of your lungs.

WHAT YOU WILL NEED
- a clean plastic gallon jug with a cap
- masking tape
- a 2-foot length of plastic tubing
- a plastic dishpan
- two plastic drinking straws
- two pens with ink in different colors

WHAT YOU WILL DO
1. Tape a strip of masking tape up the side of the plastic jug. Fill the jug with water, and put the cap on.
2. Fill a dishpan about halfway with water.

3. Have your partner turn the jug upside down into the dishpan. Keeping the opening underwater, remove the cap, being careful not to let in air bubbles.
4. Put one end of the tubing into the jug opening. Insert a drinking straw into the other end of tubing. (Use your hand to seal the top of the tubing and to hold the straw in place.)
5. Take a normal breath of air, and then exhale it into the straw. Mark the water level on the tape.
6. Refill the jug with water, and put it back into the dishpan.
7. Take a deep breath, and try to exhale all of the air from your lungs into the straw. Mark this water level on the tape.
8. Using a new drinking straw, have your partner follow the same steps. In a different color of ink, mark your partner's water levels on the tape.

IN CONCLUSION
1. Did the water level drop more when you exhaled a normal breath or a deep breath?
2. Which partner's lung capacity was greater?
3. What does this activity tell you about lung capacity during an asthma attack?

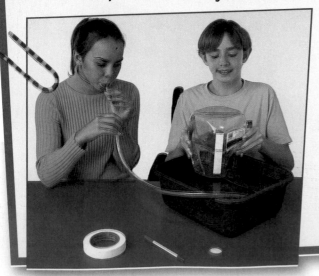

or his optimal peak flow number. By comparing future readings with the optimal peak flow number, the person will know when her or his airways are narrowing—even before symptoms start. In addition, people who have asthma can learn to recognize the warning signs of a severe attack.

- **Manage the environment.** Eliminating asthma triggers from the environment can reduce the risk of flare-ups. Floors, rugs, and carpeting should be vacuumed regularly. Bedding should be washed frequently in hot water.
- **Manage stress.** It's important for people who have asthma to manage their stress levels. Relaxation practices and special breathing techniques may also be helpful.
- **Take medication.** Two main types of medications are used to treat asthma. Controller medications help prevent asthma attacks by making the airways less sensitive to asthma triggers. Reliever medications reduce symptoms during flare-ups. **Bronchodilators** (brahng·koh·DY·lay·tuhrz), *medications that relax the muscles around the bronchial air passages,* are one type of controller medication. They are usually taken through an inhaler, a small hand-held device that dispenses the exact amount of medication needed.

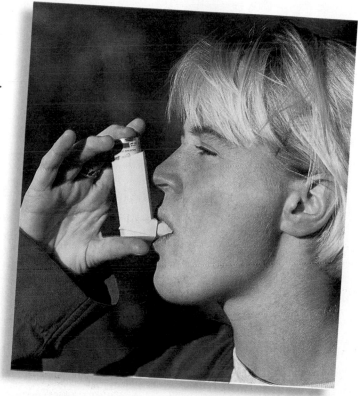

People with asthma use inhalers to take bronchodilators, medicines that open the air passages.

Lesson 1 Review

Using complete sentences, answer the following questions on a sheet of paper.

Reviewing Terms and Facts

1. **Vocabulary** Define the terms *allergy* and *allergen.*
2. **List** Name four common allergens.
3. **Distinguish** What is the difference between histamines and antihistamines?
4. **Describe** What measures can people take to manage asthma?
5. **Recall** What does a *bronchodilator* do?

Thinking Critically

6. **Compare and Contrast** In what ways is asthma different from a cold?
7. **Analyze** Why do you think it is a good idea to know whether you have an allergy?

Applying Health Skills

8. **Advocacy** Create a pamphlet that describes what asthma is and how a teen can successfully manage the condition. Also include information on how others can support the special health needs of people with asthma.

Understanding Cancer

Cancer

Cancer is the second leading cause of death in the United States, just behind heart disease. What exactly is cancer? **Cancer** is *a disease that occurs when abnormal cells grow out of control.* However, cancer isn't just one disease. It's actually a group of more than 100 diseases that affect different parts of the body.

The adult human body is made up of more than 50 trillion cells. The body's cells are continually growing and reproducing themselves. Although the majority of cells are normal, some cells are abnormal. The body's natural defenses usually destroy these abnormal cells, but sometimes an abnormal cell survives and starts to reproduce. A **tumor** (TOO·mer) is *a group of abnormal cells that forms a mass.* Tumors are either benign (bi·NYN) or malignant (muh·LIG· nuhnt). A **benign** tumor is *not cancerous* and does not spread. A **malignant** tumor is *cancerous* and may spread to other parts of the body.

Types of Cancer

Cancer can affect various parts of the body. It may begin in one area and then spread to other areas. The four most common cancers are shown in **Figure 13.4. Figure 13.5** provides more information about the various types of cancer, including their **risk factors**, or *characteristics or behaviors that increase the likelihood of developing a medical disorder or disease.*

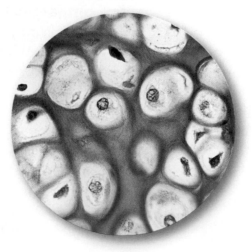
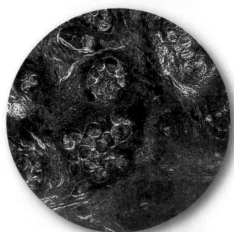

Cancer is a disease characterized by abnormal body cells growing out of control. *What differences do you see between the normal cells (left) and the cancer cells (right)?*

FIGURE 13.4

COMMON TYPES OF CANCER

Every year more than 11,000 children and teens are diagnosed with cancer in the United States. *What type of cancer caused the most deaths in the year 2000?*

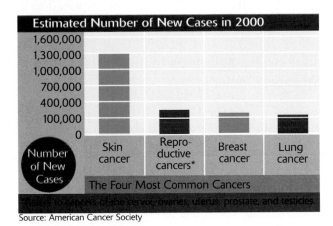

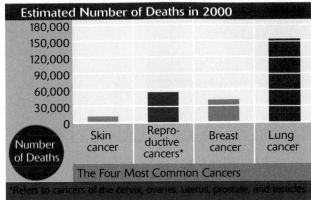

Source: American Cancer Society

Source: American Cancer Society

FIGURE 13.5

FORMS OF CANCER AND RISK FACTORS

Unhealthful behavior choices may increase the risk for developing some forms of cancer.

Form of Cancer	Risk Factors	Important Facts
Breast cancer	Family history. More common in women over age 50, but can also occur in younger women and in men.	This is the second major cause of cancer death among women.
Reproductive cancers	Vary, but include age, family history of cancer, obesity, and smoking.	In females, it can affect the cervix, ovaries, and uterus. In males, it can affect the prostate gland and testicles.
Colon and rectum cancers	A high-fat, low-fiber diet; lack of physical activity; and smoking.	Cases have declined somewhat in recent years due to increased cancer screening and better treatments.
Leukemia	Not generally known. May be linked to exposure to certain types of radiation and to certain chemicals.	This cancer causes a rise in abnormal white blood cells, hindering the body's production of healthy blood cells.
Lung cancer	Smoking.	This is the largest cause of cancer death. Nearly 80% of cases are related to smoking.
Lymphoma	Not generally known. Exposure to certain infections may play a part.	This cancer of the lymph tissue weakens the immune system, leaving the body more vulnerable to infection.
Skin cancers	Sun exposure and light skin, hair, and eye coloring.	This is the most common form of cancer in the United States. Some types are easier to treat than others.

Causes of Cancer

Like other noncommunicable diseases, some cancers can be linked to inherited traits, behavior choices, and environmental factors. **Carcinogens** (kar·SI·nuh·juhnz) are *substances in the environment that cause cancer.* Usually a person has to be exposed to a carcinogen over a long period of time for cancer to develop.

Substances and conditions that have been linked to the development of various types of cancer include

- tobacco in any form.
- ultraviolet rays from the sun.
- certain types of radiation.
- certain minerals and chemicals used in construction and manufacturing, such as asbestos, a carcinogen that is no longer used in new construction but is still present in older buildings.
- air and water pollution.
- a diet high in fat and low in fiber.

Combating Cancer

The best defense against an existing cancer is early detection. To find cancer early, doctors look for warning signs during exams.

When asbestos particles are inhaled, they can lodge in the lungs, damaging cells and increasing the risk for lung cancer.

You play the most important role in early detection. You know your body better than anyone else does. Train yourself to become aware of any unusual changes in your body. If you notice something that you think is abnormal, such as a mole or wart that changes in size or color, tell your parents or guardians and see a doctor right away.

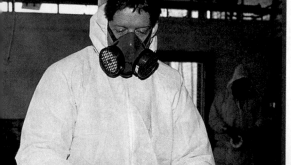

What Doctors Can Do

The most common cancer treatments are surgery, radiation therapy, and chemotherapy. Doctors often use a combination of these methods, depending on the type of cancer and how far it has progressed.

- **Surgery** is the primary treatment for many types of cancer, including breast, skin, lung, and colon cancer. In surgery, doctors remove tumors and other cancerous cells. Surgery is most effective when the cancer is confined to one area of the body.
- **Radiation therapy** is *a treatment that uses X rays or other forms of radioactivity for some types of cancer.* This therapy works best when the cancer is limited to just one area, such as the skin. It is also used to kill any cancer cells that may remain after surgery.

- **Chemotherapy** (kee·moh·THEHR·uh·pee) is *the use of powerful drugs to destroy cancer cells.* This treatment is used to stop cancers that have spread throughout the body. It is also sometimes used to shrink tumors before surgery is performed.

All of these cancer treatments have side effects, including the destruction of some healthy cells along with cancerous ones. Both radiation therapy and chemotherapy can cause nausea, fatigue, and temporary hair loss.

What You Can Do

There are no guaranteed ways to prevent cancer. However, you can make some choices that will lower your risk for developing certain cancers, such as avoiding tobacco use. You can also take action to detect cancer early, improving your chances of recovering if it does occur. Start your fight against cancer by practicing the healthful behaviors listed in the activity below and on the next page.

During radiation therapy, an X-ray machine delivers radiation to clusters of cancer cells. The radiation destroys or slows the growth of the cancerous cells.

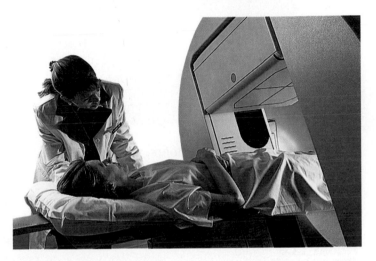

HEALTH SKILLS ACTIVITY

PRACTICING HEALTHFUL BEHAVIORS

Cancer Prevention

Food choices may be linked to as many as 33 percent of all cancer deaths. The American Institute for Cancer Research has made dietary recommendations that can help you reduce your risk for developing cancer.

- **LIMIT THE AMOUNT OF FAT YOU EAT.** Your total intake of fat should be no more than 35 percent of total calories. It's especially important to limit the amount of saturated fat to less than 10 percent of total calories.
- **EAT MORE FRUITS, VEGETABLES, AND WHOLE GRAINS.** The nutrients in these foods can help your body eliminate carcinogens before they can cause cancer.

- **GO EASY ON GRILLED MEATS.** The burnt surface of some grilled foods contains many carcinogens. However, marinating meats before grilling them can reduce the amount of carcinogens.
- **LIMIT YOUR INTAKE OF SALT.** A high salt intake has been linked to stomach cancer.

WITH A GROUP

In groups of three or four, create a puppet show for elementary school students, having your characters discuss these dietary recommendations. In the skit, show how one of the characters makes a plan to follow these guidelines.

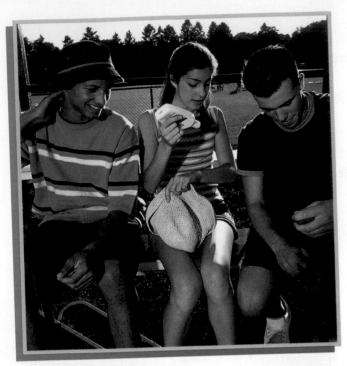

No matter what you do outdoors, you need to protect your skin from the sun's powerful UV rays. *What can you do to protect your skin from the sun?*

- **Limit sun exposure.** You can reduce your risk for developing skin cancer by protecting your skin from the sun's UV rays. The best way to protect your skin is to avoid being in the sun between 10:00 A.M. and 4:00 P.M., when the sun's rays are strongest. If you are out in the sun, wear a hat and use a sunscreen with a sun protection factor (SPF) of *at least* 15.
- **Perform self-examinations.** To check for lumps that may be cancerous, females should perform a breast self-exam once a month, and males should perform a testicular self-exam once a month. Ask a health care professional or contact the American Cancer Society for information on these self-exams. Both males and females also need to check their skin for changes in moles or other growths. Take a look at **Figure 13.6** to learn more about skin growths.

FIGURE 13.6
CHECK YOUR ABCDs

Early detection of skin cancer is important. Check your skin regularly for new growths or changes in existing growths. If you have a lot of moles, you should have them checked regularly by a dermatologist as well. The American Cancer Society recommends following the ABCD rule when you check for signs of skin cancer. *What should you do if you notice a mole that shows one of the signs of skin cancer?*

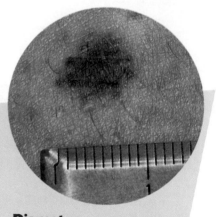

Diameter
The diameter is greater than 6 millimeters (about the size of a pencil eraser). A growth that has expanded to this size over time should be checked.

Asymmetry
One side of a mole looks different from the other side.

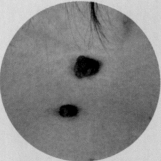

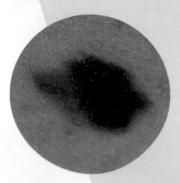

Border irregularity
The edges are jagged or blurred.

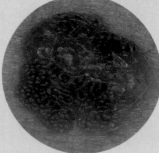

Color
The color is not uniform, or the same, throughout. If a mole is tan and brown, black, or red and white, have it checked.

- **Know the seven warning signs.** The American Cancer Society has identified seven warning signs that may signal cancer. The first letter of each warning sign spells the word *caution*. If you notice one of the signs listed in **Figure 13.7**, check with a doctor.

FIGURE 13.7

THE SEVEN WARNING SIGNS OF CANCER

Although these signs don't always mean cancer, you should see a doctor if you notice any of them. *What can you do to check for warning signs of cancer?*

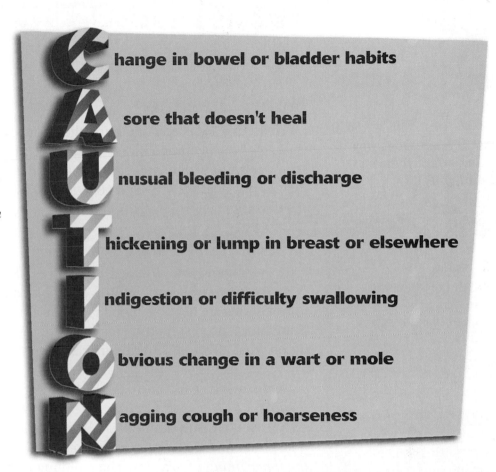

Change in bowel or bladder habits

A sore that doesn't heal

Unusual bleeding or discharge

Thickening or lump in breast or elsewhere

Indigestion or difficulty swallowing

Obvious change in a wart or mole

Nagging cough or hoarseness

Lesson 2 Review

Using complete sentences, answer the following questions on a sheet of paper.

Reviewing Terms and Facts

1. **Vocabulary** Define the term *cancer.*
2. **Recall** What is the difference between a tumor that is benign and one that is malignant?
3. **Identify** Name two forms of cancer. Then name a risk factor for each.
4. **List** What are three ways that doctors treat cancer?
5. **Recall** What is the ABCD rule? What does each letter stand for?

Thinking Critically

6. **Hypothesize** Why do you think skin cancer is the most common form of cancer in the United States?
7. **Analyze** How might knowing the seven warning signs of cancer help people protect themselves?

Applying Health Skills

8. **Communication Skills** Write a script for a public service announcement for radio or television, explaining the seven warning signs of cancer.

Understanding Heart Disease

Quick Write

List three reasons why it is important to have a healthy heart.

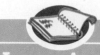

LEARN ABOUT...

- different types of heart disease.
- how heart disease is treated.
- what you can do to reduce your risk for developing heart disease.

VOCABULARY

- arteriosclerosis
- atherosclerosis
- heart attack
- hypertension
- stroke
- angioplasty

Heart Disease

Heart disease is any condition that reduces the strength or functioning of the heart and blood vessels. Heart disease kills more American adults than any other cause of death. A high-fat diet, lack of physical activity, and genetic factors may all contribute to the development of heart disease.

Types of Heart Disease

As you know, arteries are the blood vessels that carry blood away from the heart. Coronary arteries bring blood to the heart. When your arteries are healthy, blood is able to flow through them freely. Sometimes, however, problems can develop with the arteries. Conditions that affect the arteries are called arterial diseases.

Arteriosclerosis (ar·tir·ee·oh·skluh·ROH·sis) is *a group of disorders that causes a thickening and hardening of the arteries.* **Atherosclerosis** (a·thuh·roh·skluh·ROH·sis), a form of arteriosclerosis, is *a condition that occurs when fatty substances build up on the inner lining of arteries.* The buildup of fatty deposits can slow or stop the flow of blood through the arteries. This can be a serious problem if it occurs in the coronary arteries.

Because arterial diseases slow blood flow to the heart, they increase the risk of a heart attack. A **heart attack** is *a serious condition that occurs when the blood supply to the heart slows or stops and the heart muscle is damaged.* **Figure 13.8** shows what

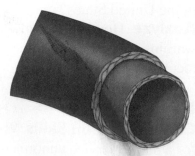
Healthy coronary artery

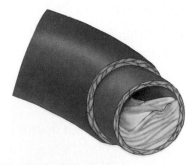
Coronary artery with atherosclerosis

For the heart to function properly, blood must be able to flow freely through the coronary arteries.

happens during a heart attack. The main symptom is often sudden pain or pressure in the chest. This pain may extend into one or both arms, the jaw, the back, or the abdomen. Other signs are shortness of breath, cold skin, vomiting, and loss of consciousness.

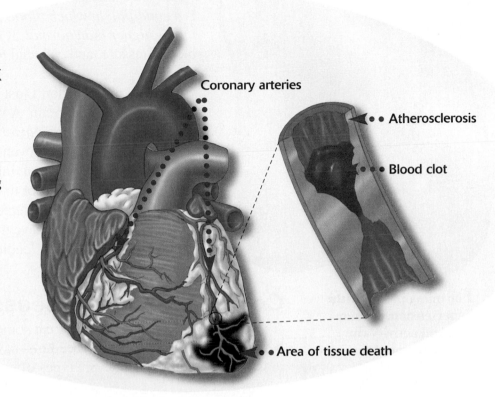

FIGURE 13.8

A HEART ATTACK

During a heart attack, a coronary artery becomes blocked, usually by a blood clot. Because the blockage prevents blood and oxygen from reaching the heart muscle tissue, the tissue dies.

Coronary arteries

Atherosclerosis

Blood clot

Area of tissue death

HEALTH SKILLS ACTIVITY

ACCESSING INFORMATION

Heart Health

You can reduce your risk of heart disease by eating healthful foods. Check out the following guidelines for some suggestions.

- **EAT FOODS THAT ARE HIGH IN FOLIC ACID, A B VITAMIN.** Good sources include leafy green vegetables, cereal, pasta, whole wheat bread, beans, and peanuts.
- **WATCH OUT FOR SATURATED FATS.** A high intake of saturated fats can increase your cholesterol level and can lead to clogged arteries. Choose low-fat foods and limit the amounts of ice cream, cheese, and butter that you eat.

- **EAT PLENTY OF FIBER.** Fiber helps prevent cholesterol from building up in your arteries. Sources include fruits, vegetables, whole grains, and dry beans and peas.
- **LIMIT YOUR SALT INTAKE TO LESS THAN ONE-FOURTH TEA-SPOON A DAY.** Season foods with herbs and spices, and snack on unsalted pretzels and popcorn.

ON YOUR OWN

Many health organizations will provide recipes that promote a healthy heart. Use Internet or library resources to find two such recipes. Use this information to make a "healthy heart" cookbook with your class.

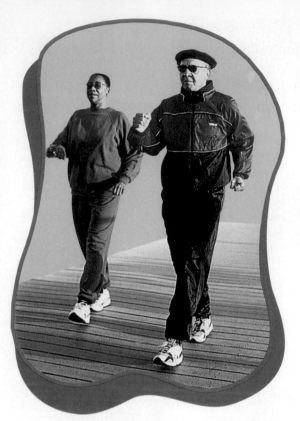

For many people with hypertension, regular physical activity can reduce the need for medication.

Related Disorders and Conditions

The force of blood pushing against the walls of the blood vessels is called blood pressure. Your blood pressure may go down when you sleep and increase when you exercise. **Hypertension** (hy·per·TEN·shuhn) is *a condition in which blood pressure stays at a level that is higher than normal*. It is also known as high blood pressure, and can lead to a heart attack or stroke.

Arterial diseases don't just affect the heart. They can also damage the brain. A **stroke** is *a serious condition that occurs when an artery of the brain breaks or becomes blocked*. This prevents the nerve cells in that part of the brain from receiving the oxygen and nutrients that they need in order to function. Depending on what part of the brain is affected, a person who has experienced a stroke may have trouble moving or speaking. Strokes are the third leading cause of death in the United States.

Combating Heart Disease

Today medications are used to treat some heart problems and help prevent others. Surgical procedures have also been developed to treat some of the more severe types of heart disease.

What Doctors Can Do

Treatment for heart disease depends on such factors as the person's age, the type of heart disease, and the extent of the problem. Possible treatments include the following:

- **Angioplasty.** Sometimes used to treat severe atherosclerosis, **angioplasty** (AN·jee·uh·plas·tee) is *a surgical procedure in which an instrument with a tiny balloon attached is inserted into an artery to clear a blockage*. When the balloon is inflated, it crushes the fatty deposit that was blocking the artery.
- **Medication.** Because blockages are often caused by blood clots, doctors may use aspirin and other medications to dissolve these clots and to stop new clots from forming.
- **Pacemaker.** People with certain types of heart disease often receive pacemakers. A pacemaker is an electronic device, surgically implanted in the chest, that sends electrical impulses to the heart. This device helps the heart to beat regularly.
- **Bypass surgery.** When a person has a blocked coronary artery, doctors may perform bypass surgery to create new paths for blood to flow around the blockage. A healthy blood vessel from another part of the body, usually from the chest or leg, is used to make a detour around the blocked part of the artery.

- **Heart transplant.** Surgeons can replace a severely diseased heart with a healthy one that has been donated. However, this type of surgery is not often used for arterial diseases.

What You Can Do

Making healthful choices now can decrease your risk of developing heart disease later. Follow these tips to keep your heart healthy.

- **Participate in regular physical activity.** Regular physical activity strengthens your heart muscle.
- **Maintain a healthy weight.** When you keep your weight within a healthy range, your heart doesn't have to work so hard. If you're overweight, consult a health care professional.
- **Manage stress.** Learn to cope with stressful situations. Effective management of stress will help you keep your blood pressure within a healthy range.
- **Avoid using tobacco.** Smokers are more than twice as likely to have heart attacks as nonsmokers. Other forms of tobacco are also linked to heart disease.

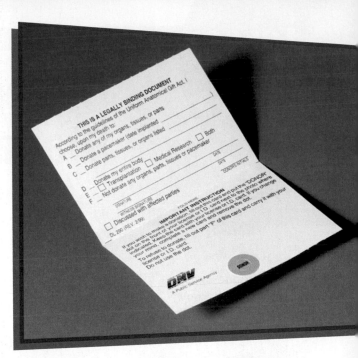

Medical technology has made it possible to transplant organs such as the heart. Adults who choose to donate their organs after death may state their wishes on a driver's license or an organ donor card.

![Lesson 3 Review]

Using complete sentences, answer the following questions on a sheet of paper.

Reviewing Terms and Facts

1. **Vocabulary** Define the terms *arteriosclerosis* and *atherosclerosis*.
2. **Recall** What causes a heart attack?
3. **Describe** What is a *stroke?*
4. **Explain** What are some habits teens can develop now to prevent heart disease later?

Thinking Critically

5. **Hypothesize** Why do you think heart disease is the number one killer in the United States?

6. **Suggest** What might you say to someone who salts food without tasting it first?

Applying Health Skills

7. **Practicing Healthful Behaviors** Demonstrate ways to use health information to help yourself: For one week, list everything you eat. Then review your list and put a plus sign next to foods that help prevent heart disease and a minus sign next to foods that increase the risk of heart disease. Identify ways to improve your eating habits.

Understanding Diabetes and Arthritis

Quick Write

Jot down one or two facts that you know about diabetes and arthritis.

LEARN ABOUT...

- what diabetes is and how it's treated.
- what arthritis is and how it's treated.

VOCABULARY

- diabetes
- insulin
- arthritis
- rheumatoid arthritis
- osteoarthritis

Diabetes

Diabetes mellitus (dy·uh·BEE·teez MEH·luh·tuhs), or **diabetes**, is *a disease that prevents the body from converting food into energy.* To get energy from food, the body must break it down into glucose (GLOO·kohs), a simple sugar. To transport glucose into cells, the body needs insulin. **Insulin** (IN·suh·lin) is *a hormone produced in the pancreas that regulates the level of glucose in the blood.* In people with diabetes, glucose cannot enter cells. Instead, it builds up in the bloodstream, causing many health problems.

There are two main types of diabetes. Type 1 diabetes usually develops during childhood or adolescence. In this type the immune system destroys the insulin-producing cells in the pancreas. The pancreas then produces little or no insulin to balance the glucose in the blood. Type 2 diabetes is strongly linked to obesity and lack of regular physical activity. It usually develops in people who are over age 40. However, more and more children and teens are developing the disease. This type occurs because the body isn't able to use effectively the insulin it produces. After several years, the body's production of insulin decreases. About 90 to 95 percent of people with diabetes have type 2 diabetes.

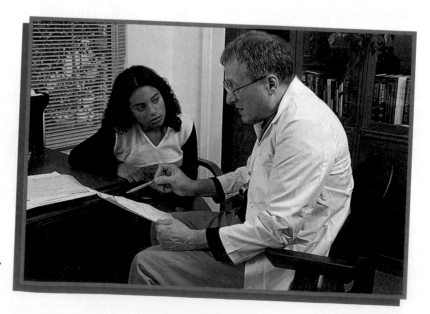

Symptoms of both types of diabetes include frequent urination, increased thirst and hunger, unexplained weight loss, blurred vision, and lack of energy. Anyone with these symptoms should see a doctor.

Most people with type 1 diabetes control the disease with insulin injections. People with type 2 diabetes, however, can sometimes control the disease by making healthful food choices and keeping physically active. Some may have to take oral medications.

Managing Diabetes

Although there is no cure for diabetes, people with the disease can keep it under control and lead normal lives. Take a look at **Figure 13.9** to find out how people who have diabetes can manage the disease.

FIGURE 13.9

MANAGING DIABETES

Diabetes affects about 17 million Americans, including 123,000 children and teens. If diabetes is not controlled, it can lead to blindness, heart disease, and kidney disorders.

Healthful Diet
People who have diabetes monitor their meals to keep the amount of glucose in their blood within safe limits. A doctor will work with the person to create a meal plan that meets her or his needs.

Insulin Injections
People with type 1 diabetes and some people with type 2 diabetes give themselves daily injections of insulin.

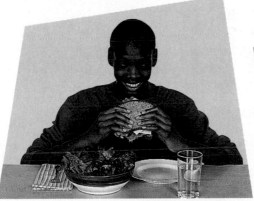

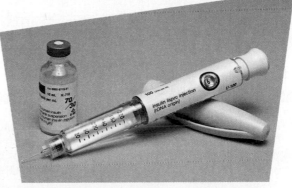

Weight Management
Doctors recommend that people with diabetes engage in regular physical activity and maintain a healthy weight.

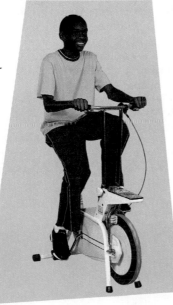

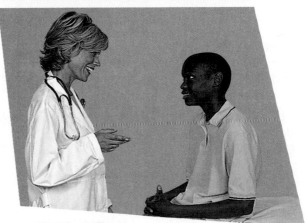

Medical Care
Anyone who has diabetes should be under a doctor's care. A doctor monitors the condition and checks for problems.

Arthritis

Arthritis (ar·THRY·tuhs) is *a disease of the joints marked by painful swelling and stiffness.* It affects about 43 million people in the United States. Arthritis is more common among older people. However, it can affect anyone, including children and teens.

Types of Arthritis

There are two main types of arthritis. **Rheumatoid** (ROO·muh·toyd) **arthritis** is *a chronic disease characterized by pain, inflammation, swelling, and stiffness of the joints.* It is the more serious and disabling form of arthritis. **Osteoarthritis** (ahs·tee·oh·ar·THRY·tuhs) is *a chronic disease that is common in older adults and results from a breakdown of cartilage in the joints.* It is the more common type of arthritis. **Figure 13.10** shows the causes, characteristics, and symptoms of both types of arthritis.

FIGURE 13.10

THE TWO MAIN TYPES OF ARTHRITIS

Although they have similarities, rheumatoid arthritis and osteoarthritis also have many differences. *Which type of arthritis is more common in children?*

Rheumatoid Arthritis	Osteoarthritis
Cause: The cause of rheumatoid arthritis is not known. The immune system attacks healthy joint tissue, leading to swelling and damage of the joints. Children with arthritis usually have this type.	**Cause:** Osteoarthritis is caused by wear and tear on the joints. Because it is more common among older people, age is considered a major risk factor. Obesity and heredity also play a role in the development of osteoarthritis.
Characteristics: Rheumatoid arthritis can affect any joints, including those of the hands, elbows, hips, knees, and feet. The disease usually progresses symmetrically—when one knee shows symptoms, the other knee will soon also show symptoms.	**Characteristics:** Osteoarthritis most often affects weight-bearing joints, such as the knees and hips. The cartilage surrounding the joints breaks down. Because cartilage normally cushions the ends of the bones, a breakdown causes bone to rub against bone.
Symptoms: The symptoms of rheumatoid arthritis include soreness, aching, and fatigue. Joints feel stiff and painful.	**Symptoms:** The symptoms of osteoarthritis include joint pain or swelling and pain and stiffness in the morning.

Managing Arthritis

Although there is no cure for arthritis, people can learn to cope with the disease. A doctor and patient can develop an effective treatment plan together. Most plans involve a combination of some or all of the following:

- **Medication.** For some types of arthritis, doctors prescribe medication to slow the spread of the disease. People who have arthritis may also take medication to ease pain and reduce swelling.
- **Diet.** A balanced eating plan helps maintain overall health and keeps weight under control.
- **Physical activity.** Regular physical activity helps to keep joints flexible and improves muscle strength.
- **Rest.** Getting enough rest is an important way to relieve stress on affected joints.
- **Heat/cold treatments.** Hot baths or heating pads help relieve pain. Cold treatments reduce swelling.
- **Joint replacement.** In severe cases a surgeon might replace a diseased joint, such as a knee or hip, with an artificial one.

This person has osteo-arthritis. You can see bony bumps around the joints, evidence that the cartilage between the joints has broken down. *What causes pain in someone who has osteo-arthritis?*

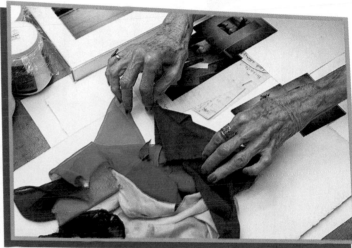

Lesson 4 Review

Using complete sentences, answer the following questions on a sheet of paper.

Reviewing Terms and Facts

1. **Vocabulary** Define the terms *diabetes* and *insulin.*
2. **Differentiate** What are the two main types of diabetes? How are they similar? How do they differ?
3. **List** Name four ways in which people with diabetes can manage their condition.
4. **Vocabulary** What is *arthritis*?
5. **Recall** What are the main differences between rheumatoid arthritis and osteoarthritis? How can people manage arthritis?

Thinking Critically

6. **Suggest** What would you say to a friend who has diabetes but who doesn't want to follow a healthful eating plan?
7. **Explain** Why might it be difficult for a person who has arthritis to play a musical instrument?

Applying Health Skills

8. **Accessing Information** Look in the Yellow Pages or on the Internet for organizations that offer support groups for people, especially young teens, who have diabetes or arthritis. Make a list of these organizations and Web sites and combine them with the findings of others in your class. Post the completed list on a bulletin board.

Waiting To Inhale

Despite having asthma, Jackie Joyner-Kersee set Olympic records in the long jump.

Some people struggling for air after exercise aren't out of shape—they have asthma.

She's considered one of the greatest female athletes of all time. Maybe that's why Jackie Joyner-Kersee thought she was simply out of shape when she gasped for air after a hard workout.

Even after a doctor told her she had asthma, Joyner-Kersee didn't want to believe it, nor did she take her medication regularly. Several years later, however, she experienced a life-threatening asthma attack and finally understood the seriousness of her condition. "I realized I was toying with my life," says Joyner-Kersee, a six-time

Olympic medalist. "I finally learned I had to respect asthma as much as I would an opponent."

Asthma is on the rise in the United States, affecting more than 17 million Americans (compared with 6.7 million in 1980). Some experts estimate that by 2020 nearly 29 million Americans could be living with the disease.

Anatomy of an Asthma Attack

Asthma is characterized by a chronic inflammation of the airways of the lungs. The figure on the next page shows an air passage (bronchiole)

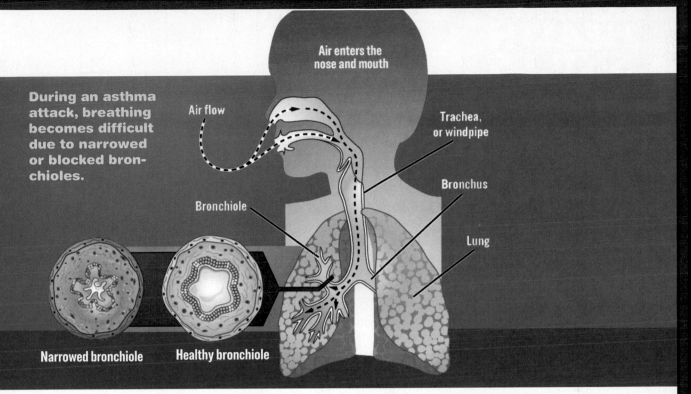

Air enters the nose and mouth

During an asthma attack, breathing becomes difficult due to narrowed or blocked bronchioles.

Air flow

Bronchiole

Trachea, or windpipe

Bronchus

Lung

Narrowed bronchiole

Healthy bronchiole

that has narrowed as a result of inflammation. An attack can occur when the air passages narrow in response to certain triggers, including a cold, cigarette smoke, allergies, stress, or excitement.

Exercise can also trigger an attack in about 80 percent of all asthma sufferers. Less common is a condition called "exercise-induced asthma." In this type of asthma, symptoms such as wheezing usually occur a few minutes after the end of a workout rather than during exercise, says Dr. Alfred Munzer of Washington Adventist Hospital in Maryland.

So how can you tell if you're experiencing an asthma attack or are just having a tough workout? "If your reaction to training seems unusual—you're unusually short of breath after a drill—get a checkup to determine if something is wrong," says Dr. Doug McKeag of the National Institute of Fitness and Sports in Indianapolis, Indiana.

Olympic swimmer Amy Van Dyken remembers feeling out of breath during a favorite training set. She didn't want to stop, even though she knew she had asthma. Halfway down the lane she was clutching the rope and gasping for air. Van Dyken, who was in the midst of a severe attack, was rushed to the hospital, where she was treated and released. She was lucky—an estimated 5,500 people die each year from asthma.

Living with Asthma

Champions like Joyner-Kersee and Van Dyken offer proof that athletes who have asthma can still excel. However, people with asthma need to stay on guard. "Asthma is a chronic condition. It requires constant monitoring," says Munzer.

The right medications can also help. If exercise is a trigger, your doctor may recommend that you use a bronchodilating inhaler, which opens air passages, about 20 minutes before working out. Anti-inflammatory compounds such as corticosteroids (not to be confused with dangerous anabolic steroids) can also provide relief. ■

TIME TO THINK...

About Asthma

Find out about other athletes and well-known people who have asthma. Create a public service announcement that mentions these celebrities as examples of people who have accomplished much despite having asthma. Using information from the chapter, include strategies that people with asthma can follow to manage the condition.

BE SMART ABOUT YOUR HEART

Model

Heart disease runs in Margaret's family. To reduce her chances of developing heart disease later in life, she has set a goal to take part in physical activities that will benefit her heart at least five days a week.

Margaret isn't sure which activities will be most helpful, so she asks her physical education teacher for advice. The teacher explains that moderate-to-vigorous physical activity and aerobic activities are excellent for the heart. Margaret already goes for walks with her mom for about an hour twice a week. She decides that she will also go in-line skating or ride her bike for at least half an hour one day a week. She also signs up for a kickboxing class that meets two nights a week. She keeps a log to ensure that she is meeting her goal. She has decided to review this log at the end of each month and to reward herself.

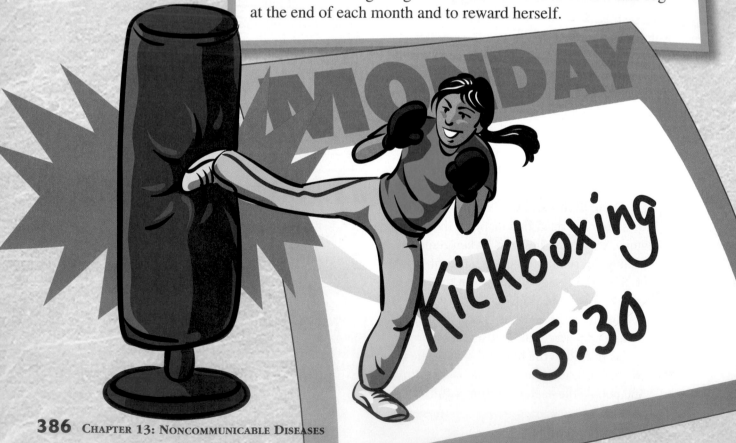

MONDAY

Kickboxing 5:30

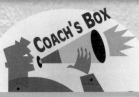

Practice

Read the scenario below and answer the questions at the end.

Like many other teens, Jeff loves to play computer games. Sometimes he gets so involved that several hours will pass without his realizing it. About twice a week, Jeff plays baseball or goes on a bike ride with his friends. He usually walks home from school and often stops at a convenience store for a soda and a hot dog or candy bar on his way.

1. Which habits might be harmful to Jeff's heart over time?

2. What goal could Jeff set to reduce his risk of heart disease?

3. What actions could Jeff take to reach this goal?

Goal Setting

1. Set a specific goal.
2. List the steps to reach your goal.
3. Get help from others.
4. Evaluate your progress.
5. Reward yourself.

Apply/Assess

You have learned about several ways to protect yourself from heart disease. They include eating healthful foods, being physically active, maintaining a healthy weight, managing stress, and avoiding tobacco.

Determine which one of these five items you most need to improve on. Then use the goal-setting steps to create a plan for developing this healthful habit. Write the goal-setting steps on a sheet of paper, explaining how you plan to follow them. For example, if you seldom eat fruits and vegetables, you might set a goal to eat five servings of them each day. Keep a log to record your progress.

Self-√Check

● Have I identified a habit that will improve my heart's health?

● Have I written a plan using the 5 goal-setting steps in order to make this habit part of my life?

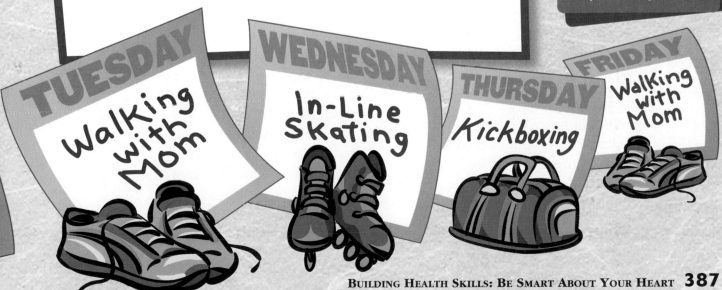

After You Read

Use your completed Foldable to review the information on allergies and asthma.

FOLDABLES™
Study Organizer

Reviewing Vocabulary and Concepts

On a sheet of paper, write the numbers 1–9. After each number, write the term from the list that best completes each sentence.

- tumor
- carcinogens
- risk factors
- pollen
- asthma
- chronic
- radiation therapy
- chemotherapy
- noncommunicable disease

Lesson 1

1. A(n) _____ is a disease that cannot be spread from person to person.

2. A(n) _____ condition is one that is present continuously or on and off over a long period of time.

3. One allergen is _____, a substance released by the flowers of some plants.

4. _____ is a chronic respiratory disease that causes air passages to narrow, making breathing difficult.

Lesson 2

5. A(n) _____ is a group of abnormal cells that forms a mass.

6. Characteristics or behaviors that increase the likelihood of developing a medical disorder or disease are known as _____.

7. Tobacco and asbestos are examples of _____.

8. Some types of cancer may be treated with X rays or other forms of radioactivity; this is called _____.

9. _____ is the use of powerful drugs to destroy cancer cells.

Lesson 3

On a sheet of paper, write the numbers 10–13. Write *True* or *False* for each statement that follows. If the statement is false, change the underlined word or phrase to make it true.

10. <u>Atherosclerosis</u> occurs when the blood supply to the heart slows or stops and the heart muscle is damaged.

11. Another term for <u>hypertension</u> is high blood pressure.

12. A stroke can occur when a blood vessel in the <u>heart</u> breaks.

13. <u>Angioplasty</u> is a procedure in which an instrument with a balloon attached is inserted into an artery to clear a blockage.

Lesson 4

On a sheet of paper, write the numbers 14–16. After each number, write the letter of the answer that best completes each statement.

14. In diabetes, the body cannot convert
    a. blood into energy.
    b. food into energy.
    c. water into energy.
    d. heat into energy.

15. Rheumatoid arthritis is
    a. one kind of diabetes.
    b. an abnormal growth of cells.
    c. the more serious and disabling form of arthritis.
    d. an allergic reaction.

16. Osteoarthritis is a chronic disease that results from a breakdown of
    a. cartilage in the joints.
    b. a coronary artery.
    c. muscle in the arms and legs.
    d. bones in the hand.

Thinking Critically

Using complete sentences, answer the following questions on a sheet of paper.

17. Hypothesize Why do you think weather reports often include pollen counts?

18. Apply Analyze risks for contracting specific diseases based on cultural, environmental, behavioral, and age factors.

19. Suggest How can you demonstrate care and concern toward someone at school or in the community who has a chronic disease? List two ways to support the special health needs of that person.

Career Corner

Osteopath A person with arthritis may seek treatment from an osteopath. Osteopaths diagnose and treat disorders of the bones, muscles, and nerves. They examine patients and advise them on ways to reduce their disease risk through physical activity and diet. These professionals complete five years of college at an osteopathic school. They also complete a one-year internship and up to seven years of residency training. If this career interests you, visit the Career Corner at health.glencoe.com to find out more.

Standardized Test Practice

Math

Read the paragraph below and then answer the questions.

Huntington's disease is an incurable brain disorder caused by heredity. The gene for this disease can be passed from parent to child. Use the figure below to answer the questions. The parent at the top of the square has an H gene, which means that he has Huntington's disease. All the small letter h's are genes that do not carry the disease.

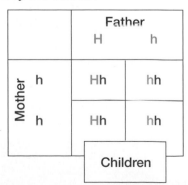

1. If the parents have one child, what is the probability that it will have Huntington's disease?

   Ⓐ 1/4
   Ⓑ 3/8
   Ⓒ 1/2
   Ⓓ 1/3

2. If the parents have two children, what is the probability that both of them will have Huntington's disease?

   Ⓐ 1/4
   Ⓑ 3/8
   Ⓒ 1/2
   Ⓓ 1/3

3. If the parents have four children, will two of them definitely have Huntington's disease? Explain.

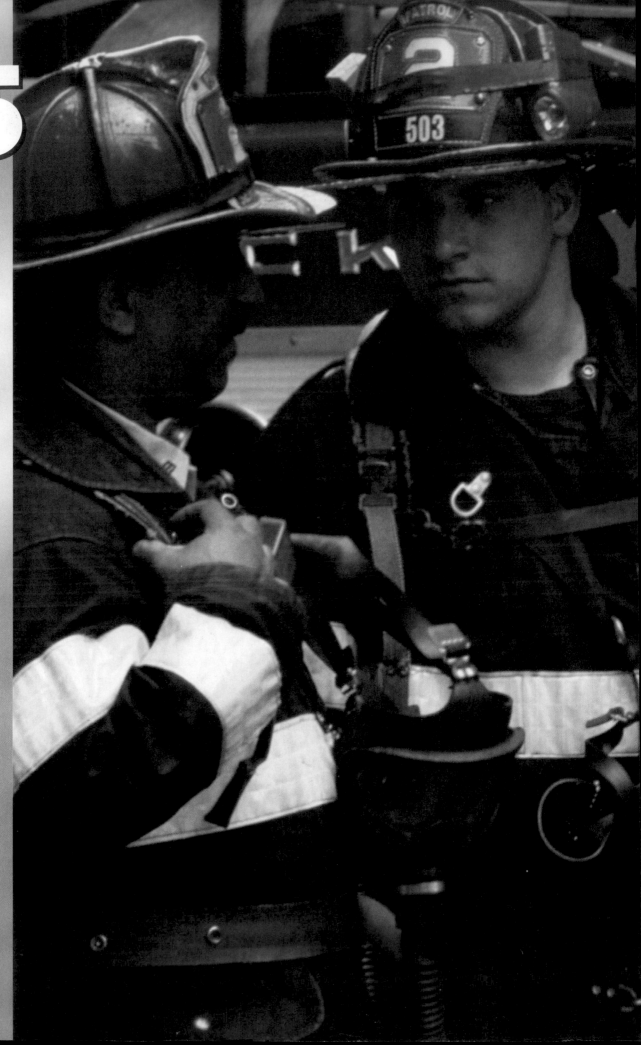

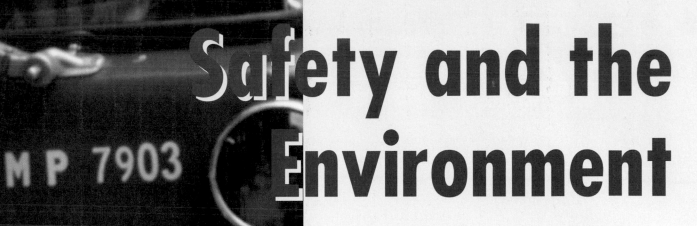

Safety and the Environment

HEALTH *in Action*

What do fighting fires and recycling have in common?

By behaving carefully, whether indoors or outdoors, you can prevent many accidents and emergencies. Being mindful of your environment and what you can do to protect it shows that you can safeguard your health and the health of others. Of course, by recycling those old newspapers, you're removing a potentially hazardous and flammable material from your home. That's like putting out a fire before it starts!

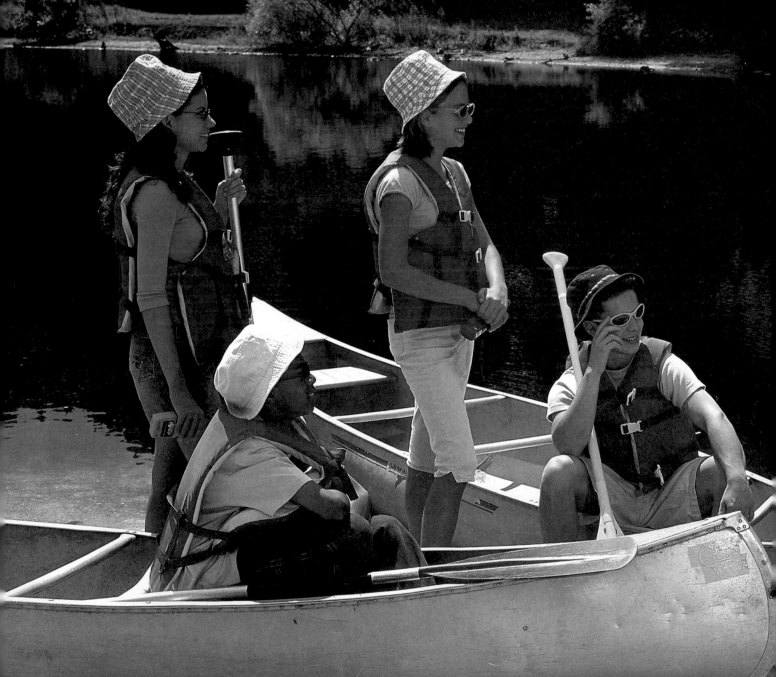

Personal Safety and Injury Prevention

HEALTH *Online*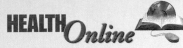

Do you know the rules for dealing with an emergency? Find out by taking the Chapter 14 Health Inventory at health.glencoe.com.

FOLDABLES™
Study Organizer

Before You Read

Make this Foldable to organize what you learn in Lesson 1 about the causes and prevention of an accident chain. Begin with three plain sheets of 8½″ × 11″ paper.

Step 1

Collect three sheets of paper, and place them 1″ apart.

Step 2

Fold up the bottom edges, stopping them 1″ from the top edges. This makes all tabs the same size.

Step 3

Crease the paper to hold the tabs in place. Staple along the fold.

Step 4

Turn and label the tabs as shown.

The Accident Chain

1. The Situation
2. The Unsafe Habit
3. The Unsafe Action
4. The Accident
5. The Result

As You Read

Under the appropriate tab, write down what you learn about each link in the accident chain.

Developing Safe Habits

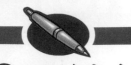

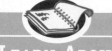

LEARN ABOUT...

- what it means to be safety conscious.
- causes of accidental injuries.
- how to prevent accidental injuries.

VOCABULARY

- safety conscious
- hazard
- accidental injuries

Safety First

"Never play with matches!" "Look both ways before you cross the street." Your parents or guardians probably began teaching you safety rules like these as soon as you were old enough to understand them. You may even repeat them to younger children.

It's not only important to learn the rules; it's also essential to be safety conscious. To be **safety conscious** means *to be aware that safety is important and to be careful to act in a safe manner.* Prevention is the best way to avoid and reduce risks. Prevention includes thinking ahead and trying to spot possible **hazards**, or *potential sources of danger,* before accidents and injuries occur. Accidents are the unexpected events that cause unintentional, or accidental, injuries. **Accidental injuries** are *injuries caused by unexpected events.*

According to the Centers for Disease Control and Prevention, adolescents are more likely to die from injuries than from all diseases combined. In the United States, accidental injuries result in more than 90,000 deaths each year. **Figure 14.1** shows the types of accidents that cause the largest number of deaths in the United States.

FIGURE 14.1

CAUSES OF DEATH FROM ACCIDENTS

In 1998 more than one-third of all deaths in motor vehicle collisions involved alcohol use by a driver or pedestrian. *Why do you think alcohol contributes to so many deaths of this kind?*

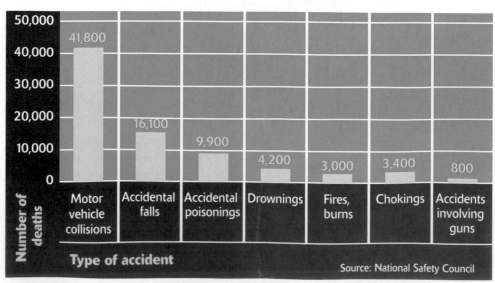

Causes of Death from Accidents (Number of deaths by Type of accident):
- Motor vehicle collisions: 41,800
- Accidental falls: 16,100
- Accidental poisonings: 9,900
- Drownings: 4,200
- Fires, burns: 3,000
- Chokings: 3,400
- Accidents involving guns: 800

Source: National Safety Council

How Accidental Injuries Occur

Being safety conscious means taking commonsense precautions, such as wearing protective gear when you go bicycling or in-line skating. Most accidental injuries happen because people become careless. They are often the result of an "accident chain," a sequence of events that leads to an unintentional injury. **Figure 14.2** demonstrates an accident chain.

FIGURE 14.2

THE ACCIDENT CHAIN

Nicole's unsafe habit and unsafe action contribute to her accidental injury. *How does each one play a role in the accident chain?*

Developing Good Character

Caring

Thinking about others' safety shows that you care. For example, keep floors and stairways at home free of clutter to help prevent falls. *What else can you do to correct unsafe situations and reduce the risk of accidents?*

1 The Situation
Nicole has overslept. She is rushing to put her jacket on and eat breakfast so that she doesn't miss the bus.

2 The Unsafe Habit
When Nicole takes off her skates, she usually leaves them on the front steps.

3 The Unsafe Action
Nicole is thinking only of getting to the bus stop. She races out the door without looking where she is going.

4 The Accident
Nicole trips over her skates and falls forward onto the sidewalk.

5 The Result
When she falls, Nicole sprains her wrist and scrapes both hands. She also misses her bus.

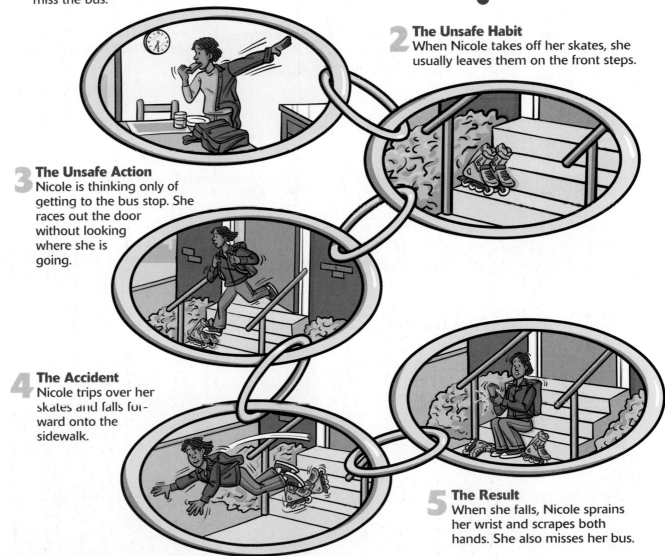

Breaking the Accident Chain

If Nicole had been safety conscious, she might not have gotten hurt. There were several points at which she could have broken the accident chain. Breaking just one link disables the accident chain and prevents accidental injuries. Take a look at the actions Nicole could have taken to break a link in the accident chain. Which one do you think she should have chosen?

- **Change the situation.** Nicole could have planned ahead. She could have set her alarm or arranged for another family member to wake her if she did not get up on time.
- **Change the unsafe habit.** Leaving your belongings on floors, steps, and other places where people have to walk is a careless habit that can lead to injury. Nicole could have put her skates in her closet, on a shelf, or in another safe place.
- **Change the unsafe action.** Although she was in a hurry, Nicole could have remained safety conscious. She could have kept her eye on the path to the bus stop to make sure that it was clear.

HEALTH SKILLS ACTIVITY

DECISION MAKING

Getting Home Safely

Brandon has basketball practice on Wednesday evenings. Because his parents work late, he usually rides his bike to and from practice. When he left his house to go to practice, it was sunny. However, by the time he got out of practice, it was raining hard. Brandon is worried that it might not be safe to ride his bike home in this weather. It's too far for him to walk home, and his parents won't be able to pick him up for at least an hour.

What Would You Do?

Suppose you were in Brandon's situation. Write a paragraph explaining what you would do and how you used the decision-making process to help you make this choice.

1. **STATE THE SITUATION.**
2. **LIST THE OPTIONS.**
3. **WEIGH THE POSSIBLE OUTCOMES.**
4. **CONSIDER VALUES.**
5. **MAKE A DECISION AND ACT.**
6. **EVALUATE THE DECISION.**

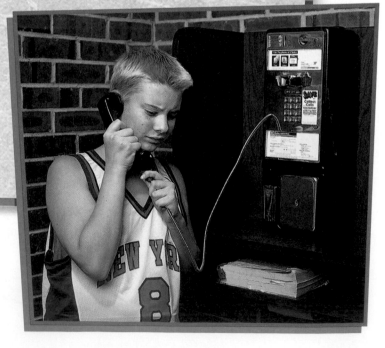

By changing the situation, the unsafe habit, or the unsafe action, Nicole could have prevented her accident and injury. If Nicole had gotten up on time, she would not have had to rush. If Nicole had put the skates in a safe place, she would not have tripped over them. If she had been paying attention, she would have stepped around the skates or pushed them out of the way. Not only would Nicole have prevented injury, but she also would have made it to the bus stop on time.

Reading Check
Evaluate your own habits. Think about what you have done this week. How could you have been more safety conscious?

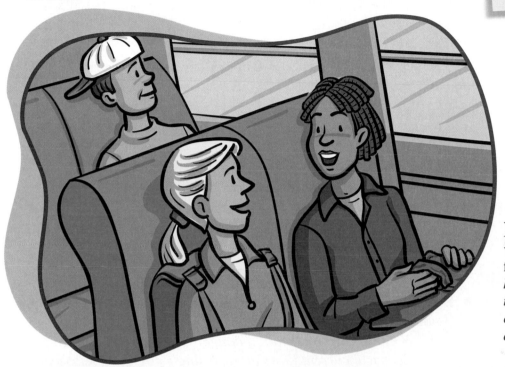

Nicole now tries to prevent accident chains from forming. *What hazards can you identify in your daily routine that could become part of an accident chain?*

Lesson 1 Review

Using complete sentences, answer the following questions on a sheet of paper.

Reviewing Terms and Facts

1. **Vocabulary** Define the term *safety conscious*. Explain how being safety conscious can help you prevent unintentional injuries.
2. **List** Name the links in an accident chain.
3. **Restate** What can you do to break an accident chain?

Thinking Critically

4. **Explain** What do you think is meant by the expression "safety first"?

5. **Hypothesize** Find a newspaper article about a motor vehicle collision. Construct an accident chain based on the events described in the article.

Applying Health Skills

6. **Goal Setting** Compile a list of strategies for preventing accidental injuries. Set a specific goal to incorporate these strategies into your daily life. Use the goal-setting steps to put your plan into action.

Safety at Home and in School

LEARN ABOUT...

- how to protect yourself and others from fires.
- ways to prevent accidental injuries at home and in school.

VOCABULARY

- flammable
- electrical overload
- smoke alarm

Fire Safety

Fire strikes more than 350,000 homes and kills more than 3,000 people a year in the United States. Here are some of the leading causes of fires in the home:

- **Careless cooking habits.** Spills can catch fire if they come into contact with the heat of an oven, stove, or open flame. Spattered grease and oil can be especially dangerous.
- **Careless cigarette smoking.** Fires can start when people fall asleep while smoking or throw smoldering cigarettes into wastebaskets.
- **Improper storage of flammable materials.** Items that are **flammable** are *able to catch fire easily.* Paint, old newspapers, and rags are all examples of flammable materials.
- **Electrical overload or damaged electrical circuits and wiring.** If you plug more than two electrical appliances into a wall outlet, you risk **electrical overload**, *a dangerous situation in which too much electrical current flows along a single circuit.* Overloaded circuits, frayed wires, and damaged cords can cause fires.

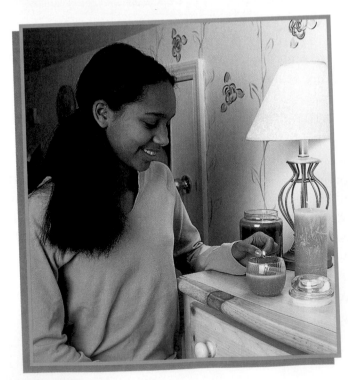

To prevent fires, never leave burning candles unattended.

Preventing Fires

Once you know how fires in the home usually start, you can learn how to prevent them by taking some simple fire safety measures.

- Keep stoves and ovens clean.
- Anyone who smokes should never smoke in bed. Wait until cigarettes and cigars in ashtrays are completely extinguished before emptying them into trash cans.
- Store matches and cigarette lighters in safe places, out of the reach of children.
- Check electrical appliances for loose or damaged cords. Repair or replace damaged appliances and broken outlets. Never run electrical cords under carpets — the movement of people and the weight of furniture can damage cords lying under the rugs.

Being Prepared for a Fire

Smoke alarms can provide a strong line of defense against injuries or deaths from fires. **Smoke alarms** are *devices that sound an alarm when they sense smoke.* Install a smoke alarm on every level of the house, preferably outside a sleeping area. To make sure that they're in working order, check smoke alarms once a month by pushing the test button, and change their batteries at least once a year.

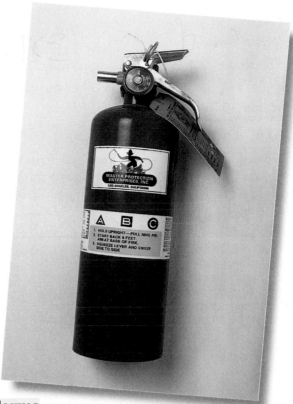

Every home should have a disposable fire extinguisher.

Water will put out fires in which paper, wood, or cloth is burning. However, you should never use water on oil, grease, or electrical fires. For this reason every home needs at least one fire extinguisher. Make sure that you read and understand the instructions so that you can operate it in an emergency. Check the pressure gauge periodically to make sure that the fire extinguisher is ready to use. Replace or recharge it as necessary.

With your family, plan escape routes in case of fire. Most fatal fires occur during the night, so every escape route should begin in a bedroom. A window with a fire escape or ladder may save a life if flames, heat, or smoke block a bedroom door. Decide on a meeting point outside so that you will know whether everyone is safe. Practice your escape plan by holding a family fire drill every six months.

Escaping a Fire

You have learned how to prevent fires. **Figure 14.3** shows what to do if a fire does break out. Knowing what to do ahead of time will help you stay calm and could save your life and the lives of other family members.

FIGURE 14.3

IN CASE OF FIRE

Memorizing the tips shown here will help you escape a fire safely. *Why do you think it is important to stay in the room with the door closed if you can't get out during a fire?*

1 If possible, leave quickly. Get out of the building *before* calling 911 or the fire department.

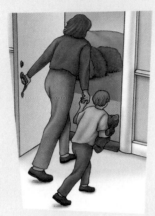

4 If you can't get out, stay in the room with the door closed. Roll up a blanket or towel and put it across the bottom of the door to keep out smoke. If there is a telephone in the room, call 911 or the fire department. If possible, open the window and yell for help.

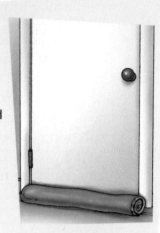

5 If your clothing catches fire, stop, drop, and roll. Rolling on the ground will smother the flames. Never run—the rush of air will fan the flames.

2 Before opening a closed door, feel it to see if it is hot. If it is, do *not* open it. There may be flames just outside the door.

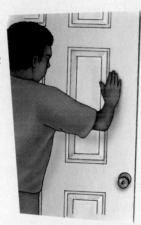

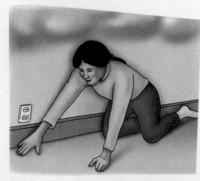

6 Once outside, go to the pre-arranged meeting place. Let everyone know that you are safe. Then someone should call 911 or the fire department. *Never* re-enter a burning building.

3 If you must exit through smoke, crawl along the floor. Because smoke and hot air rise, it is important to stay as low as possible. This will enable you to breathe in the cleaner air and ensure that you are not overcome by the smoke.

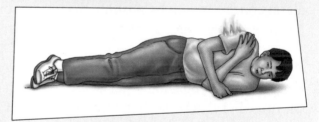

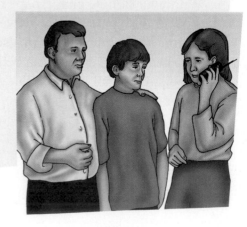

Preventing Injuries

Fires are just one type of dangerous situation. Others include falls, poisonings, electric shocks, and gun accidents. All of these situations can result in serious accidental injuries and even death.

Preventing Falls

Falls account for the largest number of nonfatal injuries among people under age 14. These safety rules can help you prevent falls:

- **Safety in the kitchen.** Clean up spills right away. Let family members know when you have washed the floor. Use a step stool—never a chair—to get items that are out of reach.
- **Safety in the bathroom.** Put a nonskid mat on the bottom of the tub or shower. In households with older adults or people who are unstable on their feet, install a secure handgrip on the side of the tub. Secure rugs with tape, or use rugs with latex backings.
- **Safety on the stairs.** Keep all staircases well lighted. Do not leave objects on the steps. Check handrails to be sure that they are stable. If small children live in the house, put gates at the top and bottom of the staircase.
- **Safety at school.** Follow school rules related to safety. For example, walk, don't run, in the hallways. Keep to the right as you walk down hallways or stairs.

Reading Check

Identify cause and effect. Write your own *If..., then...* statements about preventing falls.

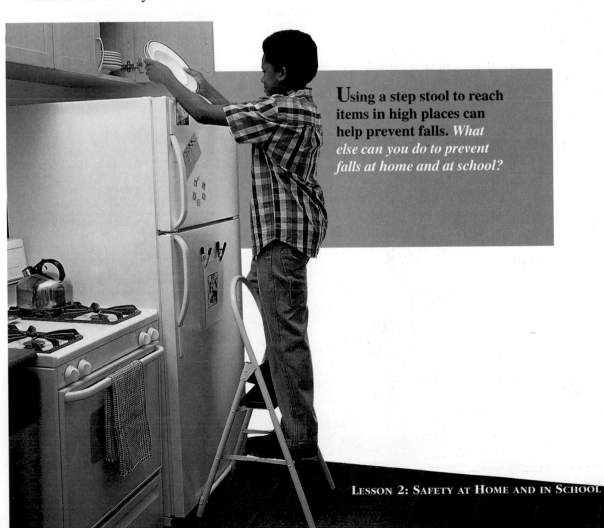

Using a step stool to reach items in high places can help prevent falls. *What else can you do to prevent falls at home and at school?*

Preventing Poisonings

Natural curiosity and the tendency to put objects into their mouths place young children at especially high risk of death by accidental poisoning. Following these rules can help you prevent such tragedies:

- Never refer to a child's medicine or vitamins as "candy."
- Make sure that all medicines have child-resistant caps.
- Put all medicines and poisonous substances away immediately after using them.
- Keep all cleaning products in their original, labeled containers.
- Store all potentially poisonous substances in high cabinets, out of children's reach. If possible, keep the cabinets locked.

Preventing Electric Shocks

Electricity can be extremely dangerous. Improper use or maintenance of electrical appliances, wiring, and outlets can cause severe electric shock. Worse yet is the danger of electrocution, or death resulting from electric shock. To avoid such dangers, follow these rules.

- Never use an electrical appliance near water, such as in a bathtub, or if you are wet.
- Unplug small appliances, such as hair dryers and toasters, when they are not in use. Repair or replace broken appliances.
- Pull out an electrical plug by the plug itself, not by the cord.
- Repair or replace loose or damaged cords.
- In homes with small children, cover unused outlets with outlet protectors.

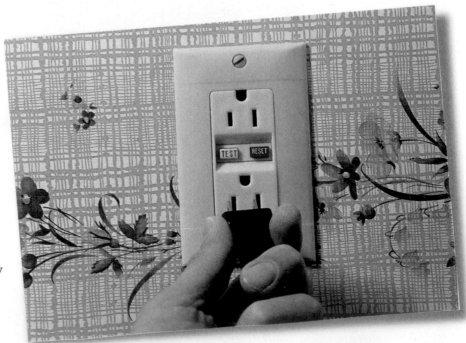

Pull on the plug to remove it from the outlet. Yanking on the cord can tear it away from the plug, possibly leading to fire or electric shock.

Gun Safety

In 1998 in the United States, 900 people died as a result of the accidental discharge of firearms. Many of these victims were children.

Observe basic gun safety rules if someone in your family, or anyone else you know, keeps guns at home. Guns should be stored unloaded, in a locked cabinet. Bullets should be stored in a different locked cabinet. A gun should never be pointed at anyone, and its barrel should aim downward when someone is carrying it. No matter what, always treat guns as if they are loaded.

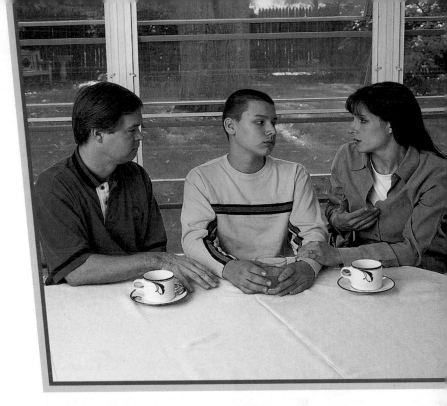

To protect yourself against weapons at school, cooperate with your school's efforts to keep them off school grounds. For example, some schools require students to go through metal detectors. Know and follow school rules prohibiting the possession of weapons. If you suspect that another student is carrying a gun or any other weapon, inform a teacher or school administrator. You can request that your name not be revealed. Some schools have established hot lines that students can call anonymously to report another student if he or she is carrying a gun or other weapon. It is everyone's responsibility to help keep schools safe.

Talk to your parents, guardians, or another trusted adult if you suspect that a teen is carrying a gun or other weapon. Discuss with them the dangers that weapons can cause to yourself and others.

Lesson 2 Review

Using complete sentences, answer the following questions on a sheet of paper.

Reviewing Terms and Facts

1. **Vocabulary** Define the term *flammable*. Give three examples of flammable materials.
2. **Identify** List three ways to prevent fires in the home.
3. **Outline** What should you do to escape if a fire breaks out in your home?
4. **List** Identify two ways to prevent falls.
5. **Identify** Name five ways to prevent electric shocks.

Thinking Critically

6. **Explain** Why is it important to establish and practice a fire escape plan at home?
7. **Infer** Explain the importance of understanding and following rules prohibiting the possession of weapons at school.

Applying Health Skills

8. **Practicing Healthful Behaviors** Create a safety checklist for your home. With your family, conduct a safety check. In a brief paragraph, discuss your findings. Add strategies for the prevention of accidental injuries.

Outdoor and Recreational Safety

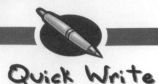
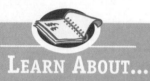
Traffic Safety

In every area of the United States, traffic laws are enforced to ensure order and safety. Almost all states require drivers and front-seat passengers to wear safety belts to prevent injuries. All drivers of motor vehicles are required to obey traffic regulations.

Bicyclists, skaters, skateboarders, and scooter riders are required to follow many of the same rules as people who are driving motor vehicles. **Pedestrians**, or *people who travel on foot,* have to obey traffic signs and take responsibility for their own safety. They cannot assume that drivers will always obey the laws or follow traffic signals and signs.

Whether you're on wheels or on foot, think about your safety and use decision-making skills to make the right choices. This will help you avoid high-risk situations involving motor vehicles and other hazards on the road.

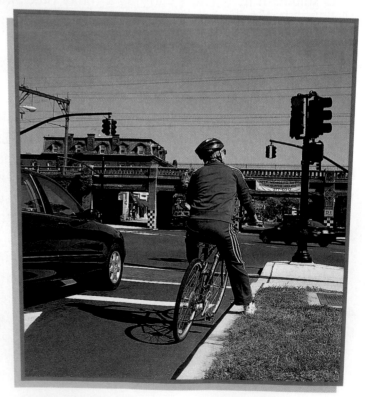

Bicyclists must ride in the same direction as traffic and stop at signals and signs just as motorists do.

Safety on Wheels

Having fun is part of bicycling, skating, skateboarding, and riding a scooter. However, these activities are not without risk. You can have fun on wheels *and* be safe by following some important guidelines. First of all, check your equipment. **Figure 14.4** explains how to check a bike for safety. Always wear a helmet. When in-line skating, skateboarding, or riding a scooter, your gear may also include wrist guards, elbow and knee pads, and light gloves. Wear athletic shoes for bicycling, skateboarding, or riding a scooter.

Always obey traffic laws. When bicycling, ride in the same direction as motor traffic. When you ride with a group, ride in a single line. Learn and use hand signals. Before turning left, look back for traffic behind you. Avoid riding in bad weather. When skating, keep your speed under control, and know how to stop and fall properly. Avoid skating at night or in traffic.

FIGURE 14.4

THE RIGHT EQUIPMENT

Maintaining and using your equipment properly will help you prevent bicycle injuries. *Why do you think it is important to check your tires?*

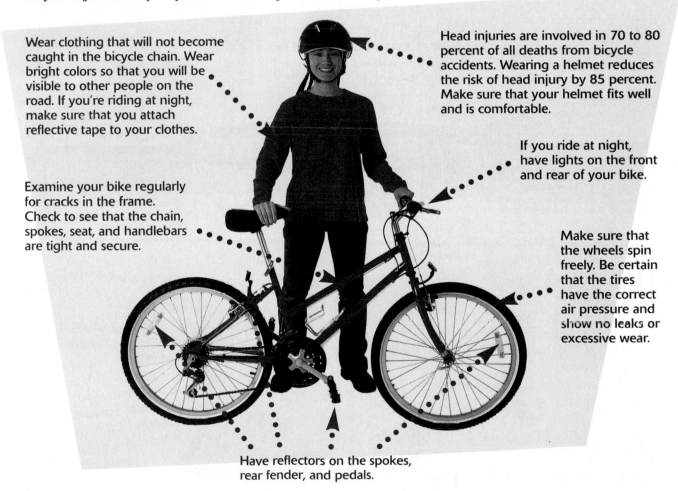

Wear clothing that will not become caught in the bicycle chain. Wear bright colors so that you will be visible to other people on the road. If you're riding at night, make sure that you attach reflective tape to your clothes.

Examine your bike regularly for cracks in the frame. Check to see that the chain, spokes, seat, and handlebars are tight and secure.

Head injuries are involved in 70 to 80 percent of all deaths from bicycle accidents. Wearing a helmet reduces the risk of head injury by 85 percent. Make sure that your helmet fits well and is comfortable.

If you ride at night, have lights on the front and rear of your bike.

Make sure that the wheels spin freely. Be certain that the tires have the correct air pressure and show no leaks or excessive wear.

Have reflectors on the spokes, rear fender, and pedals.

Safety on Foot

Pedestrians almost always have the right-of-way when they share the road with motorists. Nevertheless, when you are traveling on foot, you must obey traffic signals when crossing the street, and cross only at intersections or crosswalks. Look left, right, and left again before stepping into the street. Do not walk or run into the street from between parked cars. Finally, never assume that motorists or bicyclists

- can see you.
- know what you plan to do—such as cross the street.
- are paying attention.
- will act in a safe and capable manner.
- will signal before they turn.
- will act according to their signals.
- will obey the law.

Walking safely means following traffic rules and staying alert to the unexpected.

HEALTH SKILLS ACTIVITY

ADVOCACY

Sharing the Road

In addition to following traffic laws, safe driving requires common sense, courtesy, and alertness at all times. Some safe driving habits for motorists include

- staying a safe distance behind the motorist ahead of them.
- driving at a speed appropriate for weather and traffic conditions.
- yielding the right-of-way to pedestrians.
- slowing down for bicyclists, skaters, skateboarders, and scooter riders.

- properly maintaining the brakes, lights, and all other parts of the vehicle.
- not driving after drinking alcohol, when taking certain medications, or when tired.

ON YOUR OWN

Create a bumper sticker based on one or more of these tips. Ask permission to display your class's bumper stickers on bulletin boards in public buildings around your community.

Safety in Your Neighborhood

Violence can be a problem in any community. Although you may avoid areas where you feel unsafe, it is impossible to predict when and where an act of violence will occur. These tips will help you reduce your chances of becoming a victim of deliberate injury.

- **Avoid potential trouble.** At night, don't go out alone. Tell a parent where you're going and when you'll be home. Stay in well-lighted places. Leave expensive items at home, and always carry identification. Be prepared in case you need to make an emergency phone call. Don't talk to strangers.
- **Be smart and aware.** Be aware of the people around you, and move away from anyone who makes you feel uncomfortable.
- **Get help when you need it.** If anyone tries to touch you or says anything that frightens you, scream and run to the nearest public or safe place. Tell your parent or another trusted adult immediately. Ask for help or call 911 if necessary. If the person is a stranger, try to remember details about him or her, such as clothing, physical appearance, and type and color of car.

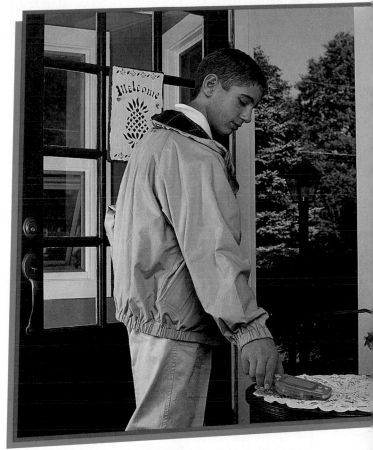

When you go out, leave valuables at home.

Recreational Safety

Most people enjoy spending time outdoors. No matter what the activity, you can stay safe by following these commonsense rules.

- **Take a buddy.** If you and a friend agree to stay together, you can help each other in case of an emergency.
- **Stay aware.** Learn the signs of weather emergencies. When necessary, move to safe shelter quickly.
- **Know your limits.** Set reasonable goals that reflect your abilities. If you're a beginning swimmer, for example, don't try to swim farther than you can handle.
- **Use good judgment.** Always ask yourself, "Do I have the equipment I need, and am I acting safely?" If you're unsure, ask a parent or other trusted adult.
- **Be sure to warm up and cool down.** Warming up and cooling down will help prevent injuries. Remember to stretch after both your warm-up and your cool-down.

Reading Check

Paraphrase. Rewrite the hiking and camping safety guidelines in your own words.

Water Safety

Once you learn to swim well, you've taken the most important step toward being safe in the water. However, even the best swimmers must follow water safety rules. Always swim with a buddy and only when a lifeguard or adult is present. Don't swim when you're tired. If you're caring for young children, don't let them go in or near a pool unless you are watching them.

Check the water depth before you dive. The American Red Cross recommends a minimum depth of 9 feet. Never dive into dark or shallow water or an above-ground pool. Check for other swimmers or objects in the water or below the surface. Most important, don't try diving unless you have been taught the proper technique.

The biggest danger involved in water recreation is drowning. **Figure 14.5** shows a technique both swimmers and nonswimmers can use to keep from drowning.

FIGURE 14.5

DROWNING PREVENTION

The technique shown here can help you stay afloat in warm water. It is not recommended for use in cold water because it can cause you to lose body heat faster. In cold water it is better to tread water slowly or float on your back to save energy.

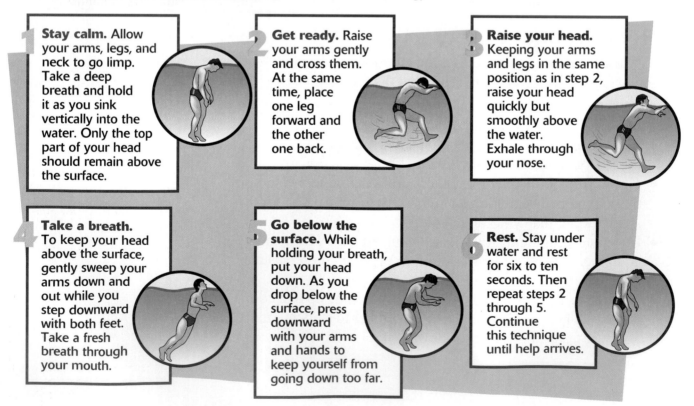

1. **Stay calm.** Allow your arms, legs, and neck to go limp. Take a deep breath and hold it as you sink vertically into the water. Only the top part of your head should remain above the surface.

2. **Get ready.** Raise your arms gently and cross them. At the same time, place one leg forward and the other one back.

3. **Raise your head.** Keeping your arms and legs in the same position as in step 2, raise your head quickly but smoothly above the water. Exhale through your nose.

4. **Take a breath.** To keep your head above the surface, gently sweep your arms down and out while you step downward with both feet. Take a fresh breath through your mouth.

5. **Go below the surface.** While holding your breath, put your head down. As you drop below the surface, press downward with your arms and hands to keep yourself from going down too far.

6. **Rest.** Stay under water and rest for six to ten seconds. Then repeat steps 2 through 5. Continue this technique until help arrives.

Hiking and Camping Safety

Hiking and camping allow you to interact with nature while enjoying physical activity. To avoid injury and illness when hiking and camping, follow these guidelines.

- **Dress for the occasion and for the weather.** Wear thick socks and comfortable, sturdy shoes. Break in your hiking boots or shoes ahead of time—you don't want blisters! You don't want insect bites or stings either, so tuck your pants into your socks, and apply an insect repellent.
- **Check your equipment.** Take along a first-aid kit, a flashlight with extra batteries, a supply of fresh water, and a compass.
- **Know where you are.** Stick to marked hiking trails and specified camping areas.
- **Never camp or hike alone.** Make sure that family members know your schedule and your route. Carry a cell phone or a walkie-talkie in case of an emergency.
- **Be plant smart.** Learn how to identify poison ivy, poison oak, and other poisonous plants so that you can stay away from them.
- **Squelch the flames.** Be sure to extinguish campfires completely. Drench them with water, or smother them with sand or dirt.

Safe camping and hiking require the right equipment.

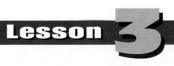 **Lesson 3 Review**

Using complete sentences, answer the following questions on a sheet of paper.

Reviewing Terms and Facts

1. **Vocabulary** Define the term *pedestrian*. Then use it in an original sentence.
2. **Recall** List three rules for safe bicycling.
3. **Restate** What are two things to remember before diving?
4. **Outline** Describe the steps you can take if you think that you are in danger of drowning.

Thinking Critically

5. **Explain** What do you think is meant by the phrase "walk defensively"? Why is this a good rule for pedestrians to follow?
6. **Justify** Why is the buddy system especially important in swimming and hiking?

Applying Health Skills

7. **Communication Skills** Select a sport or other outdoor activity mentioned in this lesson that children could participate in. Create and perform a skit to demonstrate each rule to a class of elementary school children.

Weather Emergencies and Natural Disasters

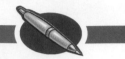

What Are Weather Emergencies?

There are certain emergency situations that no one can prevent. These include **weather emergencies**, or *dangerous situations brought on by changes in the atmosphere.* Common weather emergencies include storms, such as tornadoes, hurricanes, blizzards, and thunderstorms.

The National Weather Service (NWS) monitors the progress of storms and periodically issues bulletins about what is happening. It issues two types of advisories, or reports of advancing storms: watches and warnings. A storm watch is issued when current weather conditions indicate that a storm is likely to develop. If your area is under a storm watch, stay tuned to your radio or television for further advisories, and take steps to prepare for the storm. A storm warning is issued when an actual weather emergency is occurring and people in your area are in immediate danger. In this situation, follow the instructions of the NWS and local officials. Evacuate as quickly as possible if instructed to do so.

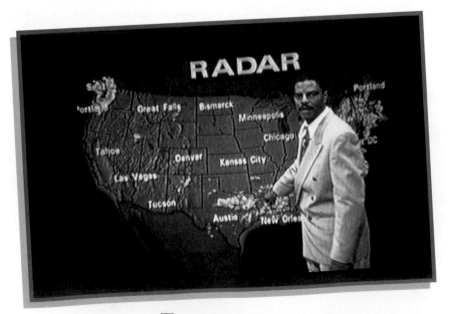

The National Weather Service monitors the progress of storms and weather emergencies.

Tornadoes

States in the Midwest and those that border the Gulf of Mexico have more tornadoes than other regions of the United States. A **tornado** is *a whirling, funnel-shaped windstorm that drops from the sky to the ground.* These storms occur most often in the spring and summer. Of all types of storms, tornadoes can cause the most severe destruction. **Figure 14.6** explains how tornadoes develop.

If a tornado watch is issued for your area, use a battery-powered radio to listen for further updates, and prepare to take shelter. If a tornado warning is issued, take shelter immediately.

- **Where to go.** You'll be safest underground in a cellar or basement. If you can't get underground, go to a windowless interior room or hallway. If you are outdoors, lie in a ditch or flat on the ground. Stay away from trees, cars, and buildings, which could fall on you.
- **What to do.** Cover yourself with whatever protection you can find, such as a mattress or heavy blanket. Then stay where you are. Tornadoes move along a narrow path at about 25 to 40 miles per hour. The storm will pass quickly.

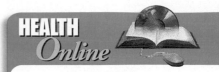

HEALTH Online

Topic: Severe weather

For a link to more information on different types of weather emergencies and natural disasters, go to **health.glencoe.com.**

Activity: Using the information provided at this link, list steps to take in the event of a specific weather emergency or natural disaster.

FIGURE 14.6

HOW A TORNADO DEVELOPS

Winds within the spiral of a tornado often swirl at more than 200 miles per hour. *What should you do if you are outside during a tornado?*

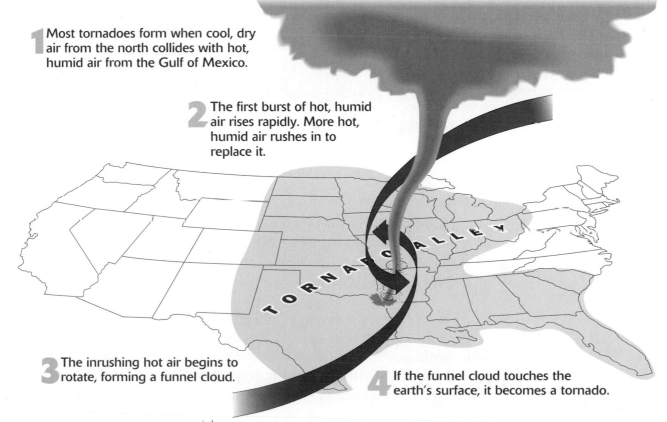

1 Most tornadoes form when cool, dry air from the north collides with hot, humid air from the Gulf of Mexico.

2 The first burst of hot, humid air rises rapidly. More hot, humid air rushes in to replace it.

3 The inrushing hot air begins to rotate, forming a funnel cloud.

4 If the funnel cloud touches the earth's surface, it becomes a tornado.

Hurricanes

People who live along the eastern and southern coastlines of the United States are no strangers to the possibility of hurricanes. A **hurricane** is *a strong windstorm with driving rain that originates at sea.* Each hurricane has a center, called its eye, where weather conditions are calm. A circular cloud mass whirls around the eye, giving the storm its fiercest strength.

Most hurricanes occur in late summer and early fall. Follow these guidelines in the event of a hurricane.

- Board up windows and doors. Bring items such as outdoor furniture and bicycles inside.
- Evacuate immediately if the NWS or local officials advise you to do so.
- If no evacuation is advised, stay indoors. Be prepared for power loss by keeping a working flashlight and battery-powered radio on hand, along with extra batteries for both items.
- Prepare an emergency kit. See **Figure 14.7** for items to include.

FIGURE 14.7

EMERGENCY SUPPLIES KIT

Keep these supplies available in the event of a weather emergency or natural disaster. Your kit should include enough supplies to last your family for three days. If you must evacuate your home, take the supplies plus sturdy walking shoes, money, and any necessary prescription medicines. *Develop personal and family emergency plans to follow in the event of a weather emergency or natural disaster. Maintain an emergency supplies kit similar to the one pictured here.*

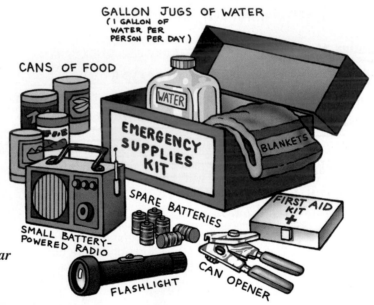

GALLON JUGS OF WATER (1 GALLON OF WATER PER PERSON PER DAY)

CANS OF FOOD

WATER

EMERGENCY SUPPLIES KIT

BLANKETS

SMALL BATTERY-POWERED RADIO

SPARE BATTERIES

FIRST AID KIT

FLASHLIGHT

CAN OPENER

Blizzards and Thunderstorms

A **blizzard** is *a very heavy snowstorm with winds of up to 45 miles per hour.* During a blizzard, stay inside if possible. Keep a flashlight and battery-powered radio on hand, both with extra batteries in case of power loss.

If you are caught outside in a blizzard, keep moving and find shelter as soon as possible. Watch for landmarks along your path to avoid getting lost. Keep your head, nose, mouth, and ears covered. This will help prevent **hypothermia**, or *a sudden and dangerous drop in body temperature.*

Thunderstorms can occur almost anywhere, but they usually cause only minor damage. Nevertheless, you still need to protect yourself, especially from the dangers of lightning. If possible, stay inside or seek shelter during the storm. Be prepared for power loss. Unplug electrical appliances, and avoid using the telephone or running water until the storm has passed. If caught outdoors, squat low to the ground in an open area. Keep away from electric poles and wires, tall trees, water, and metal objects, all of which attract lightning.

Natural Disasters

Nature can be a powerful and even destructive force. This fact becomes all too clear when a natural disaster strikes. A natural disaster is an event caused by nature that results in widespread damage, destruction, and loss. Floods and earthquakes are examples of natural disasters. To prepare for such events, put together an emergency kit of supplies like the one shown in **Figure 14.7.** Store it in a place in your home that is easily accessible.

Floods

Floods can happen almost anywhere at any time. If the NWS issues a flood watch for your area, move valuable items to higher levels of your home, and keep your emergency kit handy. Listen to radio bulletins while you watch for signs of rising water.

A flood warning means that you should evacuate your home, if so advised, and move to higher ground away from rivers, streams, and creeks. Warning of a flash flood, one that can rise suddenly and violently, requires immediate evacuation. In any flood situation, stay tuned to the radio and follow these safety rules.

- Never walk, swim, ride a bike, or drive a car through the water. Drowning is a risk. So is electrocution from downed power lines.
- Drink only bottled water. Floods can pollute the water supply.
- If an evacuation is ordered, return home only after being advised that it is safe to do so.
- Once you return home, throw away contaminated food. Disinfect anything that has come in contact with floodwaters.

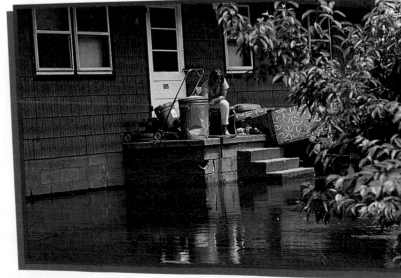

Floods are one type of natural disaster. They may be caused by heavy rainfall or by destruction of dams.

Earthquakes

An **earthquake**, *a violent shaking of the earth's surface,* can be a fearsome natural disaster. It usually is not a single event; after the initial shaking, several **aftershocks**, or *secondary earthquakes,* often occur. You can protect yourself during an earthquake by following the guidelines in **Figure 14.8**.

Although there is no reliable way to predict earthquakes, scientists use the Richter scale to record the amount of ground motion. The Richter scale rates the ground motion on a scale of 1 to 10. The most destructive quakes have a magnitude, or size, of 7 or more.

Hands-On Health

EARTH UNDER PRESSURE

Earthquakes are caused by disturbances to layers of rock underground. This activity will help you understand how rock layers change or break apart when subjected to enough pressure.

WHAT YOU WILL NEED
- paper clip
- 50 sheets of paper
- balloon
- ruler
- pencil

WHAT YOU WILL DO
1. Clip 2 sheets of paper together. Remove the paper clip, and see if it has changed shape. Repeat this procedure using 5, 20, and 50 sheets of paper. Observe the shape of the clip each time.
2. Measure the length of a balloon with a ruler. Then hold one end of the balloon against the ruler and stretch it to $1^1/_2$ times its original length. Release the balloon, and measure it to see if its length has changed. Repeat, stretching the balloon to 2, then $2^1/_2$ times its original length. Measure the balloon and note any changes in its length.

3. Grasp one end of a pencil in each hand so that your knuckles face up. Slide your thumbs toward the middle of the pencil, pushing upward gently to make it bend. Let it go, and see if it returns to its original shape.

IN CONCLUSION
1. What happened to the paper clip and the balloon when they were stretched too far?
2. What do you think would happen if the pencil were bent too far?
3. Why do you think the objects reacted to pressure in the way that they did?
4. From these experiments, what effect do you think pressure has on rock layers?

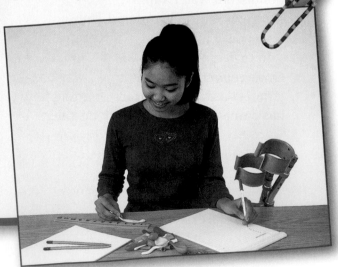

FIGURE 14.8

PROTECTING YOURSELF DURING AN EARTHQUAKE

Falling objects and crumbling buildings cause most injuries and deaths that occur during an earthquake.

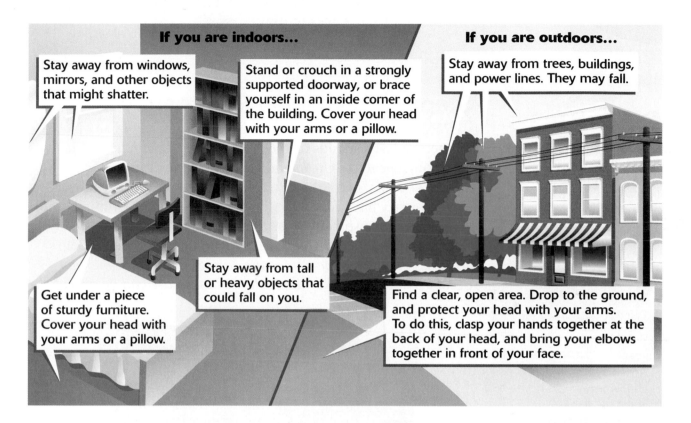

If you are indoors...

Stay away from windows, mirrors, and other objects that might shatter.

Stand or crouch in a strongly supported doorway, or brace yourself in an inside corner of the building. Cover your head with your arms or a pillow.

Get under a piece of sturdy furniture. Cover your head with your arms or a pillow.

Stay away from tall or heavy objects that could fall on you.

If you are outdoors...

Stay away from trees, buildings, and power lines. They may fall.

Find a clear, open area. Drop to the ground, and protect your head with your arms. To do this, clasp your hands together at the back of your head, and bring your elbows together in front of your face.

Lesson 4 Review

Using complete sentences, answer the following questions on a sheet of paper.

Reviewing Terms and Facts

1. **Vocabulary** Define the term *weather emergency.*
2. **Compare** Explain the difference between a storm watch and a storm warning.
3. **Recall** What is a *blizzard*?
4. **Describe** What safety rules should you follow after a flood?
5. **Identify** List two ways to protect yourself if you are indoors during an earthquake and two ways to protect yourself if you are outdoors.

Thinking Critically

6. **Compare and Contrast** How are tornadoes and hurricanes similar? How are they different?
7. **Analyze** Why is it important to be prepared *before* a weather emergency strikes?

Applying Health Skills

8. **Accessing Information** Most communities have civil defense shelters to be used during weather emergencies and natural disasters. Find out where these shelters are in your community. What qualifies a place to serve as a shelter? What have the shelters been used for in the past?

First Aid

Quick Write

On a sheet of paper, describe how you usually treat a minor cut.

LEARN ABOUT...

- steps to take in an emergency.
- how to perform CPR.
- ways to help a person who is choking.
- how to stop severe bleeding.
- treating burns.
- treatments for poisoning, fractures, sprains, and bruises.

VOCABULARY

- first aid
- cardiopulmonary resuscitation (CPR)
- rescue breathing
- abdominal thrust
- chest thrust
- first-degree burn
- second-degree burn
- third-degree burn
- fracture

Steps to Take in an Emergency

People can become injured or ill at any time and in any place. If a person has a serious or life-threatening problem, she or he will need someone to step in and provide emergency care. Time is often critical and may make the difference between life and death. If an emergency has occurred, call 911 or the emergency number in your area, or get someone else to do it. Knowing basic first-aid techniques will enable you to deal with emergencies until help arrives. **First aid** is *the immediate care given to someone who becomes injured or ill until regular medical care can be provided.*

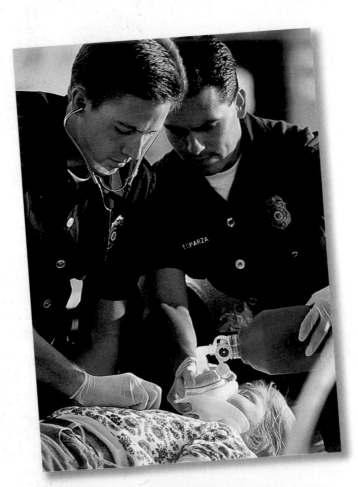

In an emergency, victims should receive professional medical care as soon as possible.

Restoring Breathing and Heartbeat

Suppose that a person's heart stopped pumping, cutting off blood flow to the brain. The victim would fall to the ground and stop breathing normally. In such a situation, a rescuer would check for responsiveness by gently shaking the victim and shouting, "Are you okay?" If the person were unresponsive, she or he might need cardiopulmonary resuscitation until professional help arrives. **Cardiopulmonary resuscitation (CPR)** is *a first aid procedure to restore breathing and circulation.* Only specially trained individuals should give CPR. If other people are around, ask passersby to find someone who has been trained in CPR. The steps involved in CPR are illustrated in **Figure 14.9** and **Figure 14.10** on page 418.

FIGURE 14.9

THE ABCs OF CPR

The first steps of CPR, as recommended by the American Heart Association, are called the ABCs. The procedure illustrated here is used for adults and older children; the procedure for infants and younger children differs somewhat.

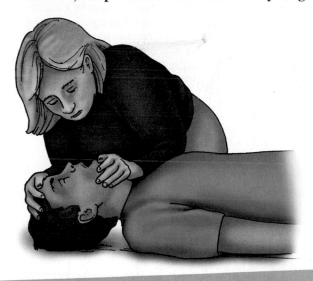
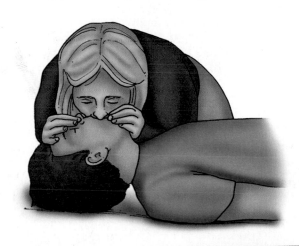

A = Airway
Look inside the victim's mouth. If you can see anything blocking the victim's airway, remove it. Gently roll the person onto his or her back. Tilt the head back as you lift up on the chin. This will open the airway.

B = Breathing
Next look, listen, and feel to find out if the victim is breathing. *Look* for the rise and fall of the chest. Place your ear next to the victim's mouth and nose and *listen* for breathing. *Feel* for the exhaled air on your cheek.

If the person is not breathing normally, perform rescue breathing. **Rescue breathing** is *a first-aid procedure in which someone forces air into the lungs of a person who is not breathing.*

1. Keeping the victim's head and chin in the proper position, pinch the person's nostrils shut.
2. Place your mouth over the victim's mouth, forming a seal. Give two slow breaths, each about 2 seconds long. The victim's chest should rise with each breath.

C = Circulation
Check for signs of circulation. These signs include normal breathing, coughing, or movement. If the victim shows no signs of circulation, start chest compressions (See **Figure 14.10**). If the victim responds (coughs or moves, for example) but is still not breathing normally, continue rescue breathing. Give one breath every 5 seconds.

FIGURE 14.10

PERFORMING THE CPR CYCLES

The full CPR cycle involves chest compressions and rescue breaths.

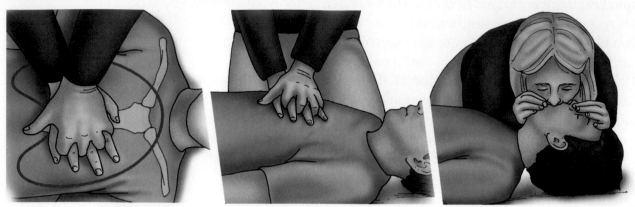

1 To perform chest compressions, kneel next to the victim's chest and position your hands properly. Find a spot on the lower half of the victim's breastbone, right between the nipples. Place the heel of one hand on that point, and interlock your fingers with the fingers of the other hand. Do not allow your fingers to rest on the victim's ribs.

2 Kneel over the victim so that your shoulders are directly over your hands and your elbows are locked. Press straight down quickly and firmly at a rate of about 100 compressions per minute. Allow the victim's chest to spring back between compressions. After every 15 compressions, give the victim two rescue breaths.

3 Complete four continuous cycles of CPR. (This should take about 1 minute.) Check for signs of circulation (normal breathing, coughing, or movement). Continue CPR, checking for signs of circulation every few minutes. If the victim begins to respond, stop chest compressions. If the victim coughs or moves but is still not breathing normally, give one rescue breath every 5 seconds until help arrives.

First Aid for Choking

Choking occurs when a person's airway becomes blocked. Food or accidentally swallowed objects create an obstruction in the airway that prevents air from entering the lungs. If the obstruction is not removed, the person can die within a few minutes.

Recognizing the signs of choking is the first step toward helping the victim. The person may clutch his or her neck, which is the universal sign for choking. The victim may also cough, gag, have high-pitched noisy breathing, or turn blue in the face. If someone appears to be choking but can cry, speak, or cough forcefully, do not attempt first aid. A strong cough can remove the object from the airway. However, if the airway is completely blocked, the victim will need immediate first aid.

For an adult or older child who is choking, use abdominal thrusts. **Abdominal thrusts** are *quick, inward and upward pulls into the diaphragm to force an obstruction out of the airway.* To perform this procedure, place your arms around the victim from the back, and use both hands to pull inward and upward. **Figure 14.11** gives a detailed illustration of how to perform abdominal thrusts. If you begin to choke when you are alone, use your fist and hand to perform the procedure on yourself. This will expel the object blocking your airway. You can also try to press your abdomen forcefully against the back or arm of a chair.

If an infant is choking, hold the infant facedown on your forearm, and hit the area between the shoulder blades five times with the heel of your other hand. Then turn the infant over and perform chest thrusts instead of abdominal thrusts. **Chest thrusts** are *quick presses into the middle of the breastbone to force an obstruction out of the airway.* **Figure 14.11** illustrates these procedures.

✓ Reading Check

Understand sentence structure. Find sentences in Figure 14.10 that do not begin with a subject. What kind of sentences are they? What parts of speech begin each sentence?

FIGURE 14.11

HELPING SOMEONE WHO IS CHOKING

Follow the choking rescue procedures shown here to help someone who is choking. *Why do you think first aid for a choking adult or child is different from first aid for a choking infant?*

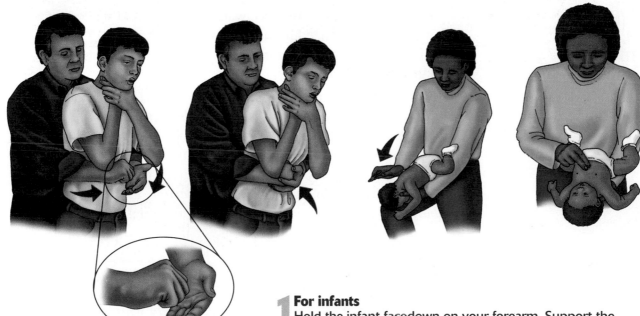

For adults and children

1 Place the thumb side of your fist against the person's abdomen, just above the navel. Grasp your fist with your other hand.

2 Give quick, inward and upward thrusts. Continue until the person coughs up the object. If the person becomes unconscious, call 911 or the local emergency number and begin CPR.

For infants

1 Hold the infant facedown on your forearm. Support the child's head and neck with your hand and point the head downward so that it is lower than the chest. With the heel of your hand, give the child five blows between the shoulder blades. If the object is not dislodged, proceed to chest thrusts (step 2).

2 Turn the infant over onto his or her back, supporting the head with one hand. With two or three fingers, press into the middle of the child's breastbone—directly between and just below the nipples—five times. Repeat steps 1 and 2 until the object is dislodged or the infant begins to breathe or cough. Make sure the infant is checked by a health care professional. If the infant becomes unconscious, call 911 or the local emergency number if you have not already done so.

FIGURE 14.12

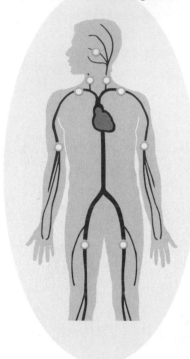

The dots show the pressure points for the main arteries. *How should you press on a pressure point?*

Stopping Severe Bleeding

Severe bleeding is a serious emergency. To stop or slow blood loss, use the following methods.

- Cover the wound with a clean cloth and press firmly against the wound with your hand. If the cloth becomes soaked with blood, add a second cloth. Do not remove the first one, however.
- Elevate the wound above the level of the heart to slow blood flow. If you think that the injury involves a broken bone, do not move it.
- If bleeding does not stop, apply pressure to a main artery leading to the wound. Squeeze the artery against the bone. **Figure 14.12** shows where these arteries are and the points where you should apply pressure.

Once the bleeding has stopped, cover the wound with a clean cloth to prevent infection. Stay with the victim until medical help arrives.

Treating Burns

If you accidentally spill hot water on your hand while you are cooking, you may need immediate medical attention. The following list explains the characteristics of the different types of burns and how to treat them:

- **First-degree burn.** *A burn in which only the outer layer of skin is burned and turns red* is called a **first-degree burn**. This type of burn can be treated by flushing the burned area with cold water (not ice) for at least 15 minutes. It should then be wrapped loosely in a clean, dry dressing. A sunburn is a type of a first-degree burn.
- **Second-degree burn.** *A moderately serious burn in which the burned area blisters* is known as a **second-degree burn**. Treatment of minor second-degree burns calls for flushing the affected area with cold water (not ice) and elevating the burned area. Wrap the cooled burn loosely in a clean, dry dressing. Do not pop blisters or peel loose skin.
- **Third-degree burn.** *A very serious burn in which all layers of the skin are damaged* is a **third-degree burn**. Such burns are usually caused by fire, electricity, or chemicals, and they require immediate medical attention. Call 911 or an ambulance at once. Do not attempt to remove burned clothing. Apply cold water (not ice) to the affected area, unless the burn was caused by electricity. In that case, just apply a dry, sterile dressing. While you are waiting for medical help to arrive, keep the victim still, and have her or him sip fluids.

Other Emergencies

You can be prepared to help out in all kinds of emergencies or accidental injuries. Always look, listen, and feel for signs of circulation. Then follow these steps for each type of emergency:

- **Poisoning.** Call 911 or a poison control center and follow the instructions you receive. Save the container of the substance responsible for the poisoning. Check the victim's breathing and pulse once a minute. Perform rescue breathing if needed. Keep the victim warm and still until help arrives.

- **Broken bones.** *A break in a bone* is called a **fracture**. Because moving broken bones can cause further injury, have the person remain still until medical assistance arrives. A trained helper can then immobilize the fractured bone.

- **Sprains and bruises.** Tell the victim not to use the injured body part. Then use the R.I.C.E. formula: **R**est, **I**ce, **C**ompression, and **E**levation.

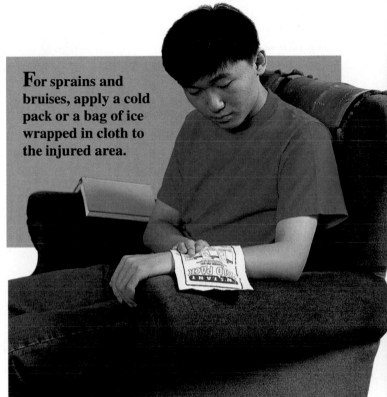

For sprains and bruises, apply a cold pack or a bag of ice wrapped in cloth to the injured area.

Lesson 5 Review

Using complete sentences, answer the following questions on a sheet of paper.

Reviewing Terms and Facts

1. **Vocabulary** Define the term *first aid.*
2. **Restate** What are the signs of circulation?
3. **Recall** Define the terms *abdominal thrust* and *chest thrust.* When would you use abdominal thrusts on a victim, and when would you use chest thrusts?
4. **Identify** List and describe the three levels of burns.

Thinking Critically

5. **Explain** Infants and toddlers are at especially high risk for choking. Make a list of foods that should not be given to very young children. Then list the kinds of toys and household objects that should be kept out of a child's reach.
6. **Hypothesize** Why do you think it is important to save the container of the substance responsible for a poisoning?

Applying Health Skills

7. **Communication Skills** With one or two classmates, create a skit about one of the following: CPR, the choking rescue, severe bleeding, burns, or poisoning. Use dialogue, narrative, and movement to demonstrate correct and effective first-aid procedures.

When Storms Spin Out Of

The storm lasted just a few seconds, but the damage was terrible. A black funnel cloud tore through town, turning 20 blocks of homes and offices in La Plata, Maryland, to rubble. The howling winds stripped bark from trees and sent roofs and cars soaring into the air.

After the twister passed, people slowly emerged into the silence that followed. They wandered, dazed, through the fallen trees, splintered wood, and broken glass. Deborah McClain, who had found shelter in her family's basement, was safe but scared. "I went upstairs, and all you could see was the sky," she says. "The roof was gone. The beds had gone out the window."

Similar scenes stretched across the eastern half of the United States on April 28, 2002. A powerful batch of tornadoes and thunderstorms hit states from Missouri to New York. Six people were killed and more than 100 were injured. At the northern edge of the storm, in Wisconsin and Minnesota, heavy snow fell.

Picking Up the Pieces

Nearly 1,000 tornadoes hit the United States each year. Unlike hurricanes, which usually can be tracked days in advance, the storms that lead to tornadoes often erupt suddenly. Although the National Weather Service issued a severe thunderstorm warning, a tornado warning did not go out until just eight minutes before the twister hit La Plata.

The storms in April 2002 were unusually severe; the system unleashed 48 tornadoes. According to the National Weather Service, the twister that hit La Plata was an F5 on the Fujita Tornado Damage Scale. An F5 rating is the worst, with fierce winds of up to 318 miles an hour. Only 1 in 1,000 tornadoes are that powerful. ■

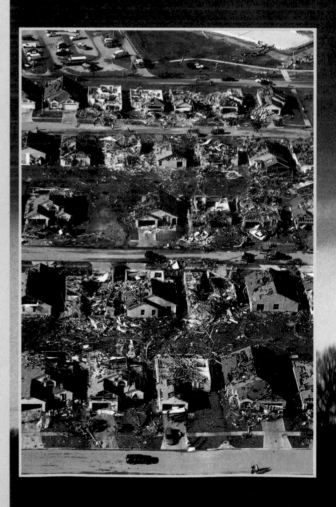

Control

How a Tornado Forms

A giant storm system made of moisture and wind is called a supercell. It is formed when warm air, rising upward, crashes into a current of downward-moving cool air. The collision can cause the wind to start spinning and form a tornado. The center of a tornado is called a vortex. It sucks in air and carries it upward. Most tornadoes are black from picking up dust.

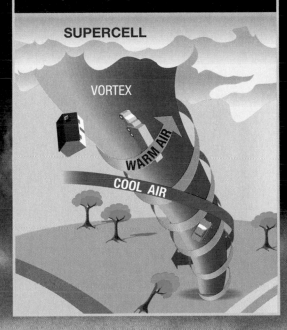

SUPERCELL

VORTEX

WARM AIR

COOL AIR

TIME TO THINK...

About Tornado Safety

Using your textbook and other reliable print and online resources, make a list of tornado-safety strategies, as well as items to include in an emergency supplies kit. Then, create a comic strip showing how one family uses the listed strategies and emergency supplies to stay safe before and during a tornado.

ESCAPING A FIRE SAFELY

Model

In the event of a household fire, it is crucial to escape immediately. Read about how one teen made sure that she and her family could escape a home fire safely.

Lynette learned about the importance of fire safety plans in health class. She and her parents drew a floor plan of their home. They identified escape routes from each room, practiced how to exit using these routes, and discussed alternatives in case their planned route was blocked. Finally, they agreed on a meeting point outside. Twice a year Lynette's family has a fire drill to rehearse how to escape safely and quickly.

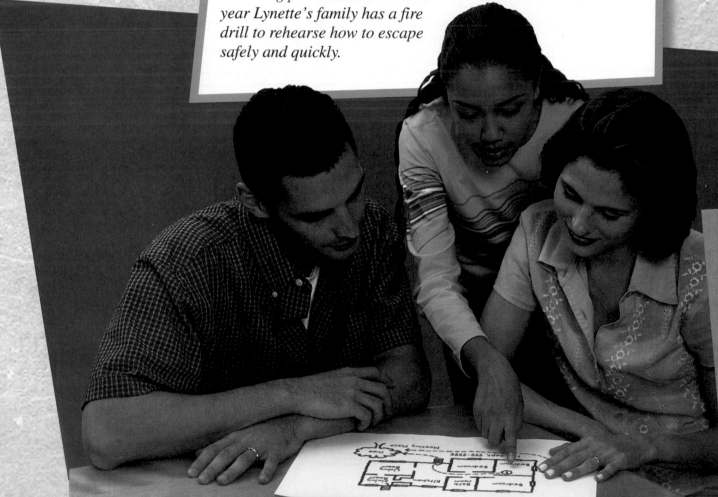

Practice

Below is a sample floor plan of a home. It shows all rooms, doors, windows, hallways, and stairs. In groups of three or four, create a fire escape plan for this home. First copy the floor plan onto a sheet of paper. Then use a colored marker to draw the best route out of the home from each room. This should be the easiest, most direct route. Use a different-colored marker to show an alternate route out of each room. This route may be longer but will allow a person to escape if the first route is blocked by flames. Remember that every escape route should begin in a bedroom. Compare your finished plans with those of the rest of the class. Did you agree on the best routes to use? Why should every family have a fire escape plan?

Apply/Assess

Using poster board and a marker, draw a floor plan of your home. If your home has two floors, use the top half of the poster board for the upper floor and the bottom half for the ground floor. Remember to include all doors, windows, and hallways. Indicate where there are staircases or ladders between floors.

Identify two escape routes from each room, using two different-colored markers—one for the best route and the other for an alternate route. Also identify a safe family meeting point outside. Share your plan with a partner and explain why each family member should learn this plan.

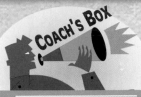

COACH'S BOX

Practicing Healthful Behaviors

The following measures can help to ensure your safety in case of a fire in your home.
- Learn the steps of escaping safely from fire, and share them with family members.
- Make a fire escape plan, including alternate escape routes.
- Hold fire drills regularly.

Self-✓Check

Does my fire safety plan
- show all rooms as well as all doors, windows, hallways, and stairs?
- include at least two possible escape routes from each room?
- include a safe meeting point outside?

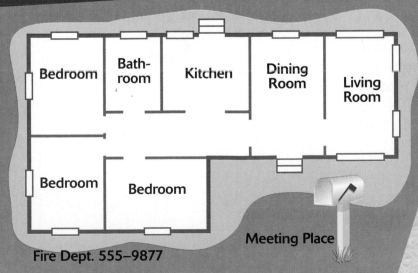

After You Read

Use your completed Foldable to review the information on the accident chain.

FOLDABLES
Study Organizer

Reviewing Vocabulary and Concepts

On a sheet of paper, write the numbers 1–6. After each number, write the term from the list that best completes each sentence.

- accident chain
- electrical overload
- smoke alarms
- step stool
- hazards
- accidental injury

Lesson 1

1. In order to prevent accidents and injuries, you must learn to spot _____, or potential sources of danger.
2. A(n) _____ is an injury caused by unexpected events.
3. Changing an unsafe habit can break the _____.

Lesson 2

4. Too many appliances plugged into an outlet can cause a fire from _____.
5. Using a(n) _____ to access items that are out of reach can help prevent falls.
6. To provide a strong line of defense against injuries or deaths from home fires, install _____ on every level of the house.

On a sheet of paper, write the numbers 7–13. Write *True* or *False* for each statement below. If the statement is false, change the underlined word or phrase to make it true.

Lesson 3

7. When bicycling, ride in the <u>opposite</u> direction of motor traffic.
8. <u>Pedestrians</u> almost always have the right-of-way when sharing the road with motorists.
9. Before crossing the street, pedestrians need to look <u>right, left, and right again</u>.

Lesson 4

10. A whirling, funnel-shaped windstorm that drops from the sky to the ground is known as a <u>tornado</u>.
11. Most hurricanes occur in <u>late spring and early summer</u>.
12. Hypothermia is a sudden and dangerous <u>rise</u> in body temperature.
13. Secondary earthquakes are known as <u>aftershocks</u>.

Lesson 5

On a sheet of paper, write the numbers 14–17. After each number, write the letter of the answer that best completes each statement.

14. Rescue breathing involves
    a. giving quick breaths every 30 seconds.
    b. placing your mouth over the victim's mouth.
    c. performing chest thrusts.
    d. applying pressure to arteries.
15. When performing CPR, one should
    a. perform chest compressions along with rescue breathing.
    b. use abdominal thrusts.
    c. apply pressure to arteries.
    d. use the R.I.C.E. formula.
16. Abdominal thrusts or chest thrusts will help a person who is
    a. bleeding.
    b. poisoned.
    c. bruised.
    d. choking.

17. When treating a fracture, do all of the following, except

    a. have the victim remain still.

    b. call 911.

    c. move the injured part.

    d. wait for help.

Thinking Critically

Using complete sentences, answer the following questions on a sheet of paper.

18. List Explain at least five precautions you could take to protect younger children from accidental injuries in your home.

19. Analyze Why is it important for as many people as possible to learn CPR?

Standardized Test Practice

Reading & Writing

Read the paragraphs below and then answer the questions.

The violent winds of a tornado whirl at speeds of up to 318 miles per hour. In the event that you are caught in a tornado, there are some steps you can take to avoid being injured.

Take shelter indoors as soon as a tornado warning is posted. If possible, hide in a basement or cellar. Crouch down under a table on the side of the room from which the tornado is approaching. If you are in a building with no basement or cellar, try to move to the center of the building, such as the hallway of a school or office building. Lie flat under a table or bed and stay away from windows. If you are outside, lie facedown in order to give yourself some protection against flying debris.

1. The words *violent* and *whirl* in the first paragraph

    A warn readers about tornadoes.

    B describe the damage of tornadoes.

    C describe what tornadoes look like.

    D explain the causes of tornadoes.

2. Which of the following best describes the organization of the second paragraph?

    A presenting the steps to take in the event of a tornado

    B comparing different ways to avoid danger during a tornado

    C explaining how to find help if a tornado strikes

    D ranking safety steps in order of importance

3. List the steps for responding to a fire or other emergency in your school.

CHAPTER 15

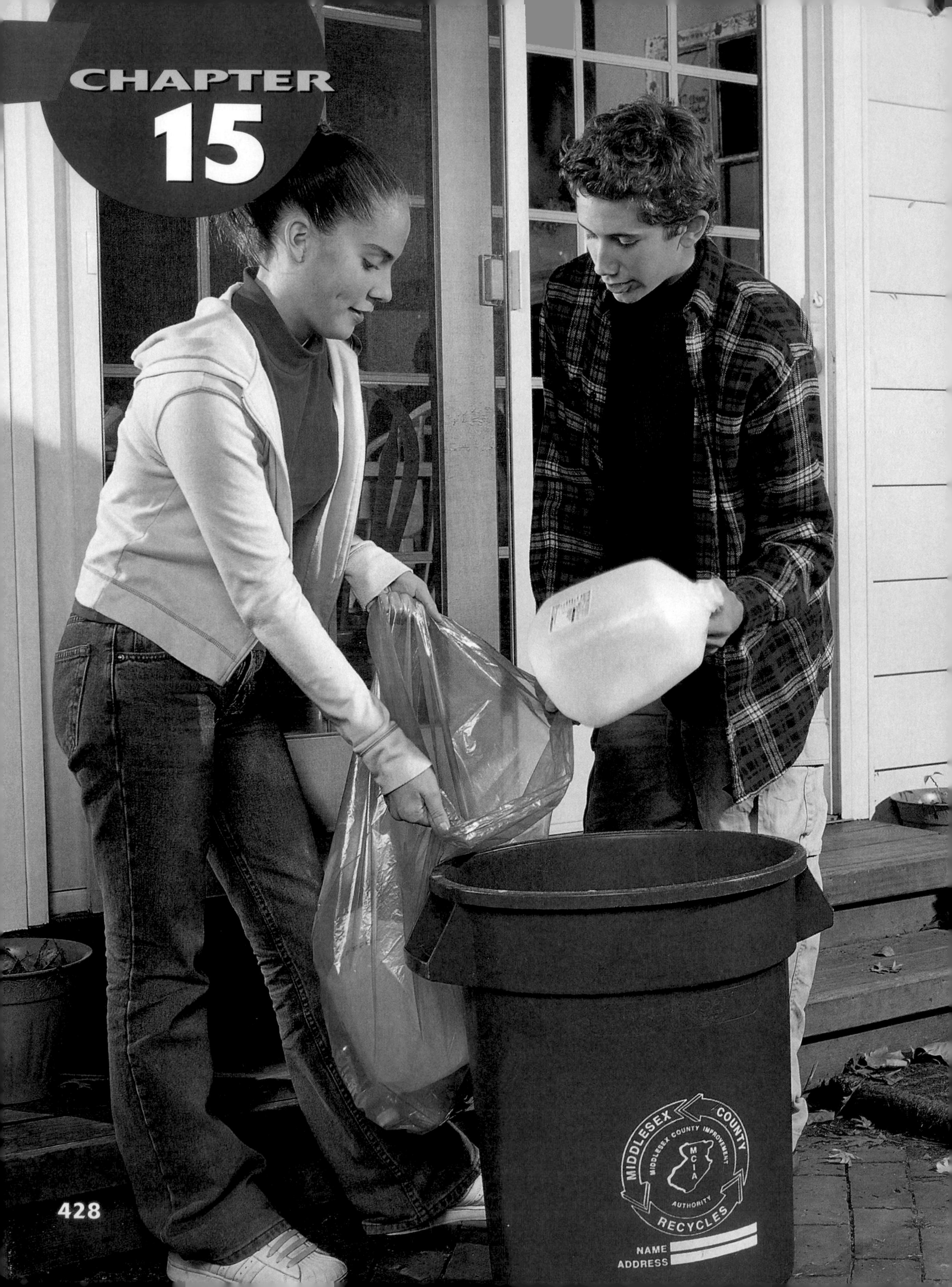
MIDDLESEX COUNTY
MIDDLESEX COUNTY IMPROVEMENT AUTHORITY
MCIA
RECYCLES
NAME
ADDRESS

The Environment and Your Health

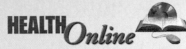
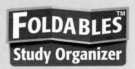

FOLDABLES™
Study Organizer

Before You Read

Make this Foldable to record the main ideas on the causes and effects of air pollution. Begin with a plain sheet of 8½" × 11" paper or a sheet of notebook paper.

Step 1

Fold the sheet of paper from top to bottom, leaving a 2" tab at the bottom.

Step 2

Fold in half from side to side.

Step 3

Unfold the paper once. Cut along the center fold line of the top layer only. This makes two tabs.

Step 4

Label the tabs as shown.

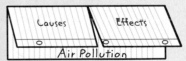

Causes   Effects
Air Pollution

As You Read

Under the appropriate tab, Take notes on the causes and effects of air pollution.

How Pollution Affects Your Health

Quick Write

List at least five places and/or objects that you associate with the word *environment*. Are your associations mostly positive or negative? Why do you think this is so?

LEARN ABOUT...

- the causes and effects of different types of pollution.
- which hazardous products may be in your home.

VOCABULARY

- pollution
- fossil fuel
- acid rain
- ozone
- smog
- groundwater
- sewage
- biodegradable
- landfill
- hazardous waste

Pollution and the Environment

Your environment consists of all the living and nonliving things around you. The people you see, your school, and your neighborhood are all part of your local environment. Your environment also includes plants, animals, air, and water.

The global environment includes forests, mountains, rivers, and the world's populations. Everyone is a citizen of the global environment, so it is everyone's job to take care of it. Humans often act in ways that harm the environment. **Pollution**, *dirty or harmful substances in the environment,* is the result of some of these actions. Pollution can pose a threat to your health.

Air Pollution

Most air pollution comes from the burning of **fossil fuels**, which are *the oil, coal, and natural gas used to provide energy.* This energy provides heat and electricity in homes and powers factories and motor vehicles. The gases that cars release into the air, including exhaust, are called automobile emissions. Because cars are one of the most widespread sources of air pollution, car manufacturers are now required to make a certain percentage of vehicles that meet strict environmental standards. Many industries and factories must also meet emission control standards.

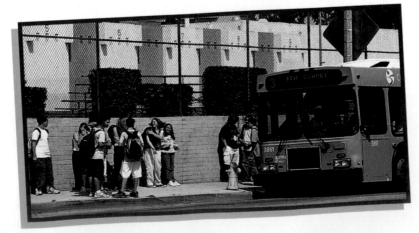

Each person who uses mass transit instead of driving keeps about 75 pounds of harmful emissions out of the air per year.

When fossil fuels burn, they release gases into the atmosphere. The gases mix with moisture in the atmosphere to form **acid rain**, which is *rain that is more acidic than normal.* Over time, acid rain can contaminate freshwater supplies. It can also harm forests by changing the chemistry of the soil.

Some gases formed by burning fossil fuels combine to produce **ozone**, *a special form of oxygen.* Ozone at ground level is a major component of smog. **Smog** is *a yellow-brown haze that forms when sunlight reacts with air pollution.* Both ozone and smog can cause many kinds of respiratory problems. In addition, people who have asthma, emphysema, or bronchitis may be affected. To help protect people from these health problems, the media and state and local agencies report the Air Quality Index regularly. See **Figure 15.1.**

Although ozone is harmful at ground level, it is very helpful in the atmosphere. Miles above the earth's surface, a protective layer of ozone shields the earth from harmful rays of the sun. In the 1970s, scientists discovered that the ozone layer was breaking down. They determined that chemicals used in homes and industries damage the ozone layer. Without its protection, people are more likely to develop skin cancer and eye damage. This is why it's especially important to protect yourself from the sun's rays with sunscreen and sunglasses. Many countries are working to help restore the ozone layer by banning the harmful substances that damage it.

Reading Check
Identify supporting details. The topic sentence of a paragraph tells the main idea. Find the supporting details for each main idea in the paragraphs on these two pages.

FIGURE 15.1

The Air Quality Index

The Air Quality Index is a guide to how safe the air is each day. *How might air quality affect the health of a community?*

Air Quality Index	Levels of Health Concern	Risk
0–50	Good	Little or none
51–100	Moderate	People who are unusually sensitive to pollution may have some symptoms. They should consider limiting the time they spend being active outdoors.
101–150	Unhealthy for sensitive groups	People who are sensitive to pollution and those who engage in outdoor physical activity are likely to have symptoms. They should limit the time they spend being active outdoors.
151–200	Unhealthy	Everyone may experience health effects and should spend only limited time being active outdoors. Sensitive people and those who engage in physical activity should avoid being outdoors for long periods.
201–300	Very unhealthy	Everyone, especially children and the elderly, may experience serious health effects and therefore should limit outdoor activity. Sensitive people and those who engage in physical activity should avoid all outdoor activity.
301–500	Hazardous	Everyone should avoid all outdoor activity.

Source: United States Environmental Protection Agency (EPA)

Water Pollution

Pollution is also a threat to all water sources. About 40 percent of the nation's rivers, lakes, and coastal waters are now too severely polluted to swim or fish in. Pollution is especially dangerous in drinking water supplies. The water that people drink comes from one of two sources. The first is surface water, such as lakes and rivers. The other is **groundwater**, or *water that collects under the earth's surface.*

Pollution can make water undrinkable. For example, lead-contaminated water can damage the brain, kidneys, nervous system, and red blood cells. Another source of water pollution is **sewage**—*garbage, detergents, and other household wastes washed down drains.* These waste materials can spread diseases such as hepatitis A, typhoid fever, and cholera.

Oil spills and chemical waste from factories also pollute water sources and cause health risks. Wastes that have been illegally dumped into waterways are another threat to water quality. Most water pollution, however, is not due to sewage, spills, or illegal dumping. Instead, it comes from chemicals and wastes on land. Runoff—rainwater or snowmelt—runs over the land and through the ground. As it moves, it picks up pollution such as pesticides, crop fertilizers, and wastes from towns and cities. It carries these chemicals to surface water or groundwater supplies.

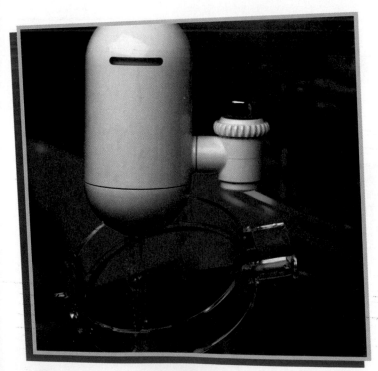

Filtration devices like the one shown here can remove some harmful substances from drinking water.
What are some other ways to keep water safe?

Solid Waste

Along with air and water, land is a natural resource that is threatened by pollution. In the United States alone, each person produces an average of 4.4 pounds of garbage per day. Some of this waste is **biodegradable**, or *easily broken down in the environment.* Biodegradable material such as newspaper or your leftovers from dinner would slowly disintegrate if you left it outside, where it would be exposed to air and rain. Nonbiodegradable material, such as plastics, would not disintegrate in these conditions.

Much of the trash Americans produce goes into **landfills**, *huge, specially designed pits where waste materials are dumped and buried.* Landfills must be carefully sealed so that toxic chemicals do not leak out and contaminate the groundwater. This means that biodegradable materials cannot easily break down inside a landfill. Some people choose to set up a compost pile—a place where biodegradable waste can break down naturally—in their yards or in other outdoor spots. Leaves, grass, shredded newspaper, some types of food, and other items can be composted.

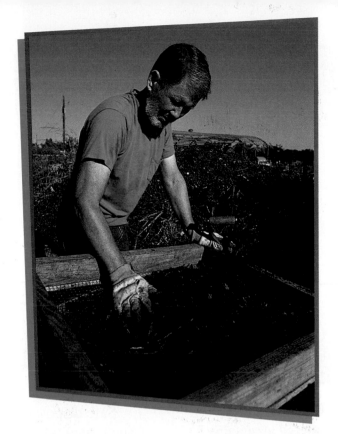

Biodegradable waste can be composted, or allowed to break down outdoors. After a few months it turns into a material that is good for fertilizing gardens. *How does composting help the environment?*

Hands-On Health

A Throwaway Society

Find out how much solid waste students and staff in your school produce in a day and in a year.

WHAT YOU WILL NEED
- pencil or pen
- paper

WHAT YOU WILL DO
1. One member of the class will ask the custodial staff how many bags of trash were thrown out on the previous school day. This would include trash collected from classrooms, restrooms, and the cafeteria.
2. Send one or two representatives to the attendance office. Find out how many students and staff members were present on the previous school day.

3. Divide the number of filled trash bags by the total number of students and staff members in attendance. The result will be the average amount of trash each person produced.
4. Multiply the number of filled trash bags by the number of school days in a year. The resulting figure is an estimate of the amount of trash your school contributes to the nation's solid wastes each year.

IN CONCLUSION
1. Brainstorm ways for students to reduce the amount of waste they produce. Prepare a list of your ideas and findings.
2. Post your list on a school bulletin board or in some other public spot.

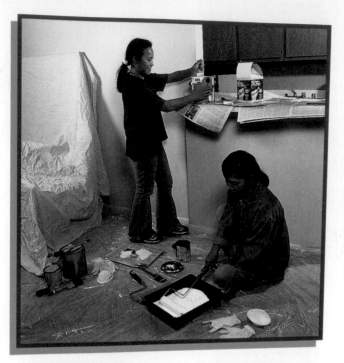

Hazardous Wastes

Some wastes produced by modern industry fall into the special category of hazardous wastes. **Hazardous wastes** are *human-made liquid, solid, or sludge wastes that may endanger human health or the environment.* Hazardous wastes can come from a variety of sources, including detergents, paint, batteries, plastics, fabrics, pesticides, and some types of insulation. These wastes can threaten individual and community health in several ways. People who are exposed to them can experience damage to the brain, liver, and kidneys. They can also develop diseases such as cancer. Hazardous wastes that are released into the environment can damage forests and farmlands.

Until 1978 it was considered acceptable for the paint used in homes to contain lead, a hazardous substance. *Why might lead-based paint still pose a health problem in some homes?*

Safe disposal of hazardous wastes requires special handling. Such materials must be stored in facilities where they will not be released into the environment. Materials in your home that may require special handling include batteries, paints, bleach, drain cleaner, motor oil, antifreeze, nail polish remover, and oven cleaner. If you need to dispose of any hazardous materials in your home, do not throw them out with the regular trash. Instead, contact your local health department or environmental agency to find out how to get these materials safely into hazardous waste storage.

Lesson 1 Review

Using complete sentences, answer the following questions on a sheet of paper.

Reviewing Terms and Facts

1. **Vocabulary** Define *pollution.*
2. **Recall** Name three fossil fuels. Explain how they are related to acid rain.
3. **Vocabulary** What is *smog?*
4. **Explain** How is ozone helpful in the earth's atmosphere?
5. **Identify** List three sources of water pollution.

Thinking Critically

6. **Evaluate** Identify the advantages and disadvantages of landfills.
7. **Synthesize** Explain how failure to dispose properly of hazardous wastes could cause drinking water to become contaminated.

Applying Health Skills

8. **Accessing Information** Exposure to pesticides and lead paint can harm health. Use reliable online and print resources to find out ways to avoid these harmful environmental conditions.

Protecting the Environment

Preventing Pollution

No individual can solve all the problems that threaten the environment. Fortunately, the governments of many nations are working to fight and prevent pollution. The **Environmental Protection Agency (EPA)**, for example, is *an agency of the United States government that is committed to protecting the environment.* Another government agency working in this area is the **Occupational Safety and Health Administration (OSHA)**, *a branch of the U.S. Department of Labor whose job is to ensure the protection of American workers.* OSHA's responsibilities include creating and enforcing regulations to lessen hazards, such as carcinogens, in workplaces.

Reducing Air Pollution

When you join in the effort to reduce air pollution, you help to protect your own health as well as that of others in your community. You can reduce air pollution in a number of ways.

- **Carpool or take public transportation.**
- **Ride your bike or walk to nearby activities.**
- **Remain tobacco free.** Tobacco smoke pollutes the body and the environment.
- **Plant trees.** Green plants filter the air as they take in carbon dioxide to make food. Trees also provide shade that cools buildings and reduces the need for air conditioning.

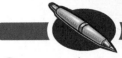

LEARN ABOUT...

- what you can do to keep air and water clean.
- how you can reduce solid wastes.
- ways in which you can conserve energy and water.

VOCABULARY

- Environmental Protection Agency (EPA)
- Occupational Safety and Health Administration (OSHA)
- recycle
- nonrenewable resources
- conservation

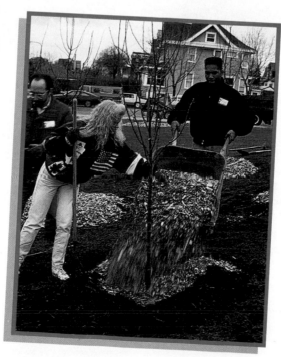

Planting trees helps clean the air, improving your physical health. *How might the beauty of trees also affect your mental health?*

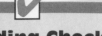

Reading Check

Make your own judgments. Use information from the text to evaluate how well you think your family or community manages waste.

Preventing Water Pollution

Keeping drinking water free of pollution protects everyone's physical health. Clean water does not carry the pathogens that cause disease. Clean water also supports agriculture and wildlife. Many people seek out the nation's lakes, streams, rivers, and oceans when they want to relax. Water that's safe for fun and recreation adds to everyone's mental and social health.

Do your part to protect or improve water quality. Use the ideas in **Figure 15.2** to keep water clean and safe.

Managing Waste

The solid waste people throw away ends up in landfills, causing environmental problems later. You can cut down on the amount of trash that you create by using the "Three Rs"—reduce, reuse, and recycle. **Figure 15.3** on the next page explains how the Three Rs can help the environment.

FIGURE 15.2

Clean Water

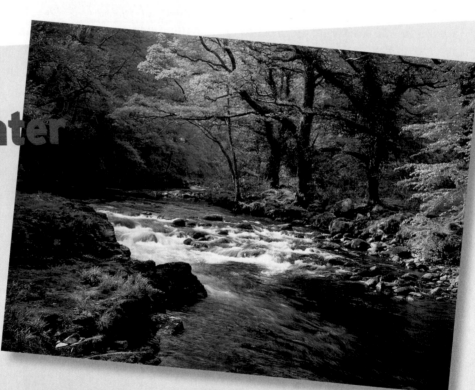

Many of your everyday actions can affect the environment. *Which of these tips could you put to use today?*

- **Reduce toxic runoff by walking pets in grassy or undeveloped areas.** Pick up pet wastes from sidewalks or other pavement.

- **Use biodegradable soaps, detergents, and bleaches.** These products break down more easily in the environment.

- **Help protect oceans, streams, rivers, and lakes.** Don't litter. Pick up litter left by others.

- **Dispose of chemicals properly.** Follow manufacturers' instructions for discarding toxic substances. Never dump such products down drains or sewers.

FIGURE 15.3

REDUCE, REUSE, RECYCLE

By reducing, reusing, and recycling, you can keep garbage out of landfills.
How do you practice the Three Rs in your household?

Strategy	Definition	Tips
Reduce	Cut down on the amount of trash you throw away	Use your own baskets or cloth bags to carry groceries home. Avoid using disposable plates, cups, tableware, or napkins. Buy products that come in bulk—they use less packaging per individual item. Do not buy items with unnecessary packaging.
Reuse	Find a practical use for an item you might otherwise throw away	Wash plastic food containers and use them for storage. Reuse plastic or paper bags when you go grocery shopping, or use them as trash bags. Donate good clothing that you no longer wear to charity. Use worn-out clothing as cleaning rags. When possible, have broken items repaired rather than throw them away.
Recycle	*Change an item in some way so that it can be used again*	Find out which items are recycled in your area, how they should be separated from other garbage, and how they are collected. When companies make new products from recycled materials, they use up less natural resources. In turn, when you buy recycled products, you are continuing to help the environment.

Many types of household waste can be recycled. These guidelines will help you prepare some common household items for recycling:

- **Aluminum.** Rinse cans and other aluminum items, such as pie pans and food trays. Crush them to save space.
- **Cardboard.** Flatten cardboard boxes and tie them together.
- **Glass.** Find out which types of glass (clear, green, and brown) your recycling center accepts. Rinse bottles and jars well, and discard caps or lids.
- **Paper.** Most types of paper and newspapers can be recycled, as long as the paper is clean, dry, and does not include any plastic components.
- **Plastic.** Many plastic items, such as water and milk containers, soda bottles, and some plastic packaging, can be recycled. Find out which types of plastics your recycling center accepts and how to prepare them for recycling.

According to the EPA, recycling kept 57 million tons of material out of landfills and incinerators (special furnaces that burn solid wastes) in 1996.

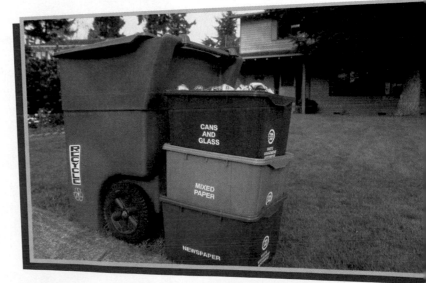

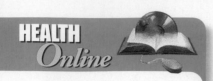
Conserving Energy and Water

Many natural materials are **nonrenewable resources**, *substances that cannot be replaced once they are used.* Fossil fuels are an example of nonrenewable resources. Once a barrel of oil is burned, it is gone forever. Some natural resources are renewable. The earth's supply of water, for example, is constantly being replenished through the water cycle. However, the amount of freshwater is limited. To protect nonrenewable resources and those in limited supply, everyone needs to practice **conservation**, or *the saving of resources.*

Guidelines for Home Conservation

The actions that you and your family take in your home have an impact on the environment. Here are some ways for you to help conserve oil, natural gas, coal, and freshwater.

Heating and cooling

- During cold weather, wear an extra layer of clothing instead of turning up the thermostat. Keep the thermostat at about 68°F.
- Seal air leaks around doors, windows, and electric sockets to prevent heat from escaping.
- Keep doors and windows closed during the air-conditioning season, and keep air conditioning at about 78°F.

Lighting and appliances

- Replace traditional lightbulbs with compact fluorescent bulbs, which use less energy and last longer.
- Switch off lights when you leave a room.
- Turn off televisions, radios, computers, and other appliances when they are not in use.
- Choose fuel-efficient appliances.

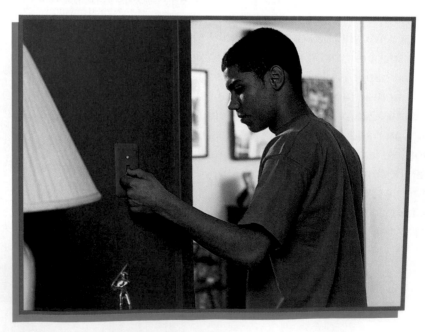

Turning off lights when you leave a room is an easy way to conserve energy. *How else can you conserve electricity in your home?*

Cooking

- When cooking a small amount of food, use a microwave or toaster oven instead of a conventional oven.
- Don't preheat a conventional oven for longer than necessary.
- Don't open the oven door unnecessarily while cooking.

Water

- Wash clothes in warm or cold, not hot, water.
- Accumulate a full load before washing laundry or running the dishwasher.
- Fix leaky faucets.
- Never let water run unnecessarily. For example, running the water while brushing your teeth uses 4.5 gallons of water per minute.
- Install low-flow showerheads.
- Fill plastic bottles with water, seal them, and place them in your toilet tank. They'll keep your tank from filling completely and will save up to a gallon of water per flush.

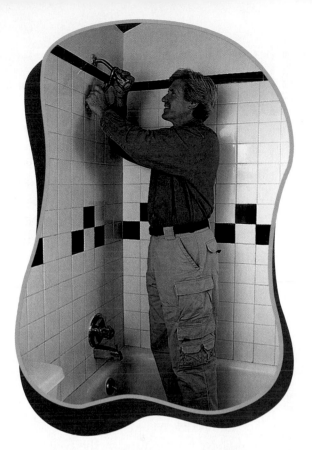

Everyone can take measures to conserve water.

Lesson 2 Review

Using complete sentences, answer the following questions on a sheet of paper.

Reviewing Terms and Facts

1. **Vocabulary** What are the functions of the *Environmental Protection Agency* and the *Occupational Safety and Health Administration*?
2. **Identify** List three ways to help reduce air pollution and three ways to help prevent water pollution.
3. **Vocabulary** Define the term *recycle*. How does recycling help people manage waste?
4. **Explain** Why are fossil fuels considered nonrenewable resources?

Thinking Critically

5. **Explain** List five ways in which people waste water, energy, or other resources each day. Why do you think people practice these behaviors? What might motivate individuals and communities to conserve?
6. **Evaluate** Suppose that you want to paint your room. Decide which one of the following paints you would buy, and explain your reasoning. Paint A does the job quickly and gives off fumes, and the label instructs you to wear rubber gloves. Paint B is environmentally safe, costs twice as much, and takes longer to use. Explain your decision.

Applying Health Skills

7. **Accessing Information** Research alternative energy sources, such as solar and wind power. Report on the advantages and disadvantages of each.

Clean

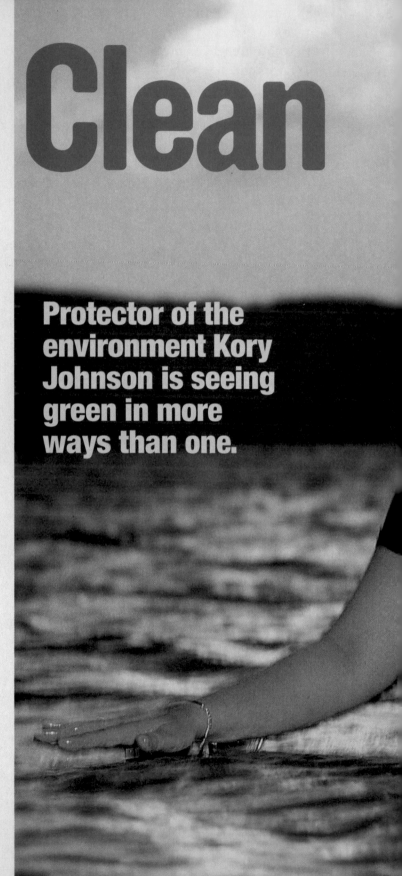

Protector of the environment Kory Johnson is seeing green in more ways than one.

Nobody helps protect the environment for the money. However, that's what Kory Johnson got—and plenty of it—when she won the Goldman Environmental Prize. Kory was studying at a friend's house when she received the telephone call telling her that she had won the $100,000 prize. "I was shocked," she says. "They said, 'You can't tell anybody.'" Kory kept the secret until the next month. That's when she was officially honored for 10 years of environmental work. At 19, Kory was the youngest of that year's six winners.

Kory's environmental work was inspired by a tragedy: Her 16-year-old sister Amy died of a heart defect that she developed before birth. The family discovered that Amy's heart trouble could have been caused by the contaminated well water that her mother drank during her pregnancy. "That's when we decided to turn something bad into something good," says Kory.

Starting Young

Even though she was only nine at the time, Kory recruited some of her school friends and founded Children for a Safe Environment. This nationwide movement against pollution now boasts 350 members. Kory has since spear-headed several projects with the group, and she received a presidential Environmental Youth Award for her efforts.

Not everyone has been so supportive, however. A teacher once called Kory a "radical," issuing this warning: "If you keep this up, no college is going to accept you." Such criticism doesn't stop Kory. While she ponders what to do with her prize money, she's hard at work on her latest issue, environmental discrimination. This happens when industries pollute poor or minority communities, whose members don't have the political power to fight back. Each time she tackles a new cause, she's reminded of how it all started. "I try to hold on to the memories I have of Amy," Kory says. "I know she would be proud of me." ■

Living

"There's still so much more I want to do," says Kory Johnson, who plans to donate $10,000 of her prize to an environmental cause.

TIME TO THINK...

About Protecting the Environment

In a small group, conduct research on a local or national environmental issue, using reliable online and print resources. Then, present your findings to the class in the form of a news broadcast. One group member should act as the "anchor," with others delivering information as reporters in the field. For visuals, create large, easy-to-understand informational and statistical charts, or posters featuring images that relate to the theme of the news report.

THE THREE Rs: REDUCE, REUSE, RECYCLE

Model

The decisions people make about what to buy affect the amounts and types of waste that are left over. One day David and a few of his friends stopped at the deli to buy something to eat. As they were waiting in line, David realized that each of them had chosen single-serving bags of chips and cans of soda. "Hey," he said, "it's really wasteful to buy all this stuff. All of this packaging is going to end up in the trash. Why don't we get a 2-liter bottle and a big bag of chips to share? It'll cost less, and we won't have to throw out a lot of junk."

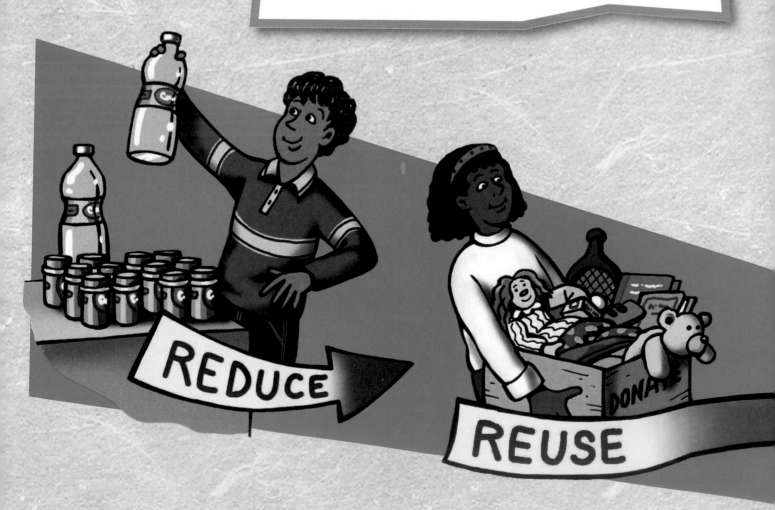

REDUCE

REUSE

Practice

Becky is moving, and her friend Sarita is helping her pack. By the end of the day there is a huge pile of things that Becky plans to get rid of—books, toys, clothes, and other items. "Well," Becky says, "I'd better start packing these up for the trash. Mom says that she wants this stuff out of here." To Sarita it seems wasteful to throw these things out. Many of the items are still in good condition. How can Sarita use her advocacy skills to persuade Becky to find a better use for her old belongings and to protect the environment?

Apply/Assess

Become an advocate for the global environment. As a class, brainstorm a list of places in your homes where you could reduce, reuse, or recycle resources or energy. Individually, sketch each of these places on a separate sheet of paper. Under each illustration, list specific measures for your family to follow. For example, under your illustration of the kitchen sink, you might write: "Don't leave water running while doing the dishes—use a dishpan instead." Bind your pages into a book, and show the book to the members of your household. Use your advocacy skills to encourage them to take care of the environment. After you've shown your book to everyone, leave it out at home as a reminder to reduce, reuse, and recycle.

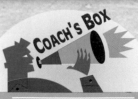

COACH'S BOX

Advocacy

The skill of advocacy asks you to
- take a clear stand on an issue.
- persuade others to make healthy choices.
- be convincing.

Self-√Check

- Have I sketched all the places in my home where I can help to protect the environment?
- Did I use my advocacy skills to make the members of my household aware of how to reduce, reuse, and recycle?
- Are the suggestions in my book realistic and practical?

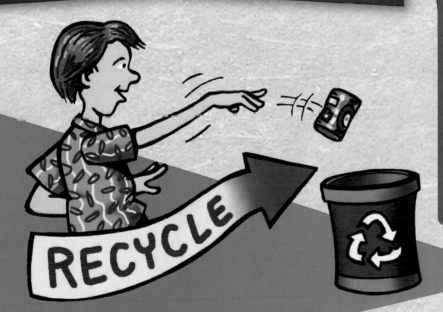

After You Read

Use your completed Foldable to review the information on causes and effects of air pollution.

FOLDABLES™
Study Organizer

Reviewing Vocabulary and Concepts

On a sheet of paper, write the numbers 1–9. After each number, write the term from the list that best completes each sentence.

- landfills
- biodegradable
- acid rain
- sewage
- runoff
- groundwater
- fossil fuels
- hazardous wastes
- ozone

Lesson 1

1. The burning of _____ causes most air pollution.
2. When gases mix with moisture in the atmosphere, the result is _____.
3. _____, a special form of oxygen, is a major component of smog.
4. Drinking water comes from either surface water or _____.
5. _____ includes garbage, detergents, and other household wastes washed down drains.
6. Pollution from pesticides and fertilizers can be carried to the water supply by _____.
7. _____ materials are easily broken down in the environment.
8. Solid wastes are commonly deposited in huge, specially designed pits known as _____.

9. Human-made liquid, solid, or sludge wastes that may endanger human health or the environment are known as _____.

Lesson 2

On a sheet of paper, write the numbers 10–14. After each number, write the letter of the answer that best completes each statement.

10. Green plants filter the air as they take in
    a. ozone.
    b. oxygen.
    c. smog.
    d. carbon dioxide.
11. Using plastic containers to store food instead of discarding them is an example of
    a. reducing.
    b. reusing.
    c. recycling.
    d. renewing.
12. All of the following items can be recycled, *except*
    a. paper with plastic components.
    b. glass bottles.
    c. cardboard boxes.
    d. aluminum cans.
13. Each of the following is an example of a nonrenewable resource, *except*
    a. natural gas.
    b. coal.
    c. water.
    d. oil.
14. To conserve energy, replace traditional light bulbs with ones that are
    a. incandescent.
    b. fluorescent.
    c. ultraviolet.
    d. infrared.

Thinking Critically

Using complete sentences, answer the following questions on a sheet of paper.

15. **Relate** Could the destruction of forests in another part of the world affect the environment where you live? Explain.

16. **Explain** How can conserving energy help keep the environment clean?

17. **Apply** Think of a product that is available in disposable and reusable forms. Develop a list of reasons to persuade people to use the reusable version of this product.

18. **Analyze** Why is everyone responsible for protecting the environment?

Career Corner

Public Health Specialist Would you like to help people stay healthy and safe in their environment? If so, consider a career as a public health specialist. These professionals plan ways to help protect and improve the health of a community. To work in this field you'll need a four-year college degree in public health. You'll also need excellent communication skills. Find out more about this and other health careers by clicking on Career Corner at health.glencoe.com.

Standardized Test Practice

Reading & Writing

Read the paragraphs below and then answer the questions.

Garbage. It smells bad, it looks terrible, and there is too much of it. Many of you might not want to think about this problem. Reconsider this type of thinking and give your attention to building a recycling center here in Dutton.

What is in the garbage that we toss out every day? It includes paper, glass, metal, plastic, rubber, food waste, and yard waste. More than 60 percent of this trash can be recycled. This would help conserve resources such as trees, water, and energy. Recycling would improve the pollution problem caused by the mountains of garbage that are accumulating in our landfills. Our valuable land would not have to be given up to create more landfills. Do something good for the earth and for the town by supporting recycling.

1. Which phrase or sentence from the passage represents an opinion?

   (A) Many of you might not want to think about this problem.

   (B) It includes paper, glass, metal, plastic, rubber, food waste, and yard waste.

   (C) This would help conserve resources such as trees, water, and energy.

   (D) Our valuable land would not have to be given up to create more landfills.

2. The last sentence of the passage appeals to the reader's sense of

   (A) humor.

   (B) responsibility.

   (C) justice.

   (D) anger.

3. Write an editorial urging people to support an issue that is important to you.

Glossary

The Glossary contains all the important terms used throughout the text. It includes the **boldfaced** terms that appear in the "Vocabulary" lists at the beginning of each lesson and in text and art.

The Glossary lists the term, the pronunciation (in the case of difficult terms), the definition, and the page on which the term is defined. The pronunciations here and in the text follow the system outlined below. The column headed "Symbol" shows the spelling used in this book to represent the letter sounds.

PRONUNCIATION KEY

Sound	As In	Symbol	Example
ă	h*a*t, m*a*p	a	abscess (AB·ses)
ā	*a*ge, f*a*ce	ay	atrium (AY·tree·uhm)
a	c*a*re, th*ei*r	eh	capillaries (KAP·uh·lehr·eez)
ä, ŏ	f*a*ther, h*o*t	ah	biopsy (BY·ahp·see)
ar	f*ar*	ar	cardiac (KAR·dee·ak)
ch	*ch*ild, mu*ch*	ch	barbiturate (bar·BI·chuh·ruht)
ĕ	l*e*t, b*e*st	e	vessel (VE·suhl)
ē	b*ea*t, s*ee*, cit*y*	ee	acne (AK·nee)
er	t*er*m, st*ir*, p*urr*	er	nuclear (NOO·klee·er)
g	*g*row	g	malignant (muh·LIG·nuhnt)
ĭ	*i*t, h*y*mn	i	bacteria (bak·TIR·ee·uh)
ī	*i*ce, f*i*ve	y	benign (bi·NYN)
		eye	iris (EYE·ris)
j	pa*g*e, fun*gi*	j	cartilage (KAR·tuhl·ij)
k	*c*oat, loo*k*, *ch*orus	k	defect (DEE·fekt)
ō	*o*pen, c*oa*t, gr*ow*	oh	aerobic (ehr·OH·bik)
ô	*or*der	or	organ (OR·guhn)
ȯ	fl*aw*, *a*ll	aw	palsy (PAWL·zee)
oi	v*oi*ce	oy	goiter (GOY·ter)
ou	*ou*t	ow	fountain (FOWN·tuhn)
s	*s*ay, ri*c*e	s	dermis (DER·mis)
sh	*sh*e, atten*ti*on	sh	conservation (kahn·ser·VAY·shuhn)
ŭ	c*u*p, fl*oo*d	uh	bunion (BUHN·yuhn)
u	p*u*t, w*oo*d, c*ou*ld	u	pulmonary (PUL·muh·nehr·ee)
ü	r*u*le, m*o*ve, y*ou*	oo	attitudes (AT·i·toodz)
w	*w*in	w	warranty (WAWR·uhn·tee)
y	*y*our	yu	urethra (yu·REE·thruh)
z	say*s*	z	hormones (HOR·mohnz)
zh	plea*s*ure	zh	transfusion (trans·FYOO·zhuhn)
ə	*a*bout, c*o*llide	uh	asthma (AZ·muh)

A

Abdominal thrust A quick inward and upward pull into the diaphragm to force an obstruction out of a person's airway. (page 418)

Abstinence Not participating in unsafe behaviors or activities. (page 16 and page 232)

Abuse (uh·BYOOS) The physical, emotional, or mental mistreatment of another person. (page 258)

Accidental injuries Injuries caused by unexpected events. (page 394)

Acid rain Rain that is more acidic than normal. (page 431)

Addiction (uh·DIK·shuhn) A psychological or physical need for a drug or other substance. (page 282)

Adolescence (a·duhl·EH·suhns) The stage of life between childhood and adulthood, usually beginning somewhere between the ages of 11 and 15. (page 154)

Adrenaline (uh·DRE·nuhl·in) A hormone that increases the level of sugar in your blood, thereby giving your body extra energy. (page 199)

Advertising Messages designed to cause consumers to buy a product or service. (page 133)

Advocacy Taking action in support of a cause. (page 41)

Aerobic (ehr·OH·bik) **exercise** Rhythmic, non-stop, moderate-to-vigorous activity that requires large amounts of oxygen and works the heart. (page 57)

Aftershock Secondary earthquake. (page 414)

AIDS (acquired immunodeficiency syndrome) A deadly disease that interferes with the body's ability to fight infection. (page 348)

Alcohol A drug created by a chemical reaction in some foods, especially fruits and grains. (page 304)

Alcoholism An illness characterized by a physical and psychological need for alcohol. (page 308)

Allergen (AL·er·juhn) A substance that causes an allergic reaction. (page 365)

Allergy An extreme sensitivity to a substance. (page 365)

Alveoli (al·VEE·oh·ly) Fragile, elastic, microscopic air sacs in the lungs where carbon dioxide from body cells and fresh oxygen from the air are exchanged. (page 276)

Amphetamine (am·FE·tuh·meen) A strong stimulant drug that speeds up the nervous system. (page 310)

Anabolic steroids (a·nuh·BAH·lik STIR·oydz) Synthetic compounds that cause muscle tissue to develop at an abnormally high rate. (page 79)

Anaerobic (AN·ehr·oh·bik) **exercise** Intense physical activity that requires little oxygen but involves short bursts of energy. (page 57)

Angioplasty (AN·jee·uh·plas·tee) A surgical procedure in which an instrument with a tiny balloon attached is inserted into an artery to clear a blockage. (page 378)

Anorexia nervosa (a·nuh·REK·see·uh nuhr·VOH·suh) An eating disorder in which a person has an intense fear of weight gain and starves herself or himself. (page 110)

Antibodies Proteins that attach to antigens, keeping them from harming the body. (page 338)

Antigens (AN·ti·jenz) Substances that send the immune system into action. (page 338)

Antihistamine A medication that relieves the symptoms of allergic reactions by suppressing the production of histamines. (page 366)

Anxiety disorder A disorder in which intense anxiety or fear keeps a person from functioning normally. (page 203)

Arteriosclerosis (ar·tir·ee·oh·skluh·ROH·sis) A group of disorders that causes a thickening and hardening of the arteries. (page 376)

Artery A type of blood vessel that carries blood away from the heart to all parts of the body. (page 64)

Arthritis (ar·THRY·tuhs) A disease of the joints marked by painful swelling and stiffness. (page 382)

Assault A physical attack or a threat of an attack for the purpose of inflicting bodily injury. (page 252)

Glossary

Assertive Willing to stand up for yourself in a firm but positive way. (page 323)

Asthma (AZ·muh) A chronic respiratory disease that causes air passages to become narrow or blocked, making breathing difficult. (page 367)

Astigmatism (uh·STIG·muh·tiz·uhm) An eye condition in which images are distorted, causing objects to appear wavy or blurry. (page 128)

Atherosclerosis (a·thuh·roh·skluh·ROH·sis) A condition that occurs when fatty substances build up on the inner lining of arteries. (page 376)

Bacteria Tiny one-celled organisms that live nearly everywhere. (page 333)

Battery The beating, hitting, or kicking of another person. (page 259)

Benign (bi·NYN) Not cancerous. (page 370)

Binge eating disorder An eating disorder in which a person repeatedly eats large amounts of food at one time. (page 110)

Biodegradable Easily broken down in the environment. (page 432)

Blizzard A very heavy snowstorm with winds of up to 45 miles per hour. (page 412)

Blood pressure The force of blood pushing against the walls of the blood vessels. (page 66)

Body composition The proportions of fat, bones, muscle, and fluid that make up body weight. (page 69)

Body language A type of nonverbal communication that includes posture, gestures, and facial expressions. (page 217)

Body Mass Index (BMI) A way to assess your body size, taking your height and weight into account. (page 108)

Body system A group of organs that work together to carry out related tasks. (page 168)

Brain The command center, or coordinator, of the nervous system. (page 314)

Bronchi (BRAHNG·ky) Two tubes that branch from the trachea; one tube leads to each lung. (page 278)

Bronchodilator (brahng·koh·DY·lay·tuhr) A medication that relaxes the muscles around the bronchial air passages. (page 369)

Bulimia nervosa (boo·LEE·mee·uh ner·VOH·suh) An eating disorder in which a person repeatedly eats large amounts of food and then purges. (page 110)

Bully Someone who uses threats, taunts, or violence to intimidate people who appear helpless. (page 256)

Calorie (KA·luh·ree) A unit of heat that measures the energy available in foods. (page 97)

Cancer A disease that occurs when abnormal cells grow out of control. (page 370)

Capillary A type of blood vessel that provides body cells with blood and connects arteries with veins. (page 64)

Carbohydrates (kar·boh·HY·drayts) The starches and sugars that provide energy. (page 88)

Carbon monoxide (KAR·buhn muh·NAHK·syd) A colorless, odorless, poisonous gas produced when tobacco burns. (page 274)

Carcinogen (kar·SI·nuh·juhn) A substance in the environment that causes cancer. (page 372)

Cardiopulmonary resuscitation (CPR) A first-aid procedure to restore breathing and circulation. (page 417)

Cartilage A type of connecting tissue that allows joints to move easily, cushions bones, and supports soft tissues, such as those in the nose and ear. (page 60)

Cell The basic unit of life. (page 168)

Central nervous system (CNS) The brain and the spinal cord. (page 314)

Character The way in which you think, feel, and act. (page 40)

Chemotherapy (kee·moh·THEHR·uh·pee) The use of powerful drugs to destroy cancer cells. (page 373)

Chest thrust A quick press into the middle of the breastbone to force an obstruction out of a person's airway. (page 419)

Chlamydia (kluh·MI·dee·uh) A bacterial STD that may affect the reproductive organs, urethra, and anus. (page 347)

Cholesterol (kuh·LES·tuh·rawl) A waxy substance used by the body to build cells and make other substances. (page 91)

Chromosomes (KROH·muh·sohmz) Threadlike structures that carry the codes for inherited traits. (page 170)

Chronic (KRAH·nik) Present continuously or on and off over a long period of time. (page 365)

Circulatory system The group of organs and tissues that transport essential materials to body cells and remove their waste products. (page 64)

Cirrhosis (suh·ROH·suhs) Scarring and destruction of liver tissue. (page 305)

Colon (KOH·luhn) A storage tube for solid wastes. (page 105)

Communicable (kuh·MYOO·ni·kuh·buhl) **disease** A disease that can be spread to a person from another person, an animal, or an object. (page 332)

Communication An exchange of thoughts, feelings, and beliefs among people. (page 216)

Comparison shopping Accessing information, comparing products, evaluating their benefits, and choosing products that offer the best value. (page 137)

Compromise To give up something in order to reach a solution that satisfies everyone. (page 227)

Conditioning Training to get into shape. (page 78)

Conflict A disagreement between people with opposing viewpoints. (page 30 and page 244)

Conflict resolution Finding a solution to a disagreement or preventing it from becoming a larger conflict. (page 30)

Consequences The results of actions. (page 13)

Conservation The saving of resources. (page 438)

Consumer (kuhn·SOO·mer) Anyone who buys products and services. (page 132)

Contagious period The length of time that a particular disease can be spread from person to person. (page 342)

Cool-down Gentle exercises that let your body adjust to ending a workout. (page 71)

Coping skills Ways of dealing with and overcoming problems. (page 201)

Criteria (kry·TIR·ee·uh) Standards on which to base your decisions. (page 33)

Culture The beliefs, customs, and traditions of a specific group of people. (page 10)

Cumulative (KYOO·myuh·luh·tiv) **risks** Related risks that increase in effect with each added risk. (page 14)

 D

Dandruff A flaking of the outer layer of dead skin cells on the scalp. (page 125)

Decibel The unit for measuring the loudness of sound. (page 130)

Decision making The process of making a choice or solving a problem. (page 31)

Dehydration The excessive loss of water from the body. (page 77)

Deliberate injury An injury that results when one person intentionally harms another. (page 253)

Depressant (di·PRE·suhnt) A drug that slows down the body's functions and reactions, including heart and breathing rates. (page 311)

Depression A mood disorder involving feelings of hopelessness, helplessness, worthlessness, guilt, and extreme sadness that continue for periods of weeks. (page 204)

Dermis (DER·mis) The skin's inner layer, which contains blood vessels, nerve endings, hair follicles, sweat glands, and oil glands. (page 122)

Diabetes (dy·uh·BEE·teez) A disease that prevents the body from converting food into energy. (page 380)

Diaphragm (DY·uh·fram) Large, dome-shaped muscle below the lungs that expands and relaxes to produce breathing. (page 278)

Digestion (dy·JES·chuhn) The process by which the body breaks down food into smaller components that can be absorbed by the bloodstream and sent to each cell in your body. (page 102)

Glossary

Digestive system A group of organs that work together to break down foods into substances that your cells can use. (page 102)

Disease Any condition that interferes with the proper functioning of your body or mind. (page 332)

Distress Stress that prevents you from doing what you need to do or that causes you discomfort. (page 198)

Drug A substance other than food that changes the structure or function of the body or mind. (page 300)

Drug abuse The use of a drug for nonmedical purposes. (page 309)

Earthquake A violent shaking of the earth's surface. (page 414)

Eating disorder An extreme eating behavior that can lead to serious illness or even death. (page 110)

Electrical overload A dangerous situation in which too much electrical current flows along a single circuit. (page 398)

Embryo (EM·bree·oh) The developing organism from fertilization to about the eighth week of development. (page 169)

Emotions Feelings such as love, joy, or fear. (page 194)

Empathy The ability to identify and share another person's feelings. (page 192)

Emphysema (em·fuh·ZEE·muh) A disease that destroys alveoli. (page 276)

Endocrine (EN·duh·kruhn) **system** Glands throughout the body that regulate body functions. (page 155)

Endorsement (in·DAWR·smuhnt) A statement of approval. (page 133)

Endurance (in·DUR·uhnts) The ability to perform vigorous physical activity without getting overly tired. (page 56)

Environment (en·VY·ruhn·ment) All the living and nonliving things that surround you. (page 9)

Environmental Protection Agency (EPA) An agency of the United States government that is committed to protecting the environment. (page 435)

Epidermis (e·puh·DER·mis) The outermost layer of skin. (page 122)

Eustress (YOO·stress) Stress that can help you to accomplish goals. (page 198)

Evaluate To determine the quality of. (page 11)

Excretion (ek·SKREE·shuhn) The process by which the body gets rid of waste materials. (page 104)

Excretory (EK·skruh·tohr·ee) **system** The system that removes wastes from the body and controls water balance. (page 104)

Exercise Physical activity that is planned, structured, and repetitive and that improves or maintains personal fitness. (page 54)

Family The basic unit of society. (page 220)

Fatigue Extreme tiredness. (page 200)

Fats Nutrients that supply energy, keep the skin healthy, and promote normal growth. (page 89)

Fertilization (fuhr·tuhl·uh·ZAY·shuhn) The joining of a male sperm cell and a female egg cell to form a new human life. (page 164)

Fetus (FEE·tuhs) The developing organism from the end of the eighth week until birth. (page 169)

Fiber The part of grains, fruits, and vegetables that the body cannot break down. (page 90)

First aid The immediate care given to someone who becomes injured or ill until regular medical care can be provided. (page 416)

First-degree burn A burn in which only the outer layer of skin is burned and turns red. (page 420)

Fitness The ability to handle the physical work and play of everyday life without becoming tired. (page 54)

Flammable Able to catch fire easily. (page 398)

Flexibility The ability to move joints fully and easily. (page 57)

Fluoride (FLAWR·eyed) A substance that helps prevent tooth decay. (page 120)

Follicles (FAH·li·kuhlz) Small sacs in the dermis that produce hair. (page 122)

Food Guide Pyramid A guide for making healthful daily food choices. (page 95)

Fossil fuel The oil, coal, and natural gas used to provide energy. (page 430)

Fracture A break in a bone. (page 421)

Fraud Deliberate deceit or trickery. (page 134)

Frequency With regard to physical fitness, the number of days you work out each week. (page 72)

Friendship A relationship between people who like each other and who have similar interests and values. (page 226)

Fungi (FUHN·jy) Primitive life forms, such as molds or yeasts, that cannot make their own food. (page 333)

Gang A group of people who associate with one another to take part in criminal activity. (page 254)

Generic (juh·NEHR·ik) **products** Products sold in plain packages at lower prices than brand name products. (page 137)

Genes The basic units of heredity. (page 170)

Genital herpes (JEN·i·tuhl HER·peez) A viral STD that produces painful blisters in the genital area. (page 347)

Genital (JEN·i·tuhl) **warts** Growths or bumps in the genital area caused by certain types of the human papillomavirus (HPV). (page 347)

Germs Organisms that are so small that they can be seen only through a microscope. (page 332)

Gonorrhea (gah·nuh·REE·uh) A bacterial STD that affects the mucous membranes of the body, particularly in the genital area. (page 347)

Groundwater Water that collects under the earth's surface. (page 432)

Gynecologist (gy·nuh·KAH·luh·jist) A doctor who specializes in the female reproductive system. (page 167)

Hallucinogen A drug that distorts moods, thoughts, and senses. (page 311)

Hate crime An illegal act against someone just because he or she is a member of a particular group. (page 253)

Hazard A potential source of danger. (page 394)

Hazardous waste Human-made liquid, solid, or sludge waste that may endanger human health or the environment. (page 434)

Head lice Parasitic insects that live on the hair shaft and cause itching. (page 125)

Health A combination of physical, mental/emotional, and social well-being. (page 4)

Health insurance A plan in which a person pays a set fee to an insurance company in return for the company's agreement to pay some or all medical expenses. (page 144)

Health maintenance organization (HMO) A health insurance plan that contracts with selected physicians and specialists to provide medical services. (page 144)

Heart and lung endurance The measure of how effectively your heart and lungs work during moderate-to-vigorous physical activity or exercise. (page 56)

Heart attack A serious condition that occurs when the blood supply to the heart slows or stops, causing damage to the heart muscle. (page 376)

Hepatitis (he·puh·TY·tis) An inflammation of the liver characterized by yellowing of the skin and the whites of the eyes. (page 343)

Heredity (huh·RED·i·tee) The passing on of traits from biological parents to children. (page 9)

Histamine (HIS·tuh·meen) Chemical in the body that causes the symptoms of an allergic reaction. (page 366)

HIV (human immunodeficiency virus) The virus that causes AIDS. (page 348)

Homicide (HAH·muh·syd) The killing of one human being by another. (page 252)

Hormones (HOR·mohnz) Chemical substances produced in certain glands that help to regulate the way your body functions. (page 154)

Glossary

Hurricane A strong windstorm with driving rain that originates at sea. (page 412)

Hygiene Cleanliness. (page 352)

Hypertension (hy·per·TEN·shuhn) A condition in which blood pressure stays at a level that is higher than normal. (page 378)

Hypothermia A sudden and dangerous drop in body temperature. (page 412)

Illegal drugs Substances that it is against the law for people of any age to manufacture, possess, buy, or sell. (page 309)

Immune (i·MYOON) **system** A combination of body defenses made up of cells, tissues, and organs that fight off pathogens. (page 336)

Immunity The body's ability to resist the pathogens that cause a particular disease. (page 340)

Individual sports Physical activities you can take part in by yourself or with another person, without being part of a team. (page 75)

Infancy (IN·fuhn·see) The first year of life. (page 173)

Infection A condition that occurs when pathogens enter the body, multiply, and damage body cells. (page 333)

Inflammation The body's response to injury or disease resulting in a condition of swelling, pain, heat, and redness. (page 337)

Influenza (in·floo·EN·zuh) A communicable disease characterized by fever, chills, fatigue, headache, muscle aches, and respiratory symptoms. (page 342)

Infomercial (IN·foh·mer·shuhl) A long TV commercial whose main purpose seems to be to present information rather than to sell a product. (page 133)

Inhalant (in·HAY·luhnt) A substance whose fumes are breathed in to produce mind-altering sensations. (page 311)

Insulin (IN·suh·lin) A hormone produced in the pancreas that regulates the level of glucose in the blood. (page 380)

Intensity With regard to physical fitness, how much energy you use when you work out. (page 72)

Interpersonal communication The sharing of thoughts and feelings between two or more people. (page 29)

Intoxicated (in·TAHK·suh·kay·tuhd) Drunk. (page 307)

Joint Place where two or more bones meet. (page 59)

Kidneys The organs that filter water and waste materials from the blood. (page 105)

Landfill A huge, specially designed pit where waste materials are dumped and buried. (page 433)

Ligament A type of connecting tissue that holds bones in place at the joints. (page 60)

Liver The body's largest gland, which secretes a liquid called bile that helps to digest fats. (page 104)

Long-term goal A goal that you plan to reach over an extended length of time. (page 37)

Lymphatic (lim·FA·tik) **system** A secondary circulatory system that helps the body fight pathogens and maintain its fluid balance. (page 338)

Lymphocytes (LIM·fuh·syts) Special white blood cells in the lymph. (page 338)

Mainstream smoke The smoke that a smoker inhales and then exhales. (page 290)

Malignant (muh·LIG·nuhnt) Cancerous. (page 370)

Managed care Health plans that emphasize preventive medicine and work to control the cost and maintain the quality of health care. (page 144)

Media The various methods for communicating information. (page 11)

Mediation (mee·dee·AY·shuhn) Resolving conflicts by using another person to help reach a solution that is acceptable to both sides. (page 250)

Medicine A drug that prevents or cures illness or eases its symptoms. (page 300)

Melanin (MEL·uh·nin) The substance that gives skin its color. (page 122)

Menstruation (men·stroo·WAY·shuhn) The flow of the uterine lining material from the body. (page 164)

Mental and emotional health Your ability to deal in a reasonable way with the stresses and changes of daily life. (page 188)

Metabolism The process by which the body gets energy from food. (page 155)

Minerals Nutrients that strengthen bones and teeth, help keep blood healthy, and keep the heart and other organs working properly. (page 89)

Mononucleosis (MAH·noh·noo·klee·OH·sis) A disease characterized by swelling of the lymph nodes in the neck and throat. (page 343)

Mood disorder A disorder in which a person undergoes mood changes that seem inappropriate or extreme. (page 204)

Muscle endurance The ability of a muscle to repeatedly exert a force over a prolonged period of time. (page 56)

Muscular system Tissues that move parts of the body and operate internal organs. (page 59)

Narcotic A drug that relieves pain and dulls the senses. (page 311)

Neglect The failure to meet the basic physical and emotional needs of a person. (page 259)

Negotiation (ni·goh·shee·AY·shuhn) The process of discussing problems face-to-face in order to reach a solution. (page 249)

Neighborhood Watch A widespread crime prevention effort undertaken by residents of a particular segment of the community. (page 257)

Neuron (NOO·rahn) One of the cells that make up the nervous system. (page 313)

Neutrality (noo·TRA·luh·tee) A promise not to take sides in a conflict. (page 250)

Nicotine (NIK·uh·teen) An addictive drug found in tobacco. (page 274)

Noncommunicable disease A disease that cannot be spread from person to person. (page 364)

Nonrenewable resources Substances that cannot be replaced once they are used. (page 438)

Nonverbal communication All the ways you can get a message across without using words. (page 217)

Nonviolent confrontation Resolving a conflict by peaceful methods. (page 248)

Nurture To provide for physical, mental, emotional, and social needs. (page 221)

Nutrient dense Having a high amount of nutrients relative to the number of calories. (page 100)

Nutrients (NOO·tree·ents) Substances in foods that your body needs in order to grow, have energy, and stay healthy. (page 88)

Nutrition (noo·TRI·shuhn) The process of taking in food and using it for energy, growth, and good health. (page 94)

Objective Based on facts. (page 15)

Occupational Safety and Health Administration (OSHA) A branch of the U.S. Department of Labor whose job is to ensure the protection of American workers. (page 435)

Ophthalmologist (ahf·thahl·MAH·luh·jist) A physician who specializes in the structure, functions, and diseases of the eye. (page 128)

Optometrist (ahp·TAH·muh·trist) A health care professional who is trained to examine the eyes for vision problems and to prescribe corrective lenses. (page 128)

Organ A body part made up of different tissues joined together to perform a function. (page 168)

Osteoarthritis (ahs·tee·oh·ar·THRY·tuhs) A chronic disease that is common in older adults and results from a breakdown of cartilage in the joints. (page 382)

Glossary

Ovaries (OH·vuh·reez) The female reproductive glands. (page 165)

Over-the-counter (OTC) medicine A medicine that you can buy without a doctor's prescription. (page 301)

Overtraining Exercising too hard or too often, without enough rest in between sessions. (page 78)

Ovulation (ahv·yuh·LAY·shuhn) The process by which the ovaries release a single mature egg. (page 164)

Ozone A special form of oxygen. (page 431)

Pancreas (PAN·kree·uhs) A gland that helps the small intestine by producing pancreatic juice, a blend of enzymes that breaks down proteins, carbohydrates, and fats. (page 104)

Passive smoker A nonsmoker who breathes secondhand smoke. (page 290)

Pathogens The germs that are responsible for causing disease. (page 333)

Pedestrian A person who travels on foot. (page 404)

Peer pressure The influence that people your age have on you to think and act like them. (page 228)

Peers People close to your age who are similar to you in many ways. (page 228)

Peripheral (puh·RIF·uh·ruhl) **nervous system (PNS)** The nerves that connect the central nervous system to all parts of the body. (page 314)

Personality A special mix of traits, feelings, attitudes, and habits. (page 189)

Physical activity Any kind of movement that causes your body to use energy. (page 54)

Physical dependence An addiction in which the body develops a chemical need for a drug. (page 283)

Physical fatigue Extreme tiredness of the whole body. (page 200)

Plaque (PLAK) A thin, sticky film that builds up on teeth and contributes to tooth decay. (page 122)

Plasma (PLAZ·muh) A yellowish fluid, the watery portion of blood. (page 66)

Pneumonia (nu·MOHN·yuh) A serious inflammation or infection of the lungs. (page 344)

Point-of-service (POS) plan A health insurance plan that combines the features of HMOs and PPOs. (page 144)

Pollen A powdery substance released by the flowers of certain plants. (page 365)

Pollution Dirty or harmful substances in the environment. (page 430)

Pores Tiny openings in the skin. (page 122)

Preferred provider organization (PPO) A health insurance plan that allows its members to select a physician who participates in the plan or visit the physician of their choice. (page 144)

Prejudice (PRE·juh·dis) A negative and unjustly formed opinion, usually against people of a different racial, religious, or cultural group. (page 245)

Preschooler A child between ages three and five. (page 174)

Prescription medicine A medicine that can be used safely only with a doctor's written permission. (page 301)

Prevention Taking steps to make sure that something does not happen. (page 16)

Primary care provider A health care professional who provides checkups and general care. (page 143)

Proteins (PROH·teenz) Nutrients used to repair body cells and tissues. (page 88)

Protozoa (proh·tuh·ZOH·uh) One-celled organisms that have a more complex structure than bacteria. (page 333)

Psychological (sy·kuh·LAH·ji·kuhl) **dependence** An addiction in which a person believes that he or she needs a drug in order to feel good or function normally. (page 283)

Psychological (sy·kuh·LAH·ji·kuhl) **fatigue** Extreme tiredness caused by a person's mental state. (page 200)

Puberty (PYOO·buhr·tee) The time when you develop certain physical characteristics of adults of your own gender. (page 156)

Pulmonary (PUL·muh·nehr·ee) **circulation** Circulation that carries the blood from the heart, through the lungs, and back to the heart. (page 65)

R

Radiation therapy A treatment that uses X rays or other forms of radioactivity for some types of cancer. (page 372)

Rape Forced sexual intercourse. (page 252)

Recycle To change an item in some way so that it can be used again. (page 437)

Refusal skills Ways to say no effectively. (page 29)

Reproduction (ree·pruh·DUHK·shuhn) The process by which living organisms produce others of their own kind. (page 160)

Reproductive (ree·pruh·DUHK·tiv) **system** Body organs and structures that make it possible to produce young. (page 160)

Rescue breathing A first-aid procedure in which someone forces air into the lungs of a person who is not breathing. (page 417)

Resilient Able to bounce back from a disappointment, difficulty, or crisis. (page 188)

Respiratory system The set of organs that supplies your body with oxygen and rids your body of carbon dioxide. (page 278)

Rheumatoid (ROO·muh·toyd) **arthritis** A chronic disease characterized by pain, inflammation, swelling, and stiffness of the joints. (page 382)

Risk behaviors Actions or choices that may cause injury or harm to you or to others. (page 12)

Risk factor A characteristic or behavior that increases the likelihood of developing a medical disorder or disease. (page 370)

Role model A person who inspires you to act or think in a certain way. (page 42)

S

Safety conscious Being aware that safety is important and being careful to act in a safe manner. (page 394)

Saliva (suh·LY·vuh) A digestive juice produced by the salivary glands in your mouth. (page 103)

Saturated fats Fats that are solid at room temperature. (page 89)

Second-degree burn A moderately serious burn in which the burned area blisters. (page 420)

Secondhand smoke Air that has been contaminated by tobacco smoke. (page 290)

Self-assessment Careful examination and judgment of your own patterns of behavior. (page 6)

Self-concept The view that you have of yourself. (page 190)

Self-esteem The confidence and pride you have in yourself. (page 191)

Semen (SEE·muhn) A mixture of sperm and fluids produced in the male reproductive tract. (page 161)

Sewage Garbage, detergents, and other household wastes washed down drains. (page 432)

Sexual abuse Sexual contact that is forced upon another person. (page 259)

Sexually transmitted diseases (STDs) Infections that are spread from person to person through sexual contact. (page 346)

Short-term goal A goal that you can reach in a short length of time. (page 37)

Side effect A reaction to a medicine other than the one intended. (page 302)

Sidestream smoke Smoke that comes from the burning end of a cigarette, pipe, or cigar. (page 290)

Skeletal system The framework of bones and other tissues that supports the body. (page 59)

Small intestine A coiled tube, about 20 feet long, where most of the digestive process takes place. (page 104)

Smog A yellow-brown haze that forms when sunlight reacts with air pollution. (page 431)

Smoke alarm A device that sounds an alarm when it senses smoke. (page 399)

Specialist (SPE·shuh·list) A health care professional trained to treat patients who have problems in specific areas. (page 143)

Sperm The male reproductive cells. (page 161)

Spinal cord A long bundle of neurons that relays messages to and from the brain and all parts of the body. (page 314)

Glossary

Stimulant (STIM·yuh·luhnt) A drug that speeds up the body's functions. (page 310)

Strength The ability of your muscles to exert a force. (page 55)

Strep throat A sore throat caused by streptococcal bacteria. (page 344)

Stress Your body's response to changes around you. (page 28)

Stress management Identifying sources of stress and learning how to handle them in ways that promote good mental and emotional health. (page 28)

Stressor A trigger of stress. (page 198)

Stroke A serious condition that occurs when an artery of the brain breaks or becomes blocked. (page 378)

Subjective Coming from a person's own views and beliefs, not necessarily from facts. (page 15)

Suicide The act of intentionally killing oneself. (page 206)

Support system A network of people available to help when needed. (page 205)

Syphilis (SI·fuh·lis) A bacterial STD that can affect many parts of the body. (page 347)

Systemic (sis·TE·mik) **circulation** Circulation that sends oxygen-rich blood to all the body tissues except the lungs. (page 65)

Tact The quality of knowing what to say to avoid offending others. (page 218)

Tar A thick, dark liquid that forms when tobacco burns. (page 274)

Target heart rate The number of heartbeats per minute that you should aim for during moderate to vigorous activity to benefit your circulatory system the most. (page 72)

Tartar (TAR·ter) Hardened plaque that threatens gum health. (page 122)

Team sports Organized physical activities with specific rules, played by opposing groups of people. (page 75)

Tendon A type of connecting tissue that joins muscle to muscle or muscle to bone. (page 60)

Testes The pair of glands that produce sperm. (page 161)

Third-degree burn A very serious burn in which all layers of the skin are damaged. (page 420)

Tissue A group of similar cells that do a particular job. (page 168)

Toddler A child between the ages of one and three. (page 174)

Tolerance The body's need for larger and larger doses of a drug to produce the same effect. (page 284)

Tornado A whirling, funnel-shaped windstorm that drops from the sky to the ground. (page 411)

Trachea (TRAY·kee·uh) The tube in the throat that takes air to and from the lungs. (page 278)

Tuberculosis (too·ber·kyuh·LOH·sis) A bacterial disease that usually affects the lungs. (page 343)

Tumor (TOO·mer) A group of abnormal cells that forms a mass. (page 370)

Ultraviolet (UV) rays An invisible form of radiation from the sun that can penetrate and change the structure of skin cells. (page 124)

Unsaturated fats Fats that are liquid at room temperature. (page 89)

Uterus (YOO·tuh·ruhs) A pear-shaped organ in which a developing child is nourished. (page 165)

Vaccine (vak·SEEN) A preparation of dead or weakened pathogens that is injected into the body to cause the immune system to produce antibodies. (page 340)

Values The beliefs that guide the way a person lives, such as beliefs about what is right and wrong and what is most important. (page 32)

Vein A type of blood vessel that carries blood back to the heart from all parts of the body. (page 64)

Verbal communication Using words to express yourself, either in speaking or in writing. (page 217)

Viruses (VY·ruh·suhz) The smallest and simplest disease-causing organisms. (page 333)

Vitamins Substances that help to regulate the body's functions. (page 89)

Warm-up Gentle exercise you do to prepare your muscles for moderate to vigorous activity. (page 71)

Warranty A company's or a store's written agreement to repair a product or refund your money should the product not function properly. (page 138)

Weather emergency A dangerous situation brought on by changes in the atmosphere. (page 410)

Wellness A state of well-being, or balanced health. (page 7)

Withdrawal The unpleasant symptoms that someone experiences when he or she stops using an addictive substance. (page 282)

Glosario

 A

Abdominal thrust/presión abdominal Una presión rápida, hacia adentro y arriba sobre el diafragma, para desalojar un objeto que bloquea la vía respiratoria de una persona.

Abstinence/abstinencia No participar en conductas o actividades peligrosas.

Abuse/abuso El maltrato físico, emocional o mental de otra persona.

Accidental injuries/lesiones accidentales Daños causados por sucesos inesperados.

Acid rain/lluvia ácida Lluvia que es más ácida de lo normal.

Addiction/adicción La necesidad psicológica o física de una droga u otra sustancia.

Adolescence/adolescencia El periodo de vida entre la niñez y la adultez que empieza generalmente entre los 11 y los 15 años.

Adrenaline/adrenalina Una hormona que aumenta el nivel de azúcar en la sangre, y por lo tanto, proporciona energía adicional al cuerpo.

Advertising/publicidad Mensajes públicos diseñados para hacer que los consumidores compren un producto o servicio.

Advocacy/promoción Actuar en apoyo de una causa.

Aerobic exercise/ejercicio aeróbico Actividad rítmica ininterrumpida de intensidad moderada a vigorosa que requiere grandes cantidades de oxígeno y hace que el corazón trabaje.

Aftershock/onda posterior Terremoto secundario.

AIDS (acquired immunodeficiency syndrome)/SIDA (síndrome de inmunodeficiencia adquirida) Una enfermedad mortal que interfiere con la habilidad del cuerpo para combatir infecciones.

Alcohol/alcohol Una droga producida por una reacción química en algunos alimentos, especialmente frutas y granos.

Alcoholism/alcoholismo Una enfermedad que se caracteriza por la necesidad física y psicológica de consumir alcohol.

Allergen/alergeno Una sustancia que causa una reacción alérgica.

Allergy/alergia Una sensibilidad extrema a una sustancia.

Alveoli/alveolos Cavidades frágiles, elásticas y microscópicas en los pulmones, donde se intercambian el bióxido de carbono que proviene de las células del cuerpo y el oxígeno puro que viene del aire.

Amphetamine/anfetamina Una droga estimulante fuerte que acelera el sistema nervioso.

Anabolic steroids/esteroides anabólicos Compuestos sintéticos que hacen que el tejido muscular se desarrolle con rapidez anormal.

Anaerobic exercise/ejercicio anaeróbico Actividad física intensa que requiere poco oxígeno pero exige breves brotes de energía.

Angioplasty/angioplastia Una operación quirúrgica en la que un instrumento con un globo diminuto se introduce en una arteria para remover una obstrucción.

Anorexia nervosa/anorexia nerviosa Un trastorno en la alimentación por el cual una persona sufre de un intenso temor a aumentar de peso y por consiguiente deja de comer.

Antibodies/anticuerpos Proteínas que se pegan a los antígenos, impidiendo que éstos le hagan daño al cuerpo.

Antigens/antígenos Sustancias que provocan el funcionamiento del sistema inmunológico.

Antihistamine/antihistamínico Una medicina que alivia los síntomas de una reacción alérgica mediante la supresión de la producción de las histaminas.

Anxiety disorder/trastorno de ansiedad Un trastorno en el cual la ansiedad intensa o el miedo impide que una persona funcione de manera normal.

Arteriosclerosis/arteriosclerosis Un conjunto de trastornos que provoca el engrosamiento y endurecimiento de las arterias.

Artery/arteria Un tipo de vaso sanguíneo que lleva sangre desde el corazón a las demás partes del cuerpo.

Arthritis/artritis Una enfermedad de las articulaciones caracterizada por inflamación dolorosa y anquilosamiento.

Assault/asalto Un ataque físico o la amenaza de tal con el fin de causar daño corporal.

Assertive/firme Dispuesto a defenderse de manera resuelta y positiva.

Asthma/asma Una enfermedad respiratoria crónica que causa el estrechamiento u obstrucción de las vías respiratorias y dificulta la respiración.

Astigmatism/astigmatismo Una afección del ojo que causa que las imágenes se vean distorsionadas y los objetos aparezcan ondulados o borrosos.

Atherosclerosis/aterosclerosis Una afección causada por la acumulación de sustancias grasas en las paredes internas de las arterias.

Bacteria/bacterias Organismos diminutos unicelulares que viven en casi todas partes.

Battery/agresión Dar palizas, golpear o dar puntapiés a otra persona.

Benign/benigno No canceroso.

Binge eating disorder/trastorno de la alimentación compulsiva Un trastorno en la alimentación por el cual una persona repetidamente come grandes cantidades de alimentos de una vez.

Biodegradable/biodegradable Que se descompone fácilmente en el medio ambiente.

Blizzard/ventisca Una tormenta de nieve fuerte, con vientos que llegan a 45 millas por hora.

Blood pressure/presión arterial La fuerza que ejerce la sangre contra las paredes de los vasos sanguíneos.

Body composition/composición del cuerpo La proporción de grasa, hueso, músculo y líquidos que componen el peso del cuerpo.

Body language/lenguaje corporal Un tipo de comunicación no verbal que incluye la postura, los gestos y las expresiones faciales.

Body Mass Index (BMI)/Índice de masa corporal Una manera de evaluar el tamaño del cuerpo al tomar en cuenta la estatura y el peso.

Body system/aparato o sistema corporal Un grupo de órganos que trabajan juntos para ejecutar funciones relacionadas.

Brain/cerebro El centro de mando, o el coordinador, del sistema nervioso.

Bronchi/bronquios Dos conductos que salen de la tráquea; cada conducto va a un pulmón.

Bronchodilator/broncodilatador Una medicina que relaja los músculos alrededor de los bronquios.

Bulimia nervosa/bulimia nerviosa Un trastorno en la alimentación por el cual una persona come grandes cantidades y después se induce el vómito.

Bully/bully Persona que mediante amenazas, burlas o violencia intimida a personas que parecen ser indefensas.

Calorie/caloría Una unidad de calor que mide la energía que contienen los alimentos.

Cancer/cáncer Una enfermedad causada por células anormales cuyo crecimiento está fuera de control.

Capillary/capilar Un tipo de vaso sanguíneo que proporciona sangre a las células del cuerpo y conecta las arterias con las venas.

Carbohydrates/hidratos de carbono Los almidones y azúcares que proporcionan energía.

Carbon monoxide/monóxido de carbono Un gas incoloro, inodoro y tóxico que produce el tabaco al quemarse.

Carcinogen/carcinógeno Una sustancia en el medio ambiente que produce cáncer.

Cardiopulmonary resuscitation (CPR)/resucitación cardiopulmonar Un procedimiento de primeros auxilios para restaurar la respiración y la circulación de la sangre.

Cartilage/cartílago Un tipo de tejido conjuntivo que permite que las articulaciones se muevan fácilmente, protege los huesos y sostiene los tejidos blandos como los de la nariz y la oreja.

Cell/célula La unidad básica de la vida.

Central nervous system (CNS)/sistema nervioso central El cerebro y la médula espinal.

Character/carácter La manera en que piensas, sientes y actúas.

Chemotherapy/quimioterapia El uso de drogas potentes para destruir células cancerosas.

Chest thrust/presión torácica Una presión rápida en el centro del esternón para desalojar un objeto que bloquea la vía respiratoria de una persona.

Chlamydia/clamidia Una infección de transmisión sexual bacterial que puede afectar los órganos de reproducción, la uretra y el ano.

Cholesterol/colesterol Una sustancia cerosa que el cuerpo usa para crear células y otras sustancias.

Chromosomes/cromosomas Estructuras filiformes que contienen los códigos genéticos de los rasgos hereditarios.

Chronic/crónico Que está siempre presente o reaparece repetidamente durante un largo periodo de tiempo.

Circulatory system/aparato circulatorio El conjunto de los órganos y los tejidos que transportan materias esenciales a las células del cuerpo y se llevan los desechos.

Cirrhosis/cirrosis La cicatrización y destrucción del tejido del hígado.

Colon/colon Un conducto donde se almacenan los desechos sólidos.

Communicable disease/enfermedad contagiosa Una enfermedad que se puede propagar a una persona de otra persona, un animal o un objeto.

Communication/comunicación El intercambio de pensamientos, sentimientos y creencias entre personas.

Comparison shopping/comparación de productos Obtener información, comparar productos, evaluar sus beneficios y escoger los que ofrecen el mejor valor.

Compromise/acordar Llegar a un acuerdo en el que se cede algo para alcanzar una solución que satisfaga a todos.

Conditioning/entrenamiento Preparación que se hace para ponerse en forma.

Conflict/conflicto Un desacuerdo entre personas con puntos de vista opuestos.

Conflict resolution/resolución de un conflicto Hallar una solución a un desacuerdo o impedir que se transforme en un conflicto mayor.

Consequences/consecuencias Los resultados de los actos.

Conservation/conservación La protección de los recursos naturales.

Consumer/consumidor Toda persona que compra productos y servicios.

Contagious period/periodo de contagio El periodo de tiempo en que se puede transmitir una enfermedad determinada de una persona a otra.

Cool-down/recuperación Ejercicios moderados que permiten que el cuerpo se ajuste al ir finalizando el plan de ejercicios.

Coping skills/capacidad para sobrellevar Métodos para tratar y superar los problemas.

Criteria/criterios Principios en que se basa una decisión.

Culture/cultura Las creencias, costumbres y tradiciones de un grupo específico de personas.

Cumulative risks/riesgos acumulativos Riesgos relacionados cuyos efectos aumentan con cada uno que se añade.

Dandruff/caspa Las escamas de piel muerta en la superficie del cuero cabelludo.

Decibel/decibel La unidad que se usa para medir el volumen del sonido.

Decision making/tomar decisiones El proceso de hacer una selección o de resolver un problema.

Dehydration/deshidratación La pérdida excesiva de agua del cuerpo.

Deliberate injury/Lesión deliberada Lesión que resulta cuando una persona intencionalmente daña a otra.

Depressant/depresivo Una droga que disminuye las funciones y reacciones del cuerpo, incluso el ritmo cardiaco y la respiración.

Depression/depresión Un trastorno del ánimo en el que una persona se siente sin esperanza, indefensa, despreciable, culpable y sumamente triste durante periodos que duran varias semanas.

Dermis/dermis La capa interna de la piel que contiene vasos sanguíneos, terminaciones nerviosas, folículos pilosos, glándulas sudoríparas y glándulas sebáceas.

Diabetes/diabetes Una enfermedad que impide que el cuerpo convierta alimentos en energía.

Diaphragm/diafragma Músculo grande en forma de domo, situado debajo de los pulmones, que se expande y se relaja para producir la respiración.

Digestion/digestión El proceso corporal de descomponer los alimentos en componentes más pequeños para que la sangre los pueda absorber y llevar a cada célula del cuerpo.

Digestive system/aparato digestivo Un conjunto de órganos que trabajan juntos para descomponer los alimentos en sustancias que tus células puedan usar.

Disease/enfermedad Toda afección que interfiere con el buen funcionamiento del cuerpo o de la mente.

Distress/angustia Estrés que impide que hagas lo que necesitas hacer o que te causa molestia.

Drug/droga Una sustancia no alimenticia que causa cambios en la estructura o el funcionamiento del cuerpo o la mente.

Drug abuse/abuso de drogas El uso de drogas para propósitos no médicos.

Earthquake/terremoto El sacudimiento violento de la superficie de la tierra.

Eating disorder/trastorno en la alimentación Una conducta de alimentación extrema que puede causar enfermedades graves o la muerte.

Electrical overload/sobrecarga eléctrica Una situación peligrosa en que demasiada corriente eléctrica fluye a través de un solo circuito.

Embryo/embrión El organismo en desarrollo desde la fecundación hasta aproximadamente la octava semana del desarrollo.

Emotions/emociones Sentimientos como el amor, la alegría o el miedo.

Empathy/empatía La habilidad de identificar y comprender los sentimientos de otra persona.

Emphysema/enfisema Una enfermedad que destruye los alveolos.

Endocrine system/sistema endocrino Glándulas en todo el cuerpo que regulan sus funciones.

Endorsement/aprobación Una declaración de aceptación.

Endurance/resistencia La habilidad de realizar actividades físicas vigorosas sin cansarse demasiado.

Environment/medio ambiente Todas las cosas vivas y no vivas que te rodean.

Environmental Protection Agency (EPA)/Agencia de Protección Ambiental Una agencia del gobierno de Estados Unidos a cargo de la protección del medio ambiente.

Epidermis/epidermis La capa más externa de la piel.

Eustress/estrés positivo Tensión que puede ayudarte a lograr tus metas.

Evaluate/evaluar Determinar la calidad de algo.

Excretion/excreción El proceso mediante el cual el cuerpo se deshace de los desechos.

Excretory system/sistema excretor El sistema que despide los desechos del cuerpo y controla el balance del agua.

Exercise/ejercicio Actividad física planeada, estructurada y repetitiva que mejora o mantiene la buena salud.

Family/familia La unidad básica de la sociedad.

Fatigue/fatiga Cansancio extremo.

Fats/grasas Nutrientes que proporcionan energía, mantienen la piel saludable y fomentan el desarrollo normal.

Fertilization/fecundación La unión de un espermatozoide y un óvulo para formar un nuevo ser humano.

Fetus/feto El organismo en desarrollo desde el final de la octava semana hasta el nacimiento.

Fiber/fibra La parte de los granos, frutas y vegetales que el cuerpo no puede descomponer.

First aid/primeros auxilios El cuidado inmediato que se da a una persona herida o enferma hasta que sea posible proporcionarle ayuda médica normal.

First-degree burn/quemadura de primer grado Una quemadura en que sólo la capa exterior de la piel se quema y se enrojece.

Fitness/buen estado físico La capacidad de participar en el trabajo físico y en las diversiones de la vida diaria sin cansarse demasiado.

Flammable/inflamable Que se prende fuego con facilidad.

Flexibility/flexibilidad La capacidad de mover las articulaciones completa y fácilmente.

Fluoride/fluoruro Una sustancia que ayuda a prevenir las caries dentales.

Follicles/folículos Sacos pequeños en la dermis que producen el vello.

Food Guide Pyramid/Pirámide Nutricional Una guía para realizar selecciones de alimentos sanas a diario.

Fossil fuel/combustible fósil El petróleo, carbón y gas natural que se usan para proporcionar energía.

Fracture/fractura Una rotura en un hueso.

Fraud/fraude Engaño o decepción deliberada.

Frequency/frecuencia En cuanto al estado físico, la cantidad de veces que uno hace ejercicio a la semana.

Friendship/amistad Una relación entre personas que simpatizan y tienen intereses y valores similares.

Fungi/hongos Seres vivos primitivos tales como mohos o levaduras que no pueden hacer sus propios alimentos.

Gang/pandilla Un grupo de personas que se relacionan para participar en actividades criminales.

Generic products/productos genéricos Productos que se venden en envases comunes y a menor precio que los de marca.

Genes/genes Las unidades básicas de la herencia.

Genital herpes/herpes genitales Una infección de transmisión sexual, causada por un virus, que produce ampollas dolorosas en el área genital.

Genital warts/verrugas genitales Erupciones o protuberancias en el área genital causadas por ciertos tipos del virus papiloma de los seres humanos.

Germs/gérmenes Organismos tan diminutos que se ven sólo a través de un microscopio.

Gonorrhea/gonorrea Una infección de transmisión sexual causada por bacterias que afecta las membranas mucosas del cuerpo, en particular en el área genital.

Groundwater/agua subterránea Agua acumulada debajo de la superficie de la tierra.

Gynecologist/ginecólogo Un médico que se especializa en el aparato reproductor femenino.

Hallucinogen/alucinógeno Una droga que altera el estado de ánimo, los pensamientos y los sentidos.

Hate crime/crimen por odio Un acto ilegal cometido en contra de una persona simplemente porque pertenece a un grupo en particular.

Hazard/peligro Una fuente posible de peligro.

Hazardous waste/desechos peligrosos Desechos líquidos, sólidos o fangosos, producidos por el hombre, que pueden perjudicar la salud del ser humano o el medio ambiente.

Head lice/piojos Insectos parasíticos que viven en el cabello y causan picazón.

Health/salud Una combinación de bienestar físico, mental/emocional y social.

Health insurance/seguro de salud Un plan en el que una persona paga una cantidad fija a una compañía de seguros que acuerda en cubrir parte o la totalidad de los gastos médicos.

Health maintenance organization (HMO)/organización para el mantenimiento de la salud Un plan de seguro de salud que contrata a ciertos médicos y especialistas para dar servicios médicos.

Heart and lung endurance/resistencia cardiaca y respiratoria La indicación de la eficacia del corazón y de los pulmones durante actividades físicas o ejercicios de intensidad moderada a vigorosa.

Heart attack/ataque cardiaco Una afección seria que se presenta cuando el flujo de sangre al corazón disminuye o cesa, dañando el músculo cardiaco.

Hepatitis/hepatitis Una inflamación del hígado, en que la piel y el blanco del ojo se ponen amarillos.

Heredity/herencia La transferencia de características de los padres biológicos a sus hijos.

Histamine/histamina Sustancia química en el cuerpo que provoca los síntomas de una reacción alérgica.

HIV (human immunodeficiency virus)/VIH (virus de inmunodeficiencia humana) El virus que causa el SIDA.

Homicide/homicidio Darle muerte una persona a otra.

Hormones/hormonas Sustancias químicas, producidas por ciertas glándulas que ayudan a regular las funciones del cuerpo.

Hurricane/huracán Una tormenta de vientos y lluvia torrencial que se origina en alta mar.

Hygiene/higiene Limpieza.

Hypertension/hipertensión Una afección en que la presión arterial de una persona se mantiene a niveles más altos de lo normal.

Hypothermia/hipotermia Un descenso rápido y peligroso de la temperatura del cuerpo.

Illegal drugs/drogas ilegales Sustancias cuya producción, posesión, compra o venta por personas de cualquier edad va en contra de la ley.

Immune system/sistema inmunológico Una combinación de las defensas del cuerpo, compuesta de células, tejidos y órganos que combaten agentes patógenos.

Immunity/inmunidad La habilidad del cuerpo de resistir los patógenos que causan una enfermedad en particular.

Individual sports/deportes individuales Actividades físicas en que puedes participar solo o con otra persona, sin formar parte de un equipo.

Infancy/infancia El primer año de vida.

Infection/infección Una afección que se produce cuando agentes patógenos invaden el cuerpo, se multiplican y dañan las células.

Inflammation/inflamación La reacción del cuerpo a lesiones o enfermedades que resulta en hinchazón, dolor, calor y enrojecimiento.

Influenza/influenza Una enfermedad contagiosa, que se caracteriza por fiebre, escalofríos, fatiga, dolor de cabeza, dolores musculares y síntomas respiratorios.

Infomercial/anuncio informativo Un anuncio de televisión largo cuyo propósito principal parece ser proveer información acerca de un producto en vez de vender el producto.

Inhalant/inhalante Una sustancia cuyos gases se aspiran para producir sensaciones alucinantes.

Insulin/insulina Una hormona producida en el páncreas que regula el nivel de glucosa en la sangre.

Intensity/intensidad En cuanto al estado físico, la cantidad de energía que usas cuando haces ejercicio.

Interpersonal communication/comunicación entre personas El compartir pensamientos y sentimientos entre dos o más personas.

Intoxicated/embriagado Borracho.

Joint/articulación Lugar en donde se unen dos o más huesos.

Kidneys/riñones Los órganos que filtran el agua y los desechos de la sangre.

Landfill/terraplén sanitario Un pozo enorme con diseño específico donde se arrojan y se entierran desechos.

Ligament/ligamento Un tipo de tejido conjuntivo que mantiene en su lugar los huesos en las articulaciones.

Liver/hígado La glándula más grande del cuerpo que secreta un líquido llamado bilis que ayuda a digerir las grasas.

Long-term goal/meta a largo plazo Un objetivo que planeas alcanzar en un largo periodo de tiempo.

Lymphatic system/sistema linfático Un aparato circulatorio secundario que le ayuda al cuerpo a defenderse de agentes patógenos y a mantener el equilibrio de los líquidos.

Lymphocytes/linfocitos Glóbulos blancos especiales en la linfa.

Mainstream smoke/humo directo El humo que el fumador aspira y exhala.

Malignant/maligno Canceroso.

Managed care/asistencia médica regulada Planes de salud que hacen hincapié en la medicina preventiva y tratan de controlar el costo y mantener la calidad de la asistencia médica.

Media/medios de difusión Los diversos métodos de comunicar información.

Mediation/mediación La resolución de conflictos por medio de otra persona que ayuda a llegar a una solución aceptable para ambas partes.

Medicine/medicina Una droga que previene o cura enfermedades o que alivia sus síntomas.

Melanin/melanina La sustancia que le da el color a la piel.

Menstruation/menstruación La eliminación de materia celular de la capa de la mucosa uterina.

Mental and emotional health/salud mental y emocional La habilidad de hacerle frente de manera razonable al estrés y a los cambios de la vida diaria.

Metabolism/metabolismo El proceso mediante el cual el cuerpo obtiene energía de los alimentos.

Minerals/minerales Nutrientes que fortalecen los huesos y los dientes, mantienen la salud de la sangre y el buen funcionamiento del corazón y otros órganos.

Mononucleosis/mononucleosis Una enfermedad que se caracteriza por la hinchazón de los ganglios linfáticos en el cuello y la garganta.

Mood disorder/trastorno del estado de ánimo Un trastorno en que la persona cambia de humor de manera aparentemente inapropiada o extrema.

Muscle endurance/resistencia muscular La habilidad que tiene un músculo para ejercer una fuerza repetidamente durante un largo periodo de tiempo.

Muscular system/sistema muscular Tejidos que mueven partes del cuerpo y hacen funcionar los órganos internos.

Narcotic/narcótico Una droga que alivia el dolor y entorpece los sentidos.

Neglect/abandono El no satisfacer las necesidades básicas físicas y emocionales de una persona.

Negotiation/negociación El proceso de hablar de un problema cara a cara para llegar a una solución.

Neighborhood Watch/vigilancia en el barrio Un esfuerzo colectivo y general de prevención del delito por parte de los residentes de un segmento particular de una comunidad.

Neuron/neurona Una de las células que componen el sistema nervioso.

Neutrality/neutralidad Una promesa de no tomar partido durante un conflicto entre otros.

Nicotine/nicotina Una droga adictiva que se encuentra en el tabaco.

Noncommunicable disease/enfermedad no contagiosa Una enfermedad que no se puede transmitir de una persona a otra.

Nonrenewable resources/recursos no renovables Sustancias que no se pueden reemplazar después de usarse.

Nonverbal communication/comunicación no verbal Todos los modos de comunicar un mensaje sin usar palabras.

Nonviolent confrontation/confrontación no violenta Resolver un conflicto por medios pacíficos.

Nurture/criar Proporcionar las necesidades físicas, emocionales, mentales y sociales a una persona.

Nutrient dense/denso en nutrientes Tener una alta cantidad de sustancias nutritivas en comparación con la cantidad de calorías.

Nutrients/nutrientes Sustancias en los alimentos que el cuerpo necesita para desarrollarse, tener energía y mantenerse saludable.

Nutrition/nutrición El proceso de ingerir alimentos y usarlos para la energía, el desarrollo y el mantenimiento de la buena salud.

Objective/objetivo Basado en los hechos.

Occupational Safety and Health Administration (OSHA)/Administración de Salud y Seguridad Ocupacional Una rama del Ministerio de Trabajo que protege la seguridad de los trabajadores estadounidenses.

Ophthalmologist/oftalmólogo Médico que se especializa en la estructura, funciones y enfermedades del ojo.

Optometrist/optómetra Un profesional de la salud que está preparado para examinar la vista y recetar lentes correctivos.

Organ/órgano Una parte del cuerpo que comprende distintos tejidos unidos para cumplir una función particular.

Osteoarthritis/osteoartritis Una enfermedad crónica, común en los ancianos, que es el resultado de la degeneración del cartílago de las articulaciones.

Ovaries/ovarios Las glándulas reproductoras femeninas.

Over-the-counter (OTC) medicine/ medicina sin receta Una medicina que se puede comprar sin receta de un médico.

Overtraining/entrenamiento excesivo Hacer demasiado ejercicio o con demasiada frecuencia, sin descanso suficiente entre sesiones.

Ovulation/ovulación El proceso mediante el cual los ovarios desprenden un único óvulo maduro.

Ozone/ozono Un tipo especial de oxígeno.

Pancreas/páncreas Una glándula que le ayuda al intestino delgado, a través de la producción de jugo pancreático, que está formado por una mezcla de varias enzimas que descomponen las proteínas, hidratos de carbono y grasas.

Passive smoker/fumador pasivo Una persona que no fuma pero que inhala humo secundario.

Pathogens/patógenos Los gérmenes que causan enfermedades.

Pedestrian/peatón Una persona que se traslada a pie.

Peer pressure/presión de pares La influencia que personas de la misma edad tienen sobre otra para que piense y actúe igual que ellas.

Peers/pares Personas de tu grupo de edad que se parecen a ti en muchas maneras.

Peripheral nervous system (PNS)/sistema nervioso periférico Los nervios que unen el sistema nervioso central a todas partes del cuerpo.

Personality/personalidad Una mezcla especial de rasgos, sentimientos, actitudes y hábitos.

Physical activity/actividad física Todo movimiento que cause que el cuerpo use energía.

Physical dependence/dependencia física Una adicción por la cual el cuerpo llega a tener una necesidad química de una droga.

Physical fatigue/fatiga física Cansancio extremo de todo el cuerpo.

Plaque/placa bacteriana Una película delgada y pegajosa que se acumula en los dientes y contribuye a las caries dentales.

Plasma/plasma Un líquido amarillento, la parte líquida de la sangre.

Pneumonia/pulmonía Inflamación o infección seria de los pulmones.

Point-of-service (POS) plan/plan de lugar del servicio Un plan de seguro médico que combina las características de las organizaciones para el mantenimiento de la salud y las organizaciones de proveedores preferidos.

Pollen/polen Una sustancia en forma de polvo, despedida por las flores de ciertas plantas.

Pollution/contaminación Sustancias sucias o dañinas en el medio ambiente.

Pores/poros Pequeños orificios en la piel.

Preferred provider organization (PPO)/ organización de proveedores preferidos Un plan de seguro de salud que permite que sus miembros seleccionen a un médico que participa en el plan o a uno de su preferencia.

Prejudice/prejuicio Una opinión negativa e injusta, generalmente en contra de personas de otro grupo racial, religioso o cultural.

Preschooler/niño preescolar Un niño entre las edades de tres y cinco años.

Prescription medicine/medicina bajo receta Una medicina que sólo puede usarse sin riesgo con la autorización de un médico.

Prevention/prevención Tomar medidas para asegurarse de que algo no suceda.

Primary care provider/profesional médico principal Un profesional de la salud que proporciona exámenes médicos y cuidado general.

Proteins/proteínas Nutrientes que se usan para reparar las células y tejidos del cuerpo.

Protozoa/protozoos Organismos unicelulares que tienen una estructura más compleja que las bacterias.

Psychological dependence/dependencia psicológica Una adicción en la que una persona cree que necesita una droga para sentirse bien o funcionar de manera normal.

Psychological fatigue/fatiga psicológica Cansancio extremo causado por el estado mental de una persona.

Puberty/pubertad La etapa de la vida en la cual una persona comienza a desarrollar ciertas características físicas propias de los adultos del mismo sexo.

Pulmonary circulation/circulación pulmonar La circulación que lleva la sangre desde el corazón, a través de los pulmones y de regreso al corazón.

R

Radiation therapy/radioterapia Un tratamiento que utiliza rayos X u otro tipo de radiactividad para algunos tipos de cáncer.

Rape/violación Relaciones sexuales forzadas.

Recycle/reciclar Cambiar un objeto de alguna manera para que se pueda volver a usar.

Refusal skills/destrezas de negación Modos eficaces de decir que no.

Reproduction/reproducción El proceso mediante el cual los organismos vivos producen otros de su especie.

Reproductive system/aparato reproductor Los órganos y estructuras del cuerpo que hacen posible engendrar hijos.

Rescue breathing/respiración de rescate Un procedimiento de primeros auxilios en el que una persona llena de aire los pulmones de una persona que no está respirando.

Resilient/con capacidad de recuperación Tener la habilidad de regresar a un estado normal después de una decepción, dificultad o crisis.

Respiratory system/aparato respiratorio El conjunto de órganos que proporciona oxígeno al cuerpo y que elimina el bióxido de carbono.

Rheumatoid arthritis/artritis reumatoide Una enfermedad crónica caracterizada por dolor, inflamación, hinchazón y anquilosamiento de las articulaciones.

Risk behaviors/conductas arriesgadas Actos o decisiones que pueden causar lesiones o daños a ti o a otros.

Risk factor/factor de riesgo Una característica o conducta que aumenta la posibilidad de llegar a tener un problema médico o enfermedad.

Role model/modelo de conducta Una persona que inspira a otras a que se comporten o piensen de cierta manera.

S

Safety conscious/consciente de la seguridad Que se da cuenta de la importancia de la seguridad y actúa con cuidado.

Saliva/saliva Un líquido digestivo producido por las glándulas salivales de la boca.

Saturated fats/grasas saturadas Grasas que son sólidas a la temperatura del ambiente.

Second-degree burn/quemadura de segundo grado Una quemadura moderadamente seria en la que se forman ampollas en el área quemada.

Secondhand smoke/humo secundario Aire que está contaminado por el humo del tabaco.

Self-assessment/autoevaluación Examen y valoración minuciosos de tus propios patrones de conducta.

Self-concept/autoconcepto La manera en que te ves a ti mismo.

Self-esteem/autoestima La confianza y orgullo que tienes de ti mismo.

Semen/semen Una mezcla de espermatozoides con los líquidos producidos por el sistema reproductor masculino.

Sewage/aguas cloacales Basura, detergentes y otros desechos caseros que se llevan las tuberías de desagüe.

Sexual abuse/abuso sexual El contacto sexual forzado por una persona.

Sexually transmitted diseases (STDs)/ enfermedades de transmisión sexual (ETS) Enfermedades que se propagan de una persona a otra, a través de contacto sexual.

Short-term goal/meta a corto plazo Una meta que uno puede alcanzar dentro de un breve periodo de tiempo.

Side effect/efecto colateral Una reacción inesperada de una medicina.

Sidestream smoke/humo indirecto Humo que procede de un cigarrillo, pipa o cigarro encendido.

Skeletal system/sistema osteoarticular La armazón de huesos y otros tejidos que sostiene el cuerpo.

Small intestine/intestino delgado Un conducto enrollado, de unos 20 pies de largo, donde tiene lugar la mayor parte de la digestión.

Smog/smog Una neblina de color amarillo-café que se forma cuando la luz solar reacciona con la contaminación del aire.

Smoke alarm/alarma contra incendios Un aparato que hace sonar una alarma cuando detecta humo.

Specialist/especialista Un profesional de la salud preparado para tratar pacientes con problemas en áreas específicas.

Sperm/espermatozoides Las células reproductoras masculinas.

Spinal cord/médula espinal Un largo conjunto de neuronas que transmiten mensajes entre el cerebro y todas las otras partes del cuerpo.

Stimulant/estimulante Una droga que acelera las funciones del cuerpo.

Strength/fortaleza La capacidad que tienen los músculos para ejercer una fuerza.

Strep throat/estreptococia Un dolor de garganta causado por bacterias estreptocócicas.

Stress/estrés La reacción del cuerpo a los cambios a su alrededor.

Stress management/control del éstres La identificación de lo que causa el estrés y aprender cómo reaccionar a ello de manera que permita mantener la buena salud mental y emocional.

Stressor/factor estresante Algo que provoca el estrés.

Stroke/apoplejía Una afección seria que se produce cuando una arteria en el cerebro se rompe o se obstruye.

Subjective/subjetivo Que proviene de las opiniones y creencias de una persona y no necesariamente de los hechos.

Suicide/suicidio Matarse intencionalmente.

Support system/sistema de asistencia Un grupo de personas dispuestas a ayudar cuando haya necesidad.

Syphilis/sífilis Una infección de transmisión sexual, causada por una bacteria, que puede afectar muchas partes del cuerpo.

Systemic circulation/circulación sistémica Circulación que lleva sangre rica en oxígeno a todos los tejidos del cuerpo, menos a los pulmones.

Tact/tacto La habilidad de saber lo que se debe decir para no ofender a los demás.

Tar/alquitrán Un líquido espeso y oscuro que forma el tabaco al quemarse.

Target heart rate/ritmo deseado del corazón El número de latidos del corazón, por minuto, que una persona debe tratar de alcanzar durante una actividad de intensidad moderada a vigorosa, para obtener lo máximo posible de beneficio para el aparato circulatorio.

Tartar/sarro Placa bacteriana endurecida que amenaza la salud de las encías.

Team sports/deportes en equipo Actividades físicas organizadas, con reglas específicas que juegan grupos opuestos de personas.

Tendon/tendón Un tipo de tejido conjuntivo que une un músculo a otro o un músculo a un hueso.

Testes/testículos Las dos glándulas que producen los espermatozoides.

Third-degree burn/quemadura de tercer grado Una quemadura muy seria en que todas las capas de la piel quedan dañadas.

Tissue/tejido Un grupo de células similares que tienen una función en particular.

Toddler/niño que empieza a andar Un niño entre uno y tres años.

Tolerance/tolerancia La necesidad del cuerpo de mayores cantidades de una droga para obtener el mismo efecto.

Tornado/tornado Una tormenta en forma de torbellino, que gira en grandes círculos y que cae del cielo a la tierra.

Trachea/tráquea El conducto en la garganta por donde pasa el aire mientras entra y sale de los pulmones.

Tuberculosis/tuberculosis Una enfermedad causada por bacterias que generalmente afecta a los pulmones.

Tumor/tumor Un grupo de células anormales que forma una masa.

Ultraviolet (UV) rays/rayos ultravioletas Una forma invisible de radiación solar que puede penetrar y cambiar la estructura de las células de la piel.

Unsaturated fats/grasas no saturadas Grasas que son líquidas a la temperatura del ambiente.

Uterus/útero Un órgano en forma de pera en el cual un bebé en desarrollo se nutre.

Vaccine/vacuna Un preparado de gérmenes muertos o debilitados que se inyecta en el cuerpo para hacer que el sistema inmunológico produzca anticuerpos.

Values/valores Las creencias que guían la manera en que una persona vive, tales como creencias sobre el bien y el mal y lo que tiene importancia.

Vein/vena Un tipo de vaso sanguíneo que lleva la sangre de todas partes del cuerpo de regreso al corazón.

Verbal communication/comunicación verbal El uso de palabras, escritas o habladas, para expresarse.

Viruses/virus Los organismos más pequeños y simples, que causan enfermedades.

Vitamins/vitaminas Sustancias que ayudan al cuerpo a regular sus funciones.

Warm-up/precalentamiento Ejercicios leves que se hacen a fin de preparar el cuerpo para una actividad de intensidad moderada a vigorosa.

Warranty/garantía La promesa escrita de un fabricante o una tienda de reparar un producto o devolver el dinero al comprador, si el producto no funciona debidamente.

Weather emergency/emergencia del tiempo Una situación peligrosa debido a cambios en la atmósfera.

Wellness/bienestar general Un estado de buena salud, o salud balanceada.

Withdrawal/síndrome de abstinencia Los síntomas desagradables que se producen cuando alguien deja de usar una sustancia a la que es adicto.

Index

Note: Page numbers in *italics* refer to art and marginal features.

Index

Index

Index

Index

Index

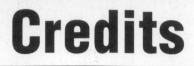

Credits

Photographs

Age fotostock: page 113. Brand X Pictures: pages 325, 356. Kwaku Alston: page 44. Kevin Birch: pages 10, 20, 55 (bottom left), 145, 158, 159, 166, 231, 266. Carson Scholars Fund: page 42. CORBIS: page 128; Philip James Corwin, page 437; Charles Gupton, page 230; Jack Hollingsworth, page 351; Richard Hutchings, page 219; Reed Kaestner, page 275; Layne Kennedy, page 432; William Manning, page 292; Richard T. Nowitz, pages 18–19; Gabe Palmer, page 373; Reuters NewMedia Inc., page 384; Pete Saloutos, pages 208–209; Kevin Schafer, page 355; Joseph Sohm/ChromoSohm, Inc., page 163; Jerry Tobias, page 146; John Welzenbach, page 174 (left); David Woods, page 174 (right). Custom Medical Stock Photos: page 356. CORBIS SYGMA: Orlando Sentinel, page 422. Bob Daemmrich Photo, Inc.: pages vii, xvi–1, 12, 33, 41 (top left), 46, 69 (both), 78, 94, 140, 177, 188, 197, 198, 226, 227, 340, 353 (right); Joel Salcido/Bob Daemmrich Associates, pages 41 (right), 73, 79. Mary Kate Denny: page 111. Envision: Zeva Oelbaum, page 178. FlashFocus: SW Productions, page 4. Tim Fuller Photography: pages 52–53, 242–243. Getty Images: page 293; Bruce Ayres/Tony Stone Images, page 416; Frank Clarkson/Tony Stone Images, page 283; Fisher/Thatcher/Tony Stone Images, page 160; Penny Gentieu/Tony Stone Images, page 174 (center); David Hanover/Tony Stone Images, page 281; Lars Klove/Image Bank, page 378; Peter Pearson/Tony Stone Images, page 9 (right); Richard Price/FPG International, page 144; Mark Scott/FPG International, page 291; Stephen Simpson, pages 80–81; Stephen Simpson/FPG International, pages 184–185, 257; Don Smetzer/Tony Stone Images, page 318; Tony Stone Images, page 164; Maria Taglienti/The Image Bank, page 96 (right); Arthur Tilley/FPG International, page 186–187; Mike Timo/Tony Stone Images, page 284; David Young-Wolff/Tony Stone Images, pages 362–363; Zigy Kaluzny/Tony Stone Images, page 288. Mark E. Gibson: pages 138, 148, 176, 244, 248, 286, 353 (left, center). Jon Gipe: page 440. Jeff Greenberg: page 190 (all). Martin Griff: page 315. The Image Works: Bob Daemmrich, pages 175 (center), 433; Sonda Dawes, page 347; W. Hill, page 225; M. Siluk, pages 46–47. Index Stock: page 112. International Stock: Dusty, page 218; Chuck Mason, page 224. Ken Karp: pages v, ix, x, xiii, 2–3, 11, 15, 24–25, 27, 28, 29, 30, 31, 32 (all), 35, 38, 43, 47, 50–51, 56 (all), 57 (both), 63, 64, 71 (all), 74, 82, 83, 86–87, 88, 91, 92, 99, 100, 106, 107, 118–119, 120, 121 (all), 124, 126, 129, 131, 132, 137, 141, 142, 149, 152–153, 157, 170, 173, 175 (left), 193, 194, 195, 200, 207, 214–215, 217, 222, 223, 234, 235, 238, 239 (all), 250, 251, 256, 263, 267, 270–271, 294, 298–299, 302, 303, 317, 326 (all), 327, 330–331, 333, 338, 344, 352, 368, 379, 380, 421, 428–429, 434, 438, 439. David Mager: pages viii, 5 (all), 7, 191, 216, 254, 300, 381 (all), 401, 409, 424–425. Eric McNatt: pages 45 (all). Masterfile: Miep van Damm, pages 236–237. Medical Images, Inc.: Frederick C. Skvara, page 370 (both). PhotoEdit: Robert Brenner, pages 390–391; Michelle D. Bridwell, page 70; Jose Carillo, page 68; Myrleen Ferguson Cate, page 262 (both); Mary Kate Denny, pages 232, 245, 308; Tony Freeman, pages 125, 206, 334; Richard Hutchings, page 290; Michael Newman, pages vi, 90, 167, 261; A. Ramey, page 289; James Shaffer, page 413; Rhoda Sidney, page 312; Steve Skjold, pages xii, 435; M. Vincent, page 342; David Young-Wolff, pages 55 (top), 154, 201, 274, 304, 383, 410, 430. Photo Researchers: Biophoto Associates, page 374 (bottom left); CNRI/Science Photo Library, page 332; Jeff Greenberg, page 282; Stephen J. Krasemann, page 374 (bottom right); Dr. P. Marazzi/Science Photo Library, page 374 (center right); Judd Pilosoff, page 110. PhotoTake: Barts Medical Library, pages 366, 374 (bottom center); Dr. Denis Kunkel, page 66. PictureQuest: Mark C. Burnett/Stock Boston, page 41 (bottom left). Michael Provost: pages xi, 39 (both), 54, 89, 277, 374 (top left), 392–393, 396, 398, 403, 404, 405, 406, 407, 414. Stock Boston: Vincent Dewitt, page 320; Laima Druskis, page 341; Thomas Fletcher, page 335; Stephen Frisch, page 399; Jim Harrison, page 58; A. Ramey, page 307; Martin Rogers, page 75 (bottom); Peter Southwick, page 17; David Ulmer, page 322; Michael Weisbrot, page 321. Stock Food: Rick Mariani Photography, page 97. SuperStock: pages 36, 96 (left), 310; Tom Rosenthal, page 75 (top). Unicorn Stock Photos: Rich Baker, page 402; Eric R. Berndt, pages 9 (left), 306; Chris Boylan, page 55 (bottom right); Dede Gilman, page 203; Martha McBride, page 372; Patti McConville, page 175 (right); Karen Mullen, page 259. Uniphoto: pages 143, 220, 436; Bill Auth, page 349; Allan Laidman, page 59; Kate Ryan, page 369. Science Source/PR: L. Miller, pages 422–423; NIBSC, pages 356–357. Kwame Zikomo: pages 272–273.

Illustrations

Art and Science, Inc.: pages 400, 417, 418, 419. Bernard Adnet: pages 8, 16, 37, 40, 180, 181, 199, 205, 246, 274. Ron Boisvert: page 313. Max Crandall: pages 102, 156, 192, 210, 211, 233, 287, 375, 386–387. Robert A. Deverell: pages 6, 14, 21, 67, 72, 77, 93, 96, 108, 109, 114, 136, 139, 148, 166, 170, 204, 253, 258, 260, 301, 332, 336, 346, 358–359, 371, 394, 415, 425, 431. Thomas J. Gagliano: page 385. Jerry Gonzalez: page 34. Illustrious Interactive: page 411. David Kelley Design: pages 61, 62, 105, 161, 339, 348, 420. Caia Koopman: pages 264–265. Alvalyn Lundgren: pages 95, 171. Mazer: page 134. Hilda Muinos: pages 39, 76, 115, 122, 249, 252, 358, 395, 397. Rick Nease: pages 147, 423. Network Graphics: pages 127, 130, 306, 408. Olivia: page 96. Parrot Graphics: page 316. Rolin Graphics: pages 65, 103, 104, 123, 155, 162, 165, 168, 169, 172, 278, 279, 305, 314, 337, 367, 376, 377. Sally Vitsky: page 276. Jerry Zimmerman: pages 13, 101, 221, 229, 255, 285, 295, 319, 349, 365, 412, 442–443.